Manual of
pulmonary function testing

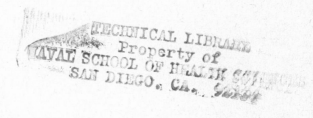

Manual of
pulmonary function testing

GREGG RUPPEL, M.Ed., R.R.T.

Director, Pulmonary Function Laboratory,
The University Hospital,
St. Louis University Medical Center;
Instructor, Forest Park Community College,
St. Louis, Missouri

FOURTH EDITION
with 85 illustrations

The C. V. Mosby Company

ST. LOUIS • WASHINGTON, D.C. • TORONTO 1986

A TRADITION OF PUBLISHING EXCELLENCE

Publisher: Thomas A. Manning
Assistant editor: Elizabeth M. Raven
Manuscript editor: Judith Bange
Book design: Kay M. Kramer
Cover design: Gail Morey Hudson
Production: Ginny Douglas

FOURTH EDITION

Printed in the United States of America

The C.V. Mosby Company
11830 Westline Industrial Drive, St. Louis, Missouri 63146

Library of Congress Cataloging-in-Publication Data

Ruppel, Gregg, 1948–
  Manual of pulmonary function testing.

  Bibliography: p.
  Includes index.
  1. Pulmonary function tests—Handbooks, manuals, etc.
I. Title. [DNLM: 1. Respiratory Function Tests.
WB 284 R946m]
RC734.P84R86 1986   616.2′4075   86-8714
ISBN 0-8016-4695-2

TS/VH/VH 9 8 7 6 5 4 3 2 1   02/B/243

TO CAROL

for her patience and encouragement

Preface

The primary function of the lung can be stated as twofold: first, the oxygenation of mixed venous blood; second, the removal of carbon dioxide from that same blood. These two functions depend on the integrity of the airways, the pulmonary vascular system, the alveolar septa, the respiratory muscles, and the respiratory control mechanisms. The ideal would be pulmonary function tests designed to assess the functional status of each of these systems separately. Most lung function tests, however, measure the status of the component systems in an overlapping way.

The evaluation of pulmonary function may be indicated for the following reasons:

1. To determine the *presence* of lung disease or abnormality of lung function
2. To determine the *extent* of abnormalities
3. To determine the *extent of impairment* caused by abnormal lung function
4. To determine the *progression* of the disease
5. To determine the *nature of the physiologic disturbance*
6. To determine a *course of therapy* for treatment of a particular lesion

This text presents, as concisely as possible, explanations of many commonly used pulmonary function studies, the testing techniques used, and the significance of individual tests in regard to pulmonary disease. Also included are sections on pulmonary exercise evaluation, testing regimens for specific purposes (disability, preoperative evaluation, etc.), pulmonary function testing equipment, computers, and quality assurance.

This fourth edition builds on the material used in earlier editions and reflects the suggestions of users of those texts. A chapter on computers in the pulmonary function laboratory has been added because of the widespread application of computers in almost every aspect of pulmonary function testing. Another new chapter covers quality assurance in the pulmonary function laboratory. Producing high-quality data is essential to accurate and consistent diagnoses; quality control and appropriate calibration techniques are more important than ever, particularly with the complexity of instrumentation found in most laboratories.

As in the previous edition, each chapter is followed by self-assessment questions and a selected bibliography. The self-assessment questions in this edition are new, and answers may be found in the Appendix. Entries in the bibliographies are separated according to specific topics in each chapter. Prediction regressions and nomograms for normal values are contained in the Appendix, along with information on the use of predicted values. Sample calculations for some of the more complicated measurements (lung volumes, plethysmography, diffusion, and exercise) are also included in the Appendix.

This manual is intended to serve as a text for students of pulmonary function testing and as a handy reference for technicians and physicians alike. Because of the diversity of testing methods and equipment currently in use, some aspects of certain tests are treated in a general way. For this reason, readers are encouraged to make use of the bibliographies provided. The presentation of the significance of various tests presumes a rudimentary knowledge of pulmonary anatomy and physiology. Again, readers are urged to refer to the general references included in the selected bibliography to refresh or support their background in lung function. The terminology used is that of the American College of Chest Physicians– American Thoracic Society Joint Committee on Pulmonary Nomenclature. In some instances test names reflect very common usage that does not follow the ACCP-ATS recommendations.

My thanks to Drs. William Kistner, John Winter, and James Wiant for their encouragement in the development of the original text. My special thanks to Drs. Roger Secker-Walker, Susan Marshall, Gerald Dolan, and Cesar Keller for comments and constructive criticisms in the preparation of the revised editions. Special thanks also go to Ronald Gilmore and Jack Tandy for their contributions to the illustrations in this and previous editions. A note of thanks also to Thomas Anderson, M.Ed., R.R.T., David Shelledy, M.A., R.R.T., Patricia Dent, B.S., M.S., R.P.T., and Barbara Disborough, M.A., R.R.T., for their reviews of and suggestions for the fourth edition. My appreciation for materials and illustrations provided goes to Warren E. Collins, Inc., Gould, Inc., Radiometer America, Jones Medical Instrument Co., Vitalograph Medical Instrumentation, Instrumentation Laboratories, Medical Graphics, Inc., and Hewlett Packard.

Gregg Ruppel

Contents

11 Quality assurance in the pulmonary function laboratory, 200

12 Case studies, 232

Appendix, 253

Manual of
pulmonary function testing

CHAPTER ONE

Lung volume tests

VITAL CAPACITY (VC)
Description

The VC is the largest volume measured on complete expiration after the deepest inspiration without forced or rapid effort (Fig. 1-1). The VC is normally recorded in either liters or milliliters, usually corrected to body temperature, body pressure, saturated with water vapor (BTPS). VC may also be referred to as slow vital capacity (SVC) in distinction to forced vital capacity (FVC), as discussed in Chapter 3.

Technique

VC is measured by having the subject inspire maximally and then exhale completely into a spirometer capable of recording change in lung volume with no time limit imposed on the maneuver. VC can also be measured from maximal expiration to maximal inspiration. This latter method is sometimes termed inspiratory vital capacity (IVC), whereas the former is simply the VC.

Significance

Normal values for VC as well as for many other lung function parameters are computed as follows according to the general form:

$$VC = AX - BY - Z$$

where

A = Height (centimeters)
B = Age (years)
X, Y, Z = Constants

Nomograms and regression equations for men, women, and children appear in the Appendix. The VC may vary as much as 20% from predicted normal values in healthy individuals and may vary from time to time in the same individual depending on the position of the body, etc. The VC in adults varies directly with height and inversely with age and is generally smaller in females than in males. Recent evidence indicates that lung volumes may differ significantly in regard to race or ethnic origin, so that interpretation of the measured volumes in regard to *predicted normal values* should consider these factors in addition to age, height, weight, and sex.

Decreases in VC can be caused by loss of distensible lung tissue, as in bronchogenic carcinoma, bronchiolar obstruction, pulmonary edema, pneumonia,

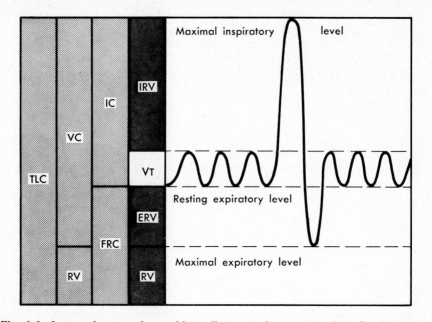

Fig. 1-1. Lung volumes and capacities—diagrammatic representation of various lung compartments, based on a typical spirogram. *TLC*, Total lung capacity; *VC*, vital capacity; *RV*, residual volume; *FRC*, functional residual capacity; *IC*, inspiratory capacity; *VT*, tidal volume; *IRV*, inspiratory reserve volume; *ERV*, expiratory reserve volume. Shaded areas indicate relationships between the subdivisions and relative sizes as compared with the TLC. The resting expiratory level should be noted, since it remains more stable than other identifiable points during repeated spirograms and hence is used as a starting point for FRC determinations, etc. (Modified from Comroe, J.H., Jr., et al.: The lung: clinical physiology and pulmonary function tests, ed. 2, Chicago, 1962, Year Book Medical Publishers, Inc.)

atelectasis, pulmonary restriction, pulmonary congestion, or surgical excisions. In general, restriction may be the result of tissue destruction, space-occupying lesions, or changes in the composition of the parenchyma itself. Tissue loss is best illustrated by resection (as in a lobectomy), wherein the decrease in VC is roughly proportional to the tissue removed. A good example of a space-occupying lesion is a tumor, which directly displaces lung tissue. Fibrotic diseases, such as silicosis, cause changes in the elastic properties of the parenchyma. There are some causes for decreases in VC not related to lung lesions, such as depression of the respiratory centers or neuromuscular diseases; reduction of available thoracic space by pleural effusion, pneumothorax, hiatus hernia, or cardiac enlargement; limitation of movement of the diaphragm by pregnancy, ascites, or tumor; and limitation of thoracic movement because of scleroderma, kyphoscoliosis, or pain.

When the VC is less than 80% of the predicted value, or is less than the 95% confidence limit (see Appendix), the interpretation of reduced VC should be correlated with the history and physical findings. The description ''mild,'' "moderate," or "severe" may be used to qualify the extent of reduction of the VC and should be based on a statistical comparison (i.e., confidence interval) of the measured VC versus the predicted VC. Spuriously low estimates of VC may result from poor subject effort or inadequate instruction in the performance of the maneuver. Reproducible values for at least three maneuvers should provide acceptable results (see Chapter 11).

INSPIRATORY CAPACITY (IC)
Description

The IC is the largest volume of gas that can be inspired from the resting expiratory level (Fig. 1-1). The IC is recorded in liters or milliliters, corrected to BTPS.

Technique

IC may be measured by having the subject breathe normally for several breaths and then inhale maximally while the changes are recorded on an appropriate spirogram and the volume inspired from the resting expiratory level measured. The IC may also be estimated by subtracting the expiratory reserve volume (ERV) from the VC. The accuracy of the measurement of IC depends on the determination of the passive end-expiratory level. This is best accomplished by recording at least three tidal breaths, across which the volume varies by less than 100 ml.

Significance

The IC normally makes up approximately 75% of the VC. Changes in the absolute volume of the IC usually parallel increases or decreases in the VC. Compensatory hyperventilation normally "dips into" the IC because both the end-inspiratory and end-expiratory levels are altered. The IC considered alone is of minimal diagnostic significance; reduction of the IC is consistent with restrictive defects.

EXPIRATORY RESERVE VOLUME (ERV)
Description

The ERV is the largest volume of gas that can be expired from the resting end-expiratory level (Fig. 1-1). Like the other lung volumes, it is recorded in liters or milliliters, corrected to BTPS.

Technique

ERV may be measured by having the subject breathe normally for several breaths and then exhale maximally while the changes are recorded on a spirogram and the volume exhaled from the average end-expiratory level measured. Likewise, the ERV may be estimated by subtracting the IC from the VC. As with the IC, accurate estimation of the ERV depends on the stability of the end-expiratory level. Erroneous estimates of ERV may confound the measurement of residual volume (RV) as described below, because the ERV is employed in the calculation of RV.

Significance

The ERV makes up approximately 25% of the VC. The ERV varies greatly in comparable subjects and in the same individual with a change of body position. As with the IC, changes in the ERV are not generally of diagnostic value, but reductions are typical in subjects with restrictive disorders. Validity often depends on the ventilatory pattern of the subject. In some obese subjects the ERV may be reduced out of proportion to the reduction in other lung volumes.

FUNCTIONAL RESIDUAL CAPACITY (FRC) AND RESIDUAL VOLUME (RV)

Description

The FRC is the volume of gas remaining in the lungs at the end-expiratory level. The RV is the volume of gas remaining in the lungs at the end of a maximal expiration (Fig. 1-1). Both are recorded in liters or milliliters, corrected to BTPS.

Technique

Open-circuit method. FRC and RV must be measured indirectly because the RV, which is a subdivision of the FRC, cannot be removed from the lungs. The concentration of nitrogen in the lungs is presumed to be in equilibrium with the atmosphere, or approximately 80%. By having the subject breathe 100% oxygen for several minutes, the nitrogen in the lungs can be gradually washed out. Since all of the N_2 cannot be washed out, the test is usually continued until the concentration of alveolar N_2 is less than 1%, and then an alveolar sample is taken. The exhaled gas is collected in a spirometer or bag (which previously has been flushed with pure O_2), and the concentration of N_2 is measured; the original volume of gas in the lungs at the end-expiratory level can be computed by the following formula (see also Fig. 1-2):

$$FRC = \frac{\%N_{2_{final}} \times \text{Expired volume} - N_{2_{tiss}}}{\%N_{2_{alveolar\ 1}} - \%N_{2_{alveolar\ 2}}}$$

where

$\%N_{2_{final}}$ = Concentration of N_2 in volume expired

$\%N_{2_{alveolar\ 1}}$ = Fraction of N_2 in alveolar gas initially

$\%N_{2_{alveolar\ 2}}$ = Fraction of N_2 in alveolar gas at end (determined from an alveolar sample)

$N_{2_{tiss}}$ = Volume of N_2 washed out of blood/tissues

Corrections for the amount of N_2 washed out of the blood and tissue and for small amounts of nitrogen in "pure" O_2 must be made when computing the FRC. For each minute of oxygen breathing, approximately 40 ml of N_2 is removed from blood and tissue, so that 0.04 multiplied by time of the test is subtracted from the volume of N_2 in the spirometer to equal $N_{2_{tiss}}$. Since not all of the N_2 in the lungs may be washed out, even after 7 minutes of O_2 breathing, the $\%N_{2_{alveolar\ 2}}$ may be measured by taking an alveolar sample near the end of the

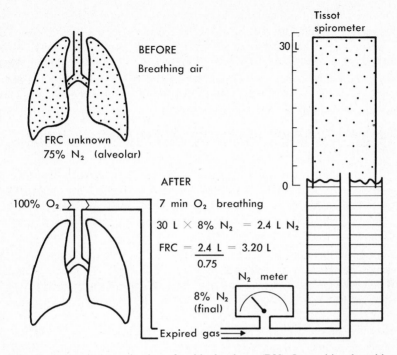

Fig. 1-2. Open-circuit determination of residual volume (RV). In a subject breathing air the alveolar nitrogen concentration is assumed to be equal to atmospheric N_2 pressure minus water vapor and CO_2, or approximately 75%. Alternatively, the fractional concentration of alveolar N_2 can be measured at the beginning and at the end of the oxygen breathing (see text). After the subject breathed 100% O_2 for 7 minutes and exhaled all gas into a large-volume spirometer (Tissot), the entire gas sample is analyzed for N_2 concentration and the FRC computed as indicated. The switch from breathing room air to pure O_2 must come at precisely the end-expiratory level to ensure that the volume actually measured is the FRC. The RV is determined by subtracting the ERV from the FRC. (Modified from Comroe, J.H., Jr., et al.: The lung: clinical physiology and pulmonary function tests, ed. 2, Chicago, 1962, Year Book Medical Publishers, Inc.)

test and subtracting this value from the alveolar N_2 present at the beginning. The FRC must be corrected to BTPS. To obtain the RV, simply subtract the ERV from the FRC as just measured.

A newer method for performing the open-circuit procedure uses a rapid N_2 analyzer coupled to a spirometer or pneumotachometer to provide a "breath-by-breath" analysis of N_2 washed out of the lungs. Analog signals proportional to N_2 concentration and volume (or flow) are integrated to derive the exhaled volume of N_2 for each breath; the values for all breaths are summed to provide the total volume of N_2 washed out. The test is continued for 7 minutes or until the %N_2 in alveolar gas has been reduced to less than 1%. The FRC is calculated by dividing the N_2 volume by the fractional concentration of alveolar N_2 at the beginning of the test and making the necessary corrections (blood/tissue washout, temperature). In addition, a breath-by-breath plot of the $\%N_2$ (or log $\%N_2$) versus volume or number of breaths can be obtained to derive indices of the distribution of ventilation (see Fig. 4-2.) In systems employing a pneumotachometer, which is sensitive to the composition of gas (see Chapter 9), corrections must be made for changes in the viscosity of the gas as oxygen replaces nitrogen in the expirate. This is usually easily accomplished by software manipulation of the analog signals.

Closed-circuit method. The FRC can also be calculated indirectly by diluting the gas in the lungs with a gas of known concentration. A suitable spirometer is filled with a known volume of gas to which helium (He) has been added. The amount (usually about 600 ml) and concentration of He (usually about 10%) are measured and recorded before the test is begun. The subject then rebreathes the gas in the spirometer, with a CO_2 absorber in place, until the concentration of He falls to a stable level; this usually takes less than 7 minutes. If the 10% He mixture is diluted in a small quantity of gas, usually 1 to 2 liters, equilibrium of the He in the lungs' rebreathing system takes place rather quickly. The final concentration of He is then recorded. The volume that was in the spirometer before the test was begun can then be calculated:

$$\text{System volume} = \frac{\text{He added (milliliters)}}{F_{He_{initial}}}$$

where

$F_{He_{initial}}$ = the %He converted to a fraction (%He/100)

Once the system volume is known, the FRC (and RV) can be computed:

$$\text{FRC} = \frac{(\%He_{initial} - \%He_{final})}{\%He_{final}} \times \text{System volume}$$

Either percent or fractional concentration of helium may be used, since the term is a ratio.

Some automated systems employ the same method to calculate the system volume; a small amount of He is added to the closed system, followed by a known volume of air. He concentrations are measured before and after the addition of the air. The dilution equation can then be applied to determine the system volume, or combined with the He concentration measurement at the end of rebreathing to solve for the FRC. Again:

$$\text{RV} = \text{FRC} - \text{ERV}$$

Rebreathing is normally continued until the He concentration changes by no more than 0.02% over 30 seconds (see Chapter 11 for criteria for acceptability of lung volumes). To correct for the volume of He absorbed by the blood during rebreathing, a volume of 50 to 100 ml is usually subtracted from the FRC. The dead space volume of the breathing valve should likewise be subtracted from the measured FRC. The FRC must be corrected to BTPS (Fig. 1-3). Sample calculations of both the open- and closed-circuit techniques can be found in the Appendix.

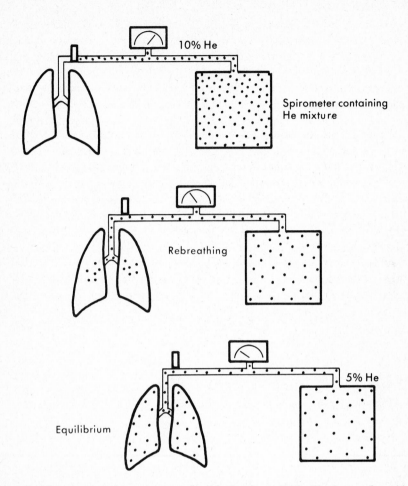

10% He

Spirometer containing
He mixture

Rebreathing

Equilibrium

5% He

Fig. 1-3. Closed-circuit determination of residual volume (RV). The lungs of a subject breathing air contain no He. The subject then rebreathes a mixture of He and air or O_2, of which the volume and He% are known. He is diluted until an equilibrium is reached. The volume of He initially present is known from the initial concentration and the volume of the rebreathing system. At the end of the test, the same volume of He is diluted in a larger-volume (rebreathing system plus lungs), and the total volume is computed from the initial He volume and the final He concentration:

$$\frac{V_{He_{initial}}}{F_{He_{final}}} = \text{Total volume of system (after rebreathing)}$$

The FRC is derived by subtracting the rebreathing system volume (see text). The switch from air to the He mixture must be made at the end-expiratory level for accurate measurement of FRC. RV is derived by subtracting the ERV. (Modified from Comroe, J.H., Jr., et al.: The lung: clinical physiology and pulmonary function tests, ed. 2, Chicago, 1962, Year Book Medical Publishers, Inc.)

Significance

In both the open- and closed-circuit techniques, the RV is measured indirectly as a subdivision of the FRC. This is the preferred method because the resting end-expiratory level is more reproducible than the points of complete inspiration or complete expiration. The end-expiratory level (and ERV) must be accurately measured; if the tidal breathing pattern is irregular, the ERV may be overestimated or underestimated, thus affecting the calculation of RV. The validity of both the open- and closed-circuit techniques depends on the assumption that all parts of the lung are reasonably well ventilated. In subjects with obstructive disease a 7-minute test period may not be long enough to wash N_2 out or mix He to a stable level in the poorly ventilated parts of the lungs. Hence the FRC, RV, and total lung capacity will appear less than the true values. Prolongation of the test improves results somewhat but will not account for *completely* trapped gas, as found in bullous emphysema. In either of the foreign gas techniques, leaks in the valving or circuitry will affect gas concentrations and tend to cause erroneous estimates of FRC. Likewise, malfunction of the gas analyzer in either method will produce spurious values. Integrity of the breathing circuit or analyzer should be questioned whenever values for FRC appear out of proportion to the subject's clinical history or other lung function parameters (spirometry, carbon monoxide diffusing capacity [D_{LCO}], etc.).

An increase in FRC is considered pathologic. An FRC increased to greater than approximately 120% of the predicted value represents hyperinflation, which may result from emphysematous changes, asthmatic or fibrotic bronchiolar obstruction, compensation for surgical removal of lung tissue, or in some instances thoracic deformity. An increase in FRC usually results in muscular and mechanical inefficiency, accompanied by increased work of breathing.

An increase in RV indicates that in spite of maximal expiratory effort, the lungs still contain an abnormally large amount of gas. This type of change may appear in young asthmatics and is usually reversible. Increases in RV are also characteristic of emphysema and chronic air trapping, as well as chronic bronchial obstruction. RV and FRC usually increase together, although this is not always true. The RV may increase without loss of ability to ventilate adequately. However, as the RV becomes larger, more ventilation is required to adequately replenish the gas concentrations normal to the lung. This usually means an increase in tidal volume (V_T), rate, or both, at the same time that the work of breathing is increased.

Table 1-1. Comparative lung volumes for a normal adult man, a subject with air trapping and a subject with restriction

Value	Normal	Air Trapping	Restriction
VC (ml)	4800	3000	3000
FRC (ml)	2400	3600	1500
RV (ml)	1200	3000	750
TLC (ml)	6000	6000	3750
RV/TLC (%)	20	50	20

FRC and RV (and the TLC derived from these) are typically decreased in restrictive diseases that interfere with the bellows action of the chest or the lungs. Decreases are typically seen in those diseases associated with extensive fibrosis such as sarcoidosis, asbestosis, and complicated silicosis. Restrictive disorders affecting the chest wall include kyphoscoliosis, pectus excavatum, neuromuscular weakness, and obesity. FRC and RV may also be decreased in diseases that occlude many alveoli, such as pneumonia.

Table 1-1 lists typical values for lung volumes for a normal adult man, a subject with air trapping (as might be seen in emphysema), and a subject with restriction (as might be seen in sarcoidosis). It should be noted that in generalized restrictive processes the lung volumes are more or less equally reduced. Thus the proportional relationship between different lung volume compartments may be relatively normal (e.g., the RV/TLC ratio). In obstructive patterns one of two changes in the proportions of the various compartments is usually observed. The RV is increased; the increase may be at the expense of a reduction in VC (Fig. 1-4), with the TLC remaining close to the expected value; or, the RV may increase with the VC being fairly well preserved, so that the TLC is actually greater than the value predicted. The term *air trapping* is sometimes used to

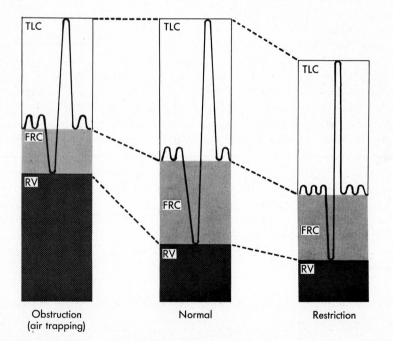

Obstruction (air trapping)   Normal   Restriction

Fig. 1-4. Lung volume alterations in obstructive and restrictive patterns. A comparison of the changes in lung volume compartments in obstruction and restriction shows the following: in obstruction (with air trapping) the FRC and RV are both increased at the expense of the VC, and hence TLC remains relatively unchanged; in restrictive patterns the FRC, RV, and VC are all decreased proportionately, resulting in a decrease in TLC (see text).

describe the increase in FRC and RV, and the term *hyperinflation* is often used to describe the absolute increase in TLC.

THORACIC GAS VOLUME (VTG)
Description

VTG measures the volume of gas contained in the thorax, whether in communication with open airways or trapped in any compartment of the thorax. The VTG is recorded in liters or milliliters.

Technique

VTG is measured using a body plethysmograph (Fig. 1-5). The technique is based on Boyle's law that the volume of gas varies inversely in proportion to the pressure to which it is subjected. At the start of the test the subject has an unknown volume of gas in the thorax (the FRC). By occluding the airway and allowing the subject to decompress the gas in the chest by making an inspiratory effort, a new volume and a new pressure are generated. The change in pulmonary gas pressure is easily measured at the airway, since mouth pressure theoretically equals alveolar pressure when there is no airflow. The change in pulmonary gas volume is measured by monitoring the pressure in the plethysmograph. The trans-

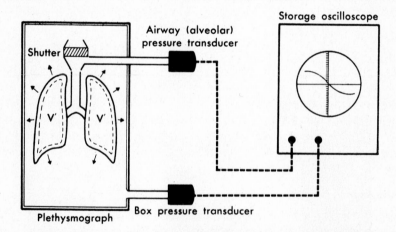

Fig. 1-5. Thoracic gas volume (VTG). A body plethysmograph is used to measure VTG. Boyle's law states that the volume varies inversely with the pressure if the temperature is held constant. A "pressure" type of plethysmograph, with pressure transducers for measurements of box pressure and airway (alveolar) pressure, is illustrated. An electronic shutter momentarily occludes the airway, so that airway pressure is approximately equal to alveolar pressure. Simultaneously, the alveolar gas is decompressed because of enlargement of the thorax, without gas flow. This change in alveolar volume is reflected by an increase in box pressure, and an estimation of the volume change can be derived by calibration. When the original pressure (P), the new pressure (P'), and the new volume (V' or V + ΔV) are known, the original volume (V or VTG) can be computed from Boyle's law (see text and Appendix).

ducer recording box pressure is calibrated directly in terms of volume change by introducing a small, known volume of gas into the plethysmograph and using the pressure change as a calibration.

As the subject breathes against the closed airway, which has been occluded by means of an electrical shutter, the air within the chest is alternately compressed and decompressed by the action of the ventilatory muscles. The transducer recording of mouth pressure (which equals alveolar pressure) is plotted on the vertical axis of an oscilloscope, while the transducer recording of box pressure (which is calibrated as volume change) is plotted on the horizontal axis (Fig. 1-5). Changes in each parameter are graphed continuously and appear as a sloping line, which is equal to $\Delta P/\Delta V$, where ΔP is the change in alveolar pressure and ΔV is the change in alveolar volume. (The change in alveolar volume is measured indirectly by noting the reciprocal change in plethysmograph volume.)

The original V_{TG} can then be obtained from the slope of the tracing by applying a derivation of Boyle's law:

$$V_{TG} = \frac{P_B}{\lambda V_{TG}}$$

where

V_{TG} = Thoracic gas volume

P_B = Barometric pressure minus water vapor pressure

λ_{TG} = Slope of the oscilloscope trace equal to $\Delta P/\Delta V$

For the complete derivation of the equation, see the Appendix.

The measurements are usually made with the subject panting shallowly at a rate of 1 to 2 breaths/sec with an open glottis. This type of breathing allows small pressure changes to be recorded at or near FRC, improves the signal-to-noise ratio, and eliminates some artifacts related to temperature fluctuations. If the mouth shutter is closed at precisely end-expiration, V_{TG} equals FRC. Several determinations can be made quickly to obtain an average for the slope of $\Delta P/\Delta V$.

Significance

The V_{TG} technique is a quick and precise means of measuring FRC and (when used in combination with simple spirometry) deriving other lung volume compartment values. The plethysmograph's obvious advantage is that it measures the volume of gas in the thoracic cavity whether or not it is in ventilatory communication with the atmosphere. Hence the V_{TG} measurement of FRC is often larger than the FRC as measured by He dilution or nitrogen washout, especially in emphysema and other diseases characterized by air trapping. When dilution tests are extended beyond 7 minutes, the results for FRC determinations approach the V_{TG} figure. Recent evidence suggests that in severe obstructive patterns the FRC may actually be overestimated when the V_{TG} technique is used. Normal lungs, however, show similar results by either method. When two or more methods of determining lung volumes are employed, it is often instructive to compare the

FRC values as determined by each method. This allows for correlation of measured lung volumes with the data produced by spirometry or D_{CO} and may elucidate whether any errors occurred in the lung volume determination.

The primary disadvantage of V_{TG} determinations is the necessity of a body plethysmograph and the requisite instrumentation. The testing maneuver itself requires that the technician carefully instruct and monitor the subject in order to obtain acceptable data (see Chapter 11). V_{TG} cannot be measured in certain subjects: those with claustrophobia, those with physical limitations that preclude entry into the box, or those unable to perform the panting maneuver acceptably.

RADIOLOGIC ESTIMATION OF TOTAL LUNG CAPACITY (TLC)
Description

Determination of TLC can be made by one of several methods using standard posteroanterior (PA) and lateral x-ray films of the chest. A commonly used procedure involves dividing the films into ellipsoid segments and estimating the volumes of each segment. A planimeter can also be used to estimate the thoracic volume.

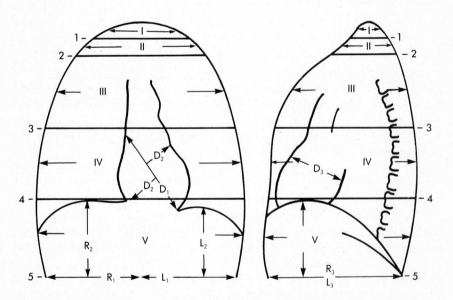

Fig. 1-6. Radiologic estimation of total lung capacity (TLC). Standard posteroanterior and lateral x-ray films are outlined as indicated with wax pencil or marker. Lines 1, 2, 3, 4, and 5 divide each film into five segments (I to V). R_1, R_2, and R_3 define the volume under the right diaphragm. L_1, L_2, and L_3 are taken from the left diaphragm; $R_1 = L_1$, $R_3 = L_3$, and L_2 is the height of the left hemidiaphragm, whereas R_2 is the height of the right side. D_1, D_2, and D_3 allow the calculation of the volume occupied by the heart. All measurements are made in centimeters, and each respective segment is measured at the points indicated by the arrows (see text).

Technique

PA and lateral chest x-ray films are shot at a standard distance of 72 inches. The borders of the lungs and heart are outlined using a china marker or similar pencil. The diaphragms are also marked. Fig 1-6 illustrates the necessary outlines for the measurements. If the lung apex is not visible on the lateral film, it can be determined after some preliminary measurements are made. The PA film is first subdivided (Fig. 1-6) as follows:

1. A horizontal line is drawn 2.75 cm from the apices (line 1).
2. A second line is drawn 2.75 cm below the first line (line 2).
3. A horizontal line is drawn through the upper diaphragm dome (line 4).
4. A horizontal line is drawn midway between lines 2 and 4 (line 3); these lines determine segments I through IV.

The lateral film is then subdivided (Fig. 1-6).

1. A horizontal line is drawn through the upper diaphragm dome (line 4).
2. The apex of the lung on the lateral view can then be determined by measuring the distance from the apex to line 4 on the PA film and transposing to the lateral.
3. Line 1 is drawn 2.75 cm below the apex.
4. Line 2 is drawn 2.75 cm below line 1.
5. Line 3 is drawn midway between lines 2 and 4, just as on the PA film.
6. A fifth horizontal line is drawn through the posterior sulcus forward to the anterior limit of the diaphragm. The distance from line 4 to line 5 is then transposed to the PA film to determine segment V (perpendicular lines are added from the margins of the diaphragms to line 5 on the PA film).

The heart is outlined as indicated on Fig. 1-6: a line, D_1, is drawn through the long axis from the right atrium to the apex. Perpendiculars (D_2) to D_1 are drawn to the farthest borders of the heart outline. A line, D_3, is drawn noting the longest distance across the heart shadow on the lateral film.

Measurements like the following are then made from each segment and recorded on a data sheet (Fig. 1-7):

1. The width and depth of each segment is recorded in centimeters, measuring from the midpoint of the segment; the height is also recorded.
2. The measurements are then multiplied (width × depth × height) and added together.
3. The sum is multiplied by a factor (0.581) derived from the formula for the volume of an ellipsoid cylinder and a correction factor for x-ray divergence. This product is the total thoracic volume (TTV).

From the TTV the non-gas volume (NGV) must be subtracted. The volume under the diaphragms is calculated separately for the right and left sides:

1. R_1 equals half the length of line 5; R_2 is the height of the right diaphragm; and R_3 is the length of line 5 on the lateral film.
2. L_1, L_2, and L_3 are measured similarly.
3. The product of these measurements is multiplied by a factor (0.381) for their volumes.
4. The heart dimensions, D_1, D_2, D_3, are treated similarly (Fig. 1-7).

Pulmonary tissue and blood volumes are derived from body measurements

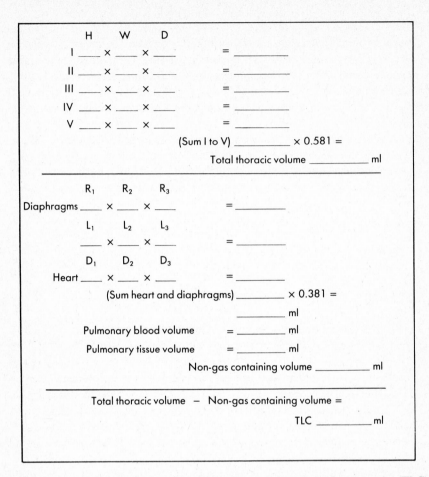

Fig. 1-7. Typical data record sheet for radiologic estimation of total lung capacity (TLC). The height *(H)*, width *(W)*, and depth *(D)* of each of the five thoracic segments (I to V) are multiplied; these five products are added and multiplied by a factor derived from the equation for the volume of an ellipsoid (see text). A similar procedure is used for the two hemidiaphragms and heart; their volumes are added to those for the pulmonary blood and tissue. The difference between the total thoracic volume and the non-gas volume is the TLC.

(see Appendix), and these volumes, as well as the heart and diaphragm volumes, are subtracted from the TTV to derive the TLC, in milliliters. It is important to note that both the PA and lateral films should be taken with the subject at TLC; specific instructions to the subject should include that he or she inspire as deeply as possible in order that the TLC be accurately estimated.

Significance

The TLC, as determined radiologically, correlates well with plethysmographic determinations in normal and obstructed subjects and may be more accurate than gas dilution techniques in moderate to severe obstruction. Radiologic determination of TLC offers a means of double-checking volumes determined by other methods and is often available in hospitals or clinics where there may not be equipment for foreign gas or plethysmographic measurements. Additionally, radiologic determination of TLC may provide lung volume information in subjects in whom other methods are impractical, such as those with a tracheostomy.

As noted above, subjects must hold their breath at TLC when each film is exposed or the TLC may be underestimated. The presence of space-occupying lesions such as masses or atelectasis may confound the routine method, but more than five segments may be created in order to subdivide around a well-defined lesion.

TOTAL LUNG CAPACITY (TLC)
Description

The TLC is the volume of gas contained in the lungs at the end of a maximal inspiration. It is recorded in liters or milliliters, corrected to BTPS.

Technique

The TLC is normally calculated by combining other specific lung volumes. The two most common are addition of the FRC and IC, and addition of the VC and RV. TLC can be calculated by the radiologic method described earlier. In addition, TLC can be calculated by several single-breath techniques (single-breath He dilution or single-breath N_2 washout). These techniques are commonly employed in conjunction with other measurements when a lung volume determination is required for the calculation of a particular parameter (e.g., alveolar volume for the calculation of $D_{L_{CO}}$). Although single-breath lung volume determinations correlate well with multiple-breath techniques in normal subjects, lung volumes tend to be underestimated in the presence of moderate to severe obstruction.

Significance

TLC may be decreased in edema, atelectasis, neoplasms, or restrictive lesions and in pulmonary congestion, pneumothorax, or thoracic restriction. Pure restrictive defects show proportional decreases in most lung compartments (Fig. 1-4), as described earlier for FRC and RV. When the TLC is less than 80% of the predicted value or less than the 95% confidence limit, a restrictive process should be suspected. TLC may be either normal or increased in bronchiolar obstruction and in emphysema (Table 1-1 and Fig. 1-4). A normal or increased TLC does not mean that ventilation or surface area for diffusion is normal. A normal TLC in conjunction with an increased RV is consistent with air trapping (RV increased, VC decreased). When the TLC is greater than 120% of the predicted value or above the 95% confidence limit as a result of an increased RV, hyperinflation is present, and the work of breathing is usually increased. (For predicted normal values, see the Appendix.)

RESIDUAL VOLUME/TOTAL LUNG CAPACITY RATIO (RV/TLC × 100)

Description

The RV/TLC ratio is a statement of the fraction of the TLC that can be defined as RV, expressed as a percentage.

Technique

The RV is divided by the TLC and multiplied by 100. Either ambient temperature, pressure, saturated with water (ATPS) or BTPS values may be used because of the ratio, but both volumes should be expressed in the same units.

Significance

In healthy young adults the RV/TLC ratio may vary from 20% to 35%. Since this is a ratio, values greater than 35% may be derived from absolute increases in RV, as in emphysema, or from a decrease in TLC, because of a loss of VC. Values greater than 35% do not indicate disability but are of greatest diagnostic value when correlated to the absolute values of RV and TLC. A large RV/TLC ratio in the presence of an increased TLC is often indicative of hyperinflation, whereas an increased RV/TLC ratio with a normal TLC indicates that air trapping is present (Table 1-1 and Fig. 1-4).

SELF-ASSESSMENT QUESTIONS

1. Calculate the FRC from the open-circuit method using the following data (refer to the Appendix):

$\%N_{2_{final}}$:	6.1% (0.061 as a fraction)
Volume expired:	33.0 L
$\%N_{2_{alveolar\ 1}}$:	80% (0.80 as a fraction)
$\%N_{2_{alveolar\ 2}}$:	2% (0.02 as a fraction)
Time:	7 min
Blood/tissue washout factor:	0.04 L/min
Breathing circuit V_D:	1.0 L
Spirometer temperature:	25° C

   FRC = _____ (BTPS)

2. A patient has these lung volumes:

	Measured	Predicted
VC	1.9	3.6
FRC	1.2	2.2
RV	0.8	1.7
TLC	2.7	5.3

   These values are consistent with:
   a. Normal lung volumes
   b. Obstructive pattern
   c. Restrictive pattern
   d. Combined obstructive and restrictive pattern

3. Calculate the FRC from the closed-circuit method using the following data (refer to the Appendix):

He added: 0.6 L
%He initial: 9.0% (0.09 as a fraction)
%He final: 6.0% (0.060 as a fraction)
He absorption correction: 0.1 L
Temperature: 25° C
FRC = _____ (BTPS)

4. A patient with severe air trapping has his FRC measured using the closed-circuit method and by plethysmography; the FRC as measured by the gas dilution method would be:
   a. Smaller than the V_{TG}
   b. Equal to the V_{TG}
   c. Much larger than the V_{TG}
   d. The two methods cannot be compared, since each measures a different lung compartment.

5. Restrictive lung disease:
   a. Interferes with airflow into or out of the lungs
   b. Interferes with the bellows action of the chest or lungs, or both
   c. Causes a proportional decrease in flows
   d. Causes a loss of elastic recoil
   e. c and d

6. In the plethysmograph, alveolar pressure is approximated:
   a. By measuring changes in box pressure
   b. By measuring flow at the mouth
   c. By measuring mouth pressure with the shutter closed
   d. From a standard nomogram

7. A subject has these lung volumes:

	Measured	Predicted
VC	1.4	2.9
FRC	3.0	2.2
RV	2.7	1.0
TLC	4.1	3.9

   These are consistent with:
   a. Normal lung volumes
   b. A restrictive pattern
   c. An obstructive pattern
   d. A combined obstructive and restrictive pattern

8. Which of the following methods of lung volume determination correlate best with the plethysmographic value in a moderate to severely obstructed individual?
   a. Radiologic method (chest x-ray film)
   b. Open-circuit method (nitrogen washout)
   c. Closed-circuit method (helium dilution)
   d. Single-breath helium dilution

9. An increased RV and RV/TLC ratio is caused by:
   a. Premature closure of small airways
   b. Air trapping
   c. Increased lung elasticity
   d. All of the above
   e. a and b

10. Body plethysmography is based directly on the principles of gas behavior as described by:
    a. Poiseuille's law
    b. Boyle's law
    c. Charles' law
    d. Graham's law
    e. All of the above
11. Which of the following are true concerning the measurement of FRC using the foreign gas techniques?
    I. The open-circuit method uses helium and nitrogen.
    II. The closed-circuit method is not affected by the evenness of ventilation.
    III. The closed-circuit method uses helium.
    IV. The open-circuit method is more accurate than the closed-circuit method because He is less dense than O_2.
    a. I, II, and IV
    b. II, III, and IV
    c. III only
    d. IV only
12. In calculating TLC from chest x-ray films, which of the following must be subtracted from the total thoracic volume?
    I. Pulmonary blood volume
    II. Volume of the heart
    III. Volume under the diaphragm
    IV. Pulmonary tissue volume
    a. I, II, III, and IV
    b. I and IV
    c. II and III
    d. III only

SELECTED BIBLIOGRAPHY
General references
Altman, P.L., and Dittmer, D.S., editors: Respiration and circulation, Bethesda, Md., 1971, Federation of American Societies for Experimental Biology.

Briscoe, W.A.: Lung volumes. In Fenn, W.O., and Rahn, H., editors: Handbook of physiology—respiration II, Washington, D.C., 1965, American Physiological Society.

Comroe, J.H., et al.: The lung: clinical physiology and pulmonary function tests, ed. 2, Chicago, 1962, Year Book Medical Publishers, Inc.

Crapo, R.O., et al.: Lung volumes in healthy nonsmoking adults, Bull. Eur. Physiopathol. Respir. **18**:419, 1982.

Goldman, H.I., and Becklake, M.R.: Respiratory function tests: normal values at median altitudes and the prediction of normal results, Am. Rev. TB Pulm. Dis. **79**:457, 1959.

Grimby, G., and Soderholm, B.: Spirometric studies in normal subjects. III. Static lung volumes and maximal voluntary ventilation in adults with a note on physical fitness, Acta Med. Scand. **173**:199, 1964.

Hepper, N.G.G., Black, L.F., and Fowler, W.S.: Relationships of lung volume to height and arm span in normal subjects and in patients with spinal deformity, Am. Rev. Respir. Dis. **91**:356, 1965.

Pare, P.D., Wiggs, B.J.R., and Coppin, C.A.: Errors in the measurement of total lung capacity in chronic obstructive lung disease, Thorax **38**:468, 1983.

West, J.B.: Respiratory physiology: the essentials, Baltimore, 1974, Williams & Wilkins.

West, J.B.: Pulmonary pathophysiology: the essentials, Baltimore, 1977, Williams & Wilkins.

Radiologic determination of TLC

Barnhard, J.H., et al.: Roentgenographic determination of total lung capacity, Am. J. Med. **28:**51, 1960.

Barrett, W.A., et al.: Computerized roentgenographic determination of total lung capacity, Am. Rev. Respir. Dis. **113:**239, 1976.

Bencowitz, H.Z.: Program for calculation of radiographic total lung capacity, Am. Rev. Respir. Dis. **128:**576, 1983.

Campbell, S.C.: Estimation of total lung capacity by planimetry of chest radiographs in children 5 to 10 years of age, Am. Rev. Respir. Dis. **127:**106, 1983.

O'Brien, R.J., and Drizd, T.A.: Roentgenographic determination of total lung capacity: normal values from a national population survey, Am. Rev. Respir. Dis. **128:**949, 1983.

Wehr, K.L., and Masferrer, R.: Clinical usefulness of planimetric estimation of total lung capacity, Respir. Care **20:**966, 1975.

Thoracic gas volume

Begin, P., and Peslin, R.: Influence of panting frequency on thoracic gas volume measurements in chronic obstructive pulmonary disease, Am. Rev. Respir. Dis. **130:**121, 1984.

Bohadana, A.B., et al.: Influence of panting frequency on plethysmographic measurements of thoracic gas volume, J. Appl. Physiol. **52:**739, 1982.

Brown, R., et al.: Influence of abdominal gas on the Boyle's law determination of thoracic gas volume, J. Appl. Physiol. **44:**469, 1978.

Dubois, A.B., et al. A rapid plethysmographic method for measuring thoracic gas volume: a comparison with a nitrogen washout method for measuring functional residual capacity, J. Clin. Invest. **35:**322, 1956.

Habib, M.P., and Engel, L.A.: Influence of the panting technique on the plethysmographic measurement of thoracic gas volume, Am. Rev. Respir. Dis. **117:**265, 1978.

Leith, D.E., and Mead, J.: Principles of body plethysmography, DLD-NHLBI, Nov. 1974.

Lourenco, R.V., and Chung, S.Y.K.: Calibration of a body plethysmograph for measurement of lung volume, Am. Rev. Respir. Dis. **95:**687, 1967.

Rodenstein, D.O., Stanescu, D.C., and Francis, C.: Demonstration of failure of body plethysmography in airway obstruction, J. Appl. Physiol. **52:**949, 1982.

Shore, S.A., et al.: Effect of panting frequency on the plethysmographic determination of thoracic gas volume in chronic obstructive pulmonary disease, Am. Rev. Respir. Dis. **128:**54, 1983.

Foreign gas lung volumes

Hathirat, S., Renzetti, A.D., and Mitchell, M.: Measurement of the total lung capacity by helium dilution in a constant volume system, Am. Rev. Respir. Dis. **102:**760, 1970.

Hickman, J.B., Blair, E., and Frayser, R.: An open-circuit helium method for measuring functional residual capacity and defective intrapulmonary gas mixing, J. Clin. Invest. **33:**1277, 1954.

Rodenstein, D.O., and Stanescu, D.C.: Reassessment of lung volume measurements by helium dilution and by body plethysmography in chronic airflow obstruction, Am. Rev. Respir. Dis. **126:**1040, 1982.

Schaaning C.G., and Gulsvik, A.: Accuracy and precision of helium dilution technique and body plethysmography in measuring lung volume, Scand. J. Clin. Invest. **32:**271, 1973.

CHAPTER TWO

Ventilation tests

TIDAL VOLUME (VT)
Description

The VT may be the volume of gas inspired or expired during each respiratory cycle and is usually measured in milliliters (Fig. 2-1). Conventionally, the expired volume is expressed as VT.

Technique

VT can be measured directly by simple spirometry (see Fig. 1-1). The subject breathes into a bellows or spirometer, or through a flow-sensing device, and the volume change is measured from the excursions directly or is integrated from the flow signal and recorded on an appropriate spirogram. Since no two breaths are identical, the VT inhaled or exhaled should be measured for at least 1 minute and then divided by the rate to determine the average VT:

$$V_T = \dot{V}/f$$

where

$\dot{V}$ = Volume expired or inspired over a given interval, usually the $\dot{V}_E$

f = Number of breaths for the same interval

Tidal ventilation may also be estimated by means of respiratory inductive plethysmography (RIP) (see Chapter 9). RIP uses coils of wire as transducers to estimate the cross-sectional area of the rib cage and abdominal compartments, and with appropriate calibration can be used to measure VT without connections to the airway.

Significance

Average values for healthy adults fall between 400 and 700 ml, but there is considerable variation even from these values. Decreased values for VT occur in many types of pulmonary disorders, particularly, severe restrictive patterns and neuromuscular diseases such as myasthenia gravis. Decreased tidal breathing is almost always accompanied by an increased respiratory rate in order to maintain alveolar ventilation. A decreased VT and rate is usually associated with respiratory center depression from drugs or brainstem lesions. Some subjects with pulmonary disease exhibit increased values for VT, particularly at rest. VT alone is not an adequate indicator of alveolar ventilation and should never be considered outside the context of rate and minute volume. Rapid rates and small VT values may suggest hypoventilation but must be correlated with arterial pH and P_{CO_2}

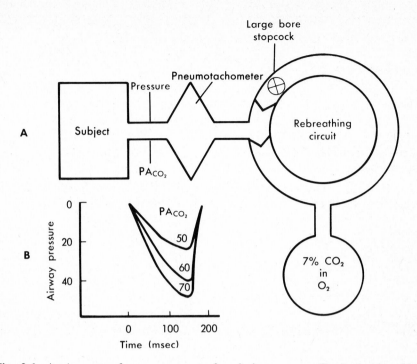

Fig. 2-1. A, Apparatus for measurement of occlusion pressure (P_{100}). A rebreathing circuit as diagrammed can be used for measurement of P_{100} and ventilation during progressive hypercapnia. Hypercapnia is produced at full arterial saturation by rebreathing 7% CO_2 in O_2 from a reservoir. Ventilation is measured by integration of the signal from the pneumotachometer. P_{ACO_2} and pressure are monitored from taps at the mouthpiece. A large-bore stopcock is placed in the inspiratory line to occlude flow for single breaths. One-way valves allow the large-bore stopcock to be closed during expiration so that the subsequent inspiration occurs against the occluded airway at FRC. **B,** Representative tracings of the airway pressure developed during occlusion at various levels of hypercapnia (P_{ACO_2} 50, 60, 70) for the first 100 msec.

values to be definitive. Many subjects with little or no pulmonary involvement display increased values for VT as a result of breathing into the pulmonary function apparatus with the nose occluded.

RATE (f)
Description

The respiratory rate (f, frequency of breathing) is the number of breaths per unit of time, usually per minute.

Technique

The rate may be determined by counting the chest movements or the excursions of a bellows or spirometer for an appropriate interval. Counting the breaths for several minutes and taking an average per minute is preferred to counting the breaths for 10 or 20 seconds and extrapolating.

Significance

An increased or decreased rate is commonly assumed to be a sign of the ventilatory status, although its value as an index of ventilation lies primarily in conjunction with measurements of V_T, minute volume, alveolar ventilation, and arterial blood gas values. Hypoxia and hypercapnia, acidosis, conditions causing decreased lung compliance, and exercise cause increases in respiratory rate, but an increased rate alone is not definitive. A decreased rate is common in central nervous system depression and in CO_2 narcosis. As with measurement of V_T, rate determinations may be artifactually elevated by connection of the subject to the unfamiliar breathing circuit, the application of the noseclip, or both.

MINUTE VOLUME EXPIRED ($\dot{V}_E$)
Description

The $\dot{V}_E$ is the total volume of gas expired in 1 minute. It includes both the alveolar and dead space ventilation and is recorded in liters per minute.

Technique

The $\dot{V}_E$ may be determined by having the subject breathe either into or out of a bellows, spirometer, or pneumotachometer or similar metering device for at least 1 minute. Measuring the expired or inspired gas volume for a period of several minutes and dividing by the time gives an average $\dot{V}_E$ or $\dot{V}_I$ (volume of gas inspired in 1 minute). The $\dot{V}_E$ is usually slightly smaller than the $\dot{V}_I$ because of the respiratory exchange ratio. Normally this difference is negligible. BTPS corrections should be made.

Significance

The $\dot{V}_E$ is the primary index of ventilation when used in conjunction with blood gas values. Since the $\dot{V}_E$ is the sum of both the dead space and effective alveolar ventilation, absolute values for $\dot{V}_E$ are not necessarily indicative of hypoventilation or hyperventilation. A large $\dot{V}_E$ may be the result of an enlarged dead space volume. Normal minute ventilation ranges from 5 to 10 L/min, with wide variations in normal subjects. $\dot{V}_E$ increases in response to hypoxia, hypercapnia, acidosis, low compliance states, anxiety, and exercise, and decreases in the opposite conditions. Subjects with an increased respiratory dead space may exhibit $\dot{V}_E$ values in excess of 20 L/min, since a large total ventilation is necessary to ensure adequate alveolar ventilation. Hypoventilation is defined as inadequate ventilation to remove CO_2 and the respiratory acidosis that results. Hyperventilation is ventilation in excess of that needed to maintain adequate CO_2 removal, with a resulting respiratory alkalosis. The diagnosis of either hyperventilation or hypoventilation requires blood gas analysis (see Chapter 6).

CHEMICAL CONTROL OF VENTILATION
Description

CO_2 response is the measurement of the increase or decrease in $\dot{V}E$ caused by breathing various concentrations of CO_2 under normoxic conditions ($Pa_{O_2} = 100$ mm Hg). It is recorded as L/min/mm Hg P_{CO_2}.

O_2 response is the measurement of the increase or decrease in minute ventilation ($\dot{V}E$) caused by breathing various concentrations of O_2 under isocapnic conditions ($Pa_{CO_2} = 40$ mm Hg).

Occlusion pressure (P_{100}) is the pressure generated in the proximal airway during the first 100 msec of breathing against an occluded airway and is measured in centimeters of water.

Technique

CO_2 response can be measured in two ways:

1. The open-circuit technique, in which various concentrations (1% to 7%) of CO_2 in air or oxygen are breathed until a steady state is reached. Measurements of end-tidal P_{CO_2}, arterial P_{CO_2}, P_{100}, and $\dot{V}E$ are then made at each concentration.

2. The closed-circuit technique, in which the subject rebreathes from a one-way circuit containing a reservoir for 7% CO_2 in O_2 (Fig. 2-1), valves and pressure taps for monitoring P_{100}, and ports for extracting gas samples for end-tidal P_{CO_2} ($P_{ET_{CO_2}}$) determinations. A pneumotachometer (see Chapter 9) is placed in line to record $\dot{V}E$. Changes in $\dot{V}E$ and $P_{ET_{CO_2}}$ are monitored and plotted to obtain a response curve.

O_2 response can be measured by either open- or closed-circuit techniques:

1. Open-circuit technique. The subject breathes gas mixtures containing oxygen concentrations from 12% to 20%, to which CO_2 is added to maintain the alveolar P_{CO_2} at a constant level. Once a steady state is reached, arterial P_{O_2}, $\dot{V}E$, and P_{100} can be measured. This procedure, often called a step test, is repeated at various O_2 concentrations to produce the response curve. Continuous monitoring of end-tidal CO_2 is necessary to titrate the addition of CO_2 to the system to maintain isocapnia (Fig. 2-2). Arterial P_{O_2} must be monitored, since it often varies from alveolar P_{O_2}. CO_2 response curves are sometimes measured at widely varying Pa_{O_2} values, and the subsequent difference in ventilation or P_{100} at any particular P_{CO_2} is attributed to the response to hypoxemia.

2. Closed-circuit technique (progressive hypoxemia). The subject rebreathes from a system similar to that used for the closed-circuit CO_2 response, but one that contains a CO_2 scrubber. CO_2 can be added to the inspired gas to maintain isocapnia, or a variable blower may be used to direct a portion of the rebreathed gas through the scrubber to maintain isocapnia. Response to decreasing inspired P_{O_2} is monitored by recording the $\dot{V}E$ or P_{100}, and the arterial P_{O_2} or saturation is measured either directly by indwelling catheter or by ear oximetry.

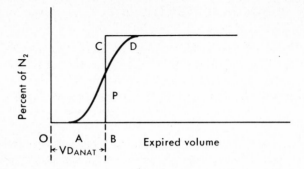

Fig. 2-2. Anatomic dead space determination. The rise in concentration of nitrogen during a single expiration, after a breath of 100% O_2, is illustrated. Only the initial portion of the breath is included. As the subject expires, the N_2 concentration rises slowly at first as pure dead space gas is exhaled; then as bronchial air is expired, the N_2 concentration rises abruptly. Since different parts of the lungs empty at different rates, the change from pure dead space air to alveolar gas appears as an S-shaped curve. By constructing a square wave front *(BC)* so that the areas *ABP* and *DCP* are equal, the anatomic dead space can be estimated as being equal to the volume expired up to point *B*.

P_{100} is measured using a system similar to that in Fig. 2-1. A pressure tap at the proximal airway records pressure changes versus time on a storage oscilloscope. A large-bore stopcock or electronic shutter mechanism is included in the inspiratory line so that inspiratory flow can be randomly occluded. The unidirectional breathing circuit allows the stopcock or shutter to be closed during expiration, so that the subsequent inspiration can occur against complete occlusion starting at FRC.

Significance

The response to an increase in P_{CO_2} in the normal individual is a linear increase in $\dot{V}E$ on the order of 3 L/min/mm Hg (P_{CO_2}). It should be noted, however, that wide variations (1 to 6 L/min) exist in normal subjects, and some variation is present in repeated testing of the same individual. The response to CO_2 in subjects with obstructive disease may be reduced; this is partially attributable to increased airway resistance, which has been shown to reduce ventilatory response in normal individuals. It is not yet clear why some subjects with obstructive disease increase ventilation to maintain a normal P_{CO_2}, whereas others tolerate an increased P_{CO_2}.

The response to a decrease in Pa_{O_2} in the normal individual appears to be exponential once the Pa_{O_2} has fallen to the range of 40 to 60 mm Hg. Again, there are wide variations in responses among individuals. The hypoxic response is increased in the presence of hypercapnia and decreased in hypocapnia. Subjects with chronic obstructive lung disease and chronic CO_2 retention receive their primary respiratory stimulus via the hypoxemic response and may suffer severe or even fatal respiratory depression if that response is obliterated by uncontrolled oxygen therapy.

Some subjects with little intrinsic lung disease show a markedly decreased response to hypoxemia or hypercapnia. These include subjects with myxedema, obesity-hypoventilation syndrome, and idiopathic hypoventilation. CO_2 and O_2 response measurements, along with tests of pulmonary mechanics, may be particularly valuable in the evaluation and treatment of these types of subjects.

P_{100} has been suggested as a measurement of ventilatory drive independent of the mechanical properties of the lungs. Since no airflow occurs during occlusion of the airway, significant interference from mechanical abnormalities, such as increased resistance or decreased compliance, is omitted. Reflexes from the airways and chest wall are also of little influence during the first 100 msec. Therefore the pressure generated can be viewed as proportional to the neural output of the medullary centers that drive the rate and depth of breathing. This proportionality may be influenced by other factors, however, such as body position and the contractile properties of the respiratory muscles.

P_{100} has been shown to increase in hypercapnia and hypoxia and appears to correlate well with the observed ventilatory responses. Some subjects with chronic airway obstruction demonstrate little or no increase in P_{100} in response to an increase in their P_{CO_2}, even with increased airway resistance, whereas normal subjects do increase their P_{100} when breathing through artificial resistance, on challenge with high P_{CO_2} or low P_{O_2}. This failure to respond to increased resistance in the airways may predispose individuals with chronic obstructive pulmonary disease (COPD) to respiratory failure when lung infections occur. Measurement of P_{100} may prove valuable in planning treatment of subjects with abnormal ventilatory responses.

RESPIRATORY DEAD SPACE (VD)
Description

The VD is that volume of the lungs that is ventilated but not perfused by pulmonary capillary blood flow. The dead space can be divided into the conducting airways, or anatomic dead space, and the nonperfused alveoli, or alveolar dead space. The combination of alveolar and anatomic dead space volumes is the physiologic dead space, or VD. The VD is recorded in milliliters or liters.

Technique

The VD can be calculated in two ways. The first uses Bohr's equation defining VD:

$$V_D = \frac{(F_{A_{CO_2}} - F_{E_{CO_2}})}{F_{A_{CO_2}}} V_E$$

where

V_E = Expired volume (tidal volume)

$F_{A_{CO_2}}$ = Fraction of CO_2 in alveolar gas

$F_{E_{CO_2}}$ = Fraction of CO_2 in expired gas

Since the concentration of CO_2 in the alveoli is difficult to measure, the partial pressures of the component gases may be substituted and the equation written thus:

$$V_D = \frac{(Pa_{CO_2} - PE_{CO_2})}{Pa_{CO_2}} V_E$$

where

Pa_{CO_2} = Arterial P_{CO_2}

PE_{CO_2} = P_{CO_2} of expired gas sample

Note that arterial P_{CO_2} may be used in place of alveolar P_{CO_2}; this presumes that equilibration is perfect between the alveoli and pulmonary capillaries, which may not be true in certain diseases. The test derives from the fact that there is practically no CO_2 in the atmosphere, and therefore the partial pressure of CO_2 in the expired gas is inversely proportional to the physiologic dead space, or V_D. By collecting gas over several respiratory cycles and obtaining simultaneous arterial P_{CO_2}, all the variables are supplied, and a reasonably accurate physiologic dead space calculation can be made by application of the equation just given. The estimation becomes more accurate as more expired gas is collected. The accuracy depends on the measurement of $\dot{V}_E$, as well as the partial pressure of CO_2.

A second method available for calculating the anatomic dead space is called the single-breath analysis method, or Fowler's method (see also Chapter 4). This technique requires continuous analysis of the concentration of nitrogen in the expired gas plus simultaneous measurement of the V_E. After inhalation of 100% O_2, the subject breathes out through the recording apparatus. During the first part of the breath pure O_2 is exhaled, and the N_2 concentration remains zero (Fig. 2-2) until a volume equal to the anatomic dead space has been exhaled. Then the N_2 concentration rises rapidly to the level of alveolar N_2, diluted with O_2. Because the conducting airways have different lengths and volumes, the curve depicting the change in N_2 concentration does not present a "square front." By numerical methods a square front can be constructed, and the anatomic dead space is the V_E up to the square front. Bohr's equation can be modified to apply to the data obtained from a single-breath analysis:

$$V_D = \frac{(F_{A_{N_2}} - F_{E_{N_2}})}{F_{A_{N_2}}} V_E$$

where

V_E = Expired volume

$F_{A_{N_2}}$ = Fraction of N_2 in alveolar gas (read from N_2 meter at end of breath)

$F_{E_{N_2}}$ = Fraction of N_2 in expired sample (computed by measuring area under %N_2 curve and dividing by V_E)

The difficulty in obtaining the $F_{E_{N_2}}$ restricts this type of calculation to more sophisticated laboratory setups.

Significance

The measurement of V_D, although difficult, yields important information regarding the status of the functional lung capacity. The anatomic dead space is larger in men than in women and becomes even larger with increases in V_T caused by exercise or pulmonary disease. The anatomic dead space increases in subjects with large FRC values and in diseases such as bronchiectasis. It may be decreased in asthma or in diseases characterized by bronchial obstruction. Because of the difficulty in measuring the anatomic dead space, estimates based on age, sex, and FRC may be used; for clinical purposes the anatomic dead space in milliliters is sometimes equated with the subject's ideal body weight in pounds.

More important is the measurement of physiologic dead space, which is accomplished reasonably well by application of the Bohr equation. The volume of ventilation that is wasted on the conducting airways and nonfunctioning alveoli is usually expressed as a fraction of the tidal volume, V_D/V_T, and is considered normal if the derived value is 0.2 to 0.4. Expressing dead space in this way eliminates the necessity of measuring the volume of expired gas in the application of the Bohr equation. Physiologic dead space measurements are a good index of ventilation/blood flow ratios, since all CO_2 in expired gas come from perfused alveoli (see Chapter 6).

ALVEOLAR VENTILATION ($\dot{V}_A$)
Description

The $\dot{V}_A$ is that volume of gas that participates in gas exchange in the lungs and can be considered equal to the V_T minus the V_D. The $\dot{V}_A$ is usually expressed as volume per unit of time, normally liters per minute.

Technique

The $\dot{V}_A$ can be calculated in two ways:

1. $$\dot{V}_A = f(V_T - V_D)$$

where

V_T = Tidal volume
V_D = Respiratory dead space
f   = Respiratory rate

Often, for the sake of convenience, the V_D is estimated as being equal to the anatomic dead space. This method is valid only when the inspired gas is uniformly distributed in relation to pulmonary blood flow.

2. Since atmospheric gas contains almost no CO_2, $\dot{V}_A$ can be calculated on the basis of CO_2 elimination from the lungs. A volume of expired gas is collected and analyzed to determine the volume of CO_2 contained. The following equation can then be used:

$$\dot{V}_A = \frac{\dot{V}_{CO_2}}{F_{A_{CO_2}}}$$

where

$\dot{V}_{CO_2}$ = Volume of CO_2 expired over a given interval

F_{ACO_2} = Fraction of alveolar gas made up of CO_2

If an end-tidal CO_2 monitor is used, a close approximation of the concentration of alveolar CO_2 is easily obtained and the equation simplified as follows:

$$\dot{V}_A = \frac{\dot{V}_{CO_2}}{\% \text{ Alveolar } CO_2} \times 100$$

The same equation can be used with a substitution of the arterial PCO_2 for the alveolar PCO_2, again presuming that the arterial blood and alveolar gas are in equilibrium. The equation then becomes:

$$\dot{V}_A = \frac{\dot{V}_{CO_2}}{Pa_{CO_2}} \times 0.863$$

where

Pa_{CO_2} = Arterial PCO_2, which was substituted for alveolar CO_2 pressure

0.863 = Factor for converting from concentration to partial pressure

The $\dot{V}_A$ and $\dot{V}_{CO_2}$ must both be corrected to BTPS for the equation to be valid.

Significance

Both of these methods are suitable for calculating the $\dot{V}_A$. The CO_2 elimination method is more accurate than the V_T, dead space, and rate equation when anatomic dead space is used in place of V_D. The difference becomes more apparent in situations where there is pronounced ventilation/blood flow imbalances. The $\dot{V}_A$ is normally about 4 to 5 L/min with wide variations in normal individuals. The adequacy of V_A can be determined only by arterial blood gas studies. Low alveolar ventilation associated with acute respiratory acidosis (Pa_{CO_2} greater than 45 and pH less than 7.35) defines *hypoventilation*. Excessive alveolar ventilation (Pa_{CO_2} less than 35 and pH greater than 7.45) defines *hyperventilation*. Chronic hypoventilation and hyperventilation are associated with abnormal PCO_2 valued, but near-normal pH values.

MAXIMUM SUSTAINED VENTILATORY CAPACITY (MSVC)
Description

The maximum sustained ventilatory capacity (MSVC) is the maximum level of ventilation that can be maintained for a specified interval, usually 15 minutes, under isocapnic conditions. Because a rebreathing circuit is used, the ventilation measurement is typically *not* corrected to BTPS (see technique). The MSVC is recorded in liters per minute.

Technique

MSVC is measured by having the subject ventilate in a rebreathing system, such as that in Fig. 2-3. A bag-in-box apparatus is connected to a spirometer or

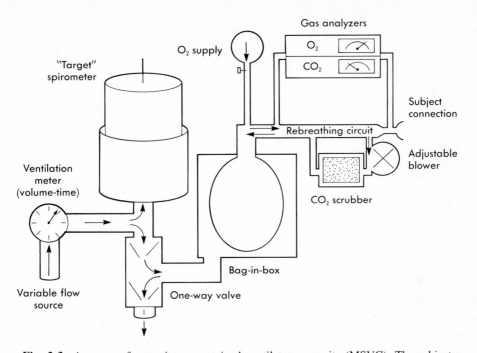

Fig. 2-3. Apparatus for maximum sustained ventilatory capacity (MSVC). The subject breathes through a rebreathing system that consists of a bag-in-box to which an O_2 supply, gas analyzers for O_2 and CO_2, and a CO_2 scrubbing device are attached. The analyzers allow continuous monitoring of the O_2 and CO_2 concentrations; the O_2 supply is adjusted to maintain a normal F_{IO_2}, while an adjustable blower on the CO_2 scrubber regulates the CO_2 concentration in the system to avoid hypercapnia or hypocapnia. Connected to the box via a one-way valve is a volume displacement spirometer. A variable flow source is adjusted to deliver a fixed volume of gas to the "target" spirometer per minute. As the subject inspires, gas is removed from the bag and the spirometer falls; on exhalation, gas is forced from the box out the one-way valve, and the spirometer rises. As long as the subject's minute ventilation matches the flow of gas entering the target spirometer, the spirometer's volume remains fairly constant. Flow is gradually adjusted to obtain the maximal flow that the subject can maintain over an extended interval (see text).

other volume transducer via a large one-way valve. A large valve is required to minimize resistance at higher flow rates. A variable flow generator supplies gas to the spirometer at selected flow rates. As the subject inspires from the bag-in-box system, gas is removed from the spirometer into the box, and then into the atmosphere on exhalation. Connected to the rebreathing circuitry are O_2 and CO_2 analyzers, as well as taps for addition of O_2, and a scrubber for CO_2 removal. Using readings from the gas analyzers, O_2 can be added to maintain an acceptable F_{IO_2} (normally greater than 15%). By attaching a variable speed blower to the CO_2 scrubber, the fraction of CO_2 in the circuit can be maintained close to baseline levels. The subject rebreathes and attempts to keep the spirometer at a "target" level. As long as the subject ventilates at a flow equal to the flow rate from the generator, the spirometer volume remains relatively constant. If the subject cannot match the flow, the spirometer rises, and the flow must be further adjusted. The subject is usually allowed to choose the most efficient tidal volume/ breathing rate combination. Several short trials may be necessary in order to establish the level of ventilation that can be maintained for the desired interval (15 minutes). Some learning may occur, so that repeat runs may be needed to establish the subject's highest ("best") MSVC.

Significance

In normal subjects maximum voluntary ventilation (MVV; see Chapter 3) ranges from 100 to 200 L/min, whereas resting ventilation is usually on the order of 5 to 10 L/min. The MSVC falls between these extremes, usually at 65% to 70% of the MVV. A subject with an MVV of 100 L/min would typically have an MSVC of about 70 L/min. The MSVC represents a level of ventilation that can be sustained for an extended period and is determined by the status of the respiratory control mechanisms, the respiratory muscles, and the total work of breathing (compliance and resistance). Knowing the MSVC is particularly useful in evaluating the endurance of the respiratory muscles, and this value has been used to assess various therapies aimed at training or reconditioning this group of muscles. MSVC is reduced in subjects with obstructive disease, because of the increased work of breathing associated with ventilation at higher flow rates. In spite of this absolute reduction, the MSVC may be above 70% of the same subject's MVV. Because of the low absolute levels of sustainable ventilation in subjects with obstruction, it is clear why exercise limitations may occur with normal activities such as walking. MSVC may also be reduced in subjects with defects influencing the neuromuscular aspects of ventilation, such as myasthenia gravis. The MSVC, as an index of respiratory muscle endurance, is often used in conjunction with maximal inspiratory/expiratory pressure (see Chapter 3), which relates to respiratory muscle strength.

SELF-ASSESSMENT QUESTIONS

1. The main difficulty in trying to assess a subject's ventilatory response to hypoxemia is:
   a. Hyperventilation normally occurs with a Pa_{O_2} of 80 to 85 mm Hg
   b. Special gas mixtures (less than 21% O_2) are needed
   c. A normal P_{CO_2} (isocapnia) must be maintained
   d. All of the above
2. A subject is given a closed-circuit CO_2 response test. The results show an increase in ventilation at the rate of 5 L/min for each mm Hg change in P_{CO_2}. This:
   a. Is markedly reduced
   b. Is only slightly reduced
   c. Is within normal limits
   d. Cannot be determined from the information provided
3. Exhaled gas is collected in a meteorologic balloon for a 5-minute interval; during this period the subject breathes 55 times. If the total volume collected is 30 liters, what is the:

V_T _____

Rate (f) _____

$\dot{V}_E$ _____

4. A subject's $\dot{V}_E$ is measured as 22.7 L/min. Blood gases in the same subject reveal a pH of 7.54 and a P_{CO_2} of 23; this level of ventilation is:
   a. Consistent with hypoventilation
   b. Consistent with a decrease in dead space V_D
   c. Consistent with hyperventilation
   d. Inconsistent with the reported blood gases

5. Which of the following parameters would be useful in assessing the response to increasing carbon dioxide tensions (CO_2 response test)?
   a. Minute ventilation ($\dot{V}_E$)
   b. Physiologic dead space (V_D)
   c. P_{100} (occlusion pressure in 100 msec)
   d. FEV_1
   e. a and c

6. The response to an increased $P_{A_{CO_2}}$ in normal individuals is:
   a. To decrease $\dot{V}_E$ slightly
   b. To increase $\dot{V}_E$ by 20 L/min for each millimeter of Hg increase in P_{CO_2}
   c. To increase $\dot{V}_E$ by 1 to 6 L/min for each millimeter of Hg increase in P_{CO_2}
   d. To maintain a constant $\dot{V}_E$ until the $P_{A_{CO_2}}$ rises to 55 to 60 mm Hg

7. The normal response to a decrease in arterial oxygen tension (Pa_{O_2}) is:
   a. A linear increase in $\dot{V}_E$ as the Pa_{O_2} drops below 100 mm Hg
   b. An exponential increase in $\dot{V}_E$ as the Pa_{O_2} drops below 100 mm Hg
   c. An exponential increase in $\dot{V}_E$ at a Pa_{O_2} of less than 60 mm Hg
   d. A linear decrease in $\dot{V}_E$ at a Pa_{O_2} of less than 60 mm Hg

8. P_{100} measures the:
   a. Output of the respiratory centers
   b. Effect of breathing high concentrations of oxygen
   c. $\dot{V}_E$ when the Pa_{O_2} is 100 mm Hg
   d. Endurance of the diaphragm

9. A subject has arterial blood drawn and expired gas collected: $\dot{V}_E$ is 12 L/min, Pa_{CO_2} is 44 mm Hg, and partial pressure of CO_2 in the expired sample ($P_{E_{CO_2}}$) is 22 mm Hg. What is the volume of V_D/min?

   $\dot{V}_D$ = _____

   If the subject has an f of 18 breaths/min, what are the following values?

   V_T = _____

   V_D = _____

   V_D/V_T = _____

10. A subject has a $\dot{V}_E$ of 10 L/min and an f of 20 breaths/min; if the subject's $\dot{V}_A$ is measured as 6 L/min, what is his V_D?

    V_D = _____ liters

11. A subject has an MSVC that is 83% of her MVV, but the MVV is only 27% of the predicted value; these findings are:
    a. Consistent with normal lung function in an older adult
    b. Consistent with an obstructive disease pattern
    c. Consistent with a mild restrictive pattern
    d. Physiologically impossible

12. A subject has his MSVC measured, but the "target" spirometer continues to rise; this could happen if:
   a. The subject is breathing too rapidly
   b. There is insufficient O_2 being added
   c. The flow generated exceeds the subject's MSVC
   d. Any of the above

SELECTED BIBLIOGRAPHY

General references

Comroe, J.H.: Physiology of respiration, Chicago, 1965, Year Book Medical Publishers, Inc.

West, J.B.: Respiratory physiology: the essentials, Baltimore, 1974, Williams & Wilkins.

West, J.B.: Pulmonary pathophysiology: the essentials, Baltimore, 1977, Williams & Wilkins.

Ventilation

Gray, J.S., Gracius, F.S., and Carter, E.T.: Alveolar ventilation and dead space problem, J. Appl. Physiol. **2:**307, 1956.

Riley, R.L., and Cournand, A.: 'Ideal' alveolar air and the analysis of ventilation-perfusion relationships in the lungs, J. Appl. Physiol. **1:**825, 1949.

Severinghaus, J.W., and Stipfel, M.: Alveolar dead space as an index of distribution of blood flow in pulmonary capillaries, J. Appl. Physiol. **10:**335, 1957.

Control of ventilation

Cherniack, N.S., et al.: Occlusion pressure as a technique in evaluating respiratory control, Chest **70**(suppl.):137, 1956.

Shaw, R.A., Schonfeld, S.A., and Whitcomb, M.E.: Progressive and transient hypoxic ventilatory drive tests in healthy subjects, Am. Rev. Respir. Dis. **126:**37, 1982.

Sullivan, T.Y., and Yu, P.L.: Reproducibility of CO_2 response curves with ten minutes separating each rebreathing test, Am. Rev. Respir. Dis. **129:**23, 1984.

Respiratory muscles

Black, L.F., and Hyatt, R.E.: Maximal respiratory pressures: normal values and relationship to age and sex, Am. Rev. Respir. Dis. **99:**696, 1976.

Brody, A.W., et al.: Correlations, normal standards, and interdependence in tests of ventilatory strength and mechanics, Am. Rev. Respir. Dis. **89:**214, 1964.

Leith, D., and Bradley, M.: Ventilatory muscle strength and endurance training, J. Appl. Physiol. **41:**508, 1976.

CHAPTER THREE

Pulmonary mechanics tests

FORCED VITAL CAPACITY (FVC)
Description

The FVC is the maximum volume of gas that can be expired as forcefully and rapidly as possible after maximal inspiration. The FVC is always an expired volume unless specifically stated otherwise. The same maneuver performed by beginning at maximal expiration and inspiring as forcefully as possible is called forced inspiratory vital capacity (FIVC). The FVC is usually recorded in liters, corrected to BTPS.

Technique

FVC is measured by having the subject, after inspiring maximally, expire as forcefully and rapidly as possible into a bellows or spirometer, or through a pneumotachometer. The volume may be read from a direct tracing such as a kymograph (Fig. 3-1) or recorded from a digital display. A spirometer that produces a hard copy report is preferred in all cases except simple screening, when a permanent spirogram is to be obtained subsequently. The spirometer must meet American Thoracic Society (ATS) requirements (see Appendix). The volume must be corrected to BTPS.

Significance

The FVC is normally equal to the VC; they may be unequal because of obstruction (FVC less than VC) or because of poor effort by the subject. The FVC may exceed the VC in instances where the subject's effort is variable. The FVC may be reduced in chronic obstructive diseases, whereas the VC appears closer to normal. The forced expiration causes higher than normal transpulmonary pressures, so that bronchiolar collapse, obstructive lesions, and air trapping are all exaggerated. Decreased FVC is common in restrictive diseases such as pulmonary fibrosis, as well as in obstructive processes such as emphysema and asthma. A lower than predicted FVC in restrictive patterns usually results from an increase in fibrotic tissue, vascular congestion, space-occupying lesions such as tumors, neuromuscular disorders such as myasthenia gravis, or chest deformities such as scoliosis. Obesity and pregnancy are common causes of reduced FVC. Decreased FVC in obstructive patterns follows loss of support for small airways (< 2 mm) as in emphysema, bronchiolar plugging accompanying mucus secretion as in bronchitis and asthma, or bronchiolar constriction as in asthma. Interpretation of the FVC in obstructive diseases requires correlation to flows, where-

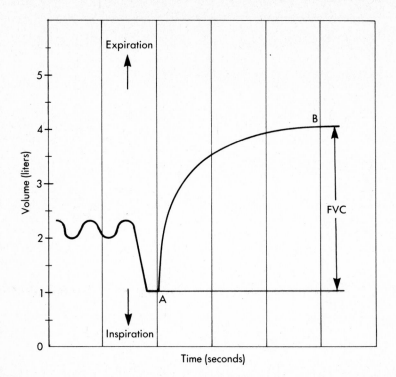

Fig. 3-1. Forced vital capacity (FVC)—typical spirogram plotting volume change against time as the subject exhales forcefully. In this tracing expiration causes an upward deflection; in some systems the tracing is inverted. The subject inspires to the maximal inspiratory level, *A,* and then expires as rapidly as possible to the maximal expiratory level, *B* (see text).

as in restrictive patterns the FVC should be considered in relation to the other lung volumes (RV, TLC, etc.) Values less than 80% of predicted values, or less than the 95% confidence limit, are considered abnormal in both obstruction and restriction; values less than 50% of predicted values denote a marked reduction in FVC and are often accompanied by exertional dyspnea.

The validity of the FVC maneuver depends largely on the subject's effort and cooperation, as well as on the instruction and coaching supplied by the technologist. Because of its central role in routine spirometry, the acceptability of the FVC should be evaluated according to specific criteria (see Chapter 11).

FORCED EXPIRATORY VOLUME (FEV$_T$)
Description

The FEV$_T$ is the volume of gas expired over a given time interval during the performance of an FVC maneuver. The interval is stated as a subscript to FEV. Those intervals in common use are FEV$_{0.5}$, FEV$_{1.0}$, FEV$_{2.0}$, and FEV$_{3.0}$. The

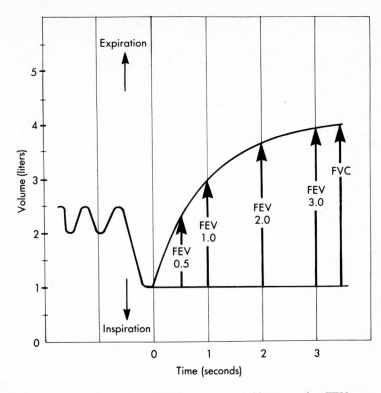

Fig. 3-2. Forced expiratory volume (FEV) maneuver—spirogram of an FEVᴛ maneuver, with the subject exhaling as forcefully and rapidly as possible. Marks indicate the FEV at the various intervals.

FEVᴛ is normally stated in liters, and ᴛ is expressed as seconds (Fig. 3-2). Of the various FEV measurements, $FEV_{1.0}$ is the most widely used.

Technique

FEVᴛ may be measured by introducing a means of timing an FVC maneuver over the described intervals. Normally this is done by recording the FVC spirogram on graph paper moving at a fixed speed, so that the volume at any interval can be read from the graph. Because accurate measurement of the FEV intervals depends on determination of the *start-of-test,* the spirometer should provide a hard copy tracing; this allows for direct measurement of the volume-time curve and back-extrapolation if necessary (see Chapter 11). Automated systems detect the start-of-test as a flow or volume change threshold and then store volume and flow data points via software. Computer-generated representations of the volume-time curve may not provide a means of assessing the start-of-test; hence inaccurate FEV values may result. Some electronic units report the FEVᴛ only in digital form from the exhaled volume or flow, but such measurements should be used only for screening when a hard copy spirogram is available for correlation. Corrections to BTPS must be made.

Significance

Since the FEV$_T$ maneuver measures a volume of gas expired over a unit of time, it is in reality a measure of the average flow over that interval. By assessing the flow at specific intervals, the severity of airway obstruction can be ascertained. Decreased values for FEV$_T$ are common in both obstructive and restrictive patterns. Airway narrowing due to mucus secretion, bronchospasm, inflammation, or loss of elastic support all result in decreased values for FEV$_T$. However, the FEV$_T$ may remain relatively normal in spite of obstruction in the small airways (< 2 mm). Fibrosis, edema, space-occupying lesions, neuromuscular disorders, and chest wall deformities may all cause the FEV$_T$ to be decreased. Distinction between obstructive and restrictive causes for reduced FEV values is made by relating the FEV$_T$ to the FVC (see below) and to other flow measurements.

Of all the FEV parameters, FEV$_1$ is the most widely used spirometric parameter, particularly for assessment of airway obstruction. FEV$_1$ is used for simple screening, for assessment of response to bronchodilators, for inhalation challenge studies, and for detection of exercise-induced bronchospasm (see Chapters 7 and 8).

The validity of the test depends largely on the cooperation and effort of the subject. Accurate measurement of FEV requires an adequate spirometer, acceptable hard copy, and attention to specific criteria defining an acceptable maneuver (see Chapter 11).

FORCED EXPIRATORY VOLUME/FORCED VITAL CAPACITY RATIO (FEV$_T$/FVC or FEV$_T$%)
Description

The FEV$_T$% is a statement of the FEV for a given interval expressed as a percentage of the subject's actual FVC.

Technique

As described for FVC and FEV$_T$, normally the FVC and FEV$_T$ are computed from the same test maneuver. However, because a subject performing an FEV maneuver cannot "overshoot" either the FVC or FEV$_T$, the best FEV$_T$ and FVC may come from different maneuvers. Thus the FEV$_T$/FVC ratio may be the product of two or more maneuvers. If instantaneous or averaged flows are to be reported, they should be obtained from that test with the largest sum of FVC and FEV$_1$ (see Chapter 11).

Significance

A normal individual can expire 50% to 60% of the FVC in 0.5 second, 75% to 85% in 1 second, 94% in 2 seconds, and 97% in 3 seconds. Slightly lower ratios may be observed in elderly adults, but in general, subjects without airway obstruction can expire their VC within 4 seconds. Conversely, subjects with obstructive disease will show a reduced $FEV_T\%$ in most cases; an FEV_1/FVC ratio lower than 65% to 70% is the hallmark of obstructive disease. Since the FEV_1/FVC is a ratio, mild to moderate obstructive disease can be identified without reference to absolute predicted values. Subjects with restrictive disease often show a normal, or supranormal, $FEV_T\%$, since flow rates may be minimally affected, and the FEV_1 and FVC are usually reduced in equal proportion. Validity again depends on the individual's effort and cooperation. Poor effort on the FVC maneuver may result in an overestimate of the $FEV_T\%$. Some clinicians prefer to use the largest VC to calculate the $FEV_T\%$, even if that VC comes from a slow vital capacity maneuver (see case studies in Chapter 12).

FORCED EXPIRATORY FLOW$_{200-1200}$ (FEF$_{200-1200}$)
Description

The $FEF_{200-1200}$ is the *average* flow rate for the liter of gas expired after the first 200 ml during an FEV maneuver. The same test is also termed maximal expiratory flow rate ($MEFR_{200-1200}$). The $FEF_{200-1200}$ is usually recorded in liters per second but may be stated in liters per minute (Fig. 3-3).

Technique

$FEF_{200-1200}$ is measured from an acceptable FEV maneuver. Normally a spirographic tracing is made, and the time interval from the 200 ml point to the 1200

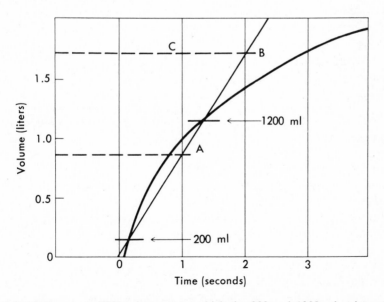

Fig. 3-3. $FEF_{200-1200}$—FEV spirogram on which the 200 and 1200 ml points of the expiration have been marked; a line connecting these two points is extended to cross two time lines 1 second apart, points *A* and *B*. The flow rate in liters per second can be read as the vertical distance between the points of intersection *(AC)* and here is about 1.0 L/sec.

ml point is divided into 1 liter to obtain the average flow rate for that interval. If the 200 and 1200 ml points are marked on the shoulder of the curve, a straight line connecting them may be extended so that it intersects two time lines 1 second apart on the graph paper. The flow rate may then be read as the distance between these two points of intersection (Fig. 3-3). Flows must be corrected to BTPS, but volume points should be marked on the uncorrected curve before BTPS corrections are applied. FEV curves that display back-extrapolated volumes (see Chapter 11) greater than 200 ml yield spurious values for $FEF_{200-1200}$.

Significance

The $FEF_{200-1200}$ measures the average flow of the early part of a forced expiration. The initial 200 ml of volume may be expired at a slower rate because of inertia of the lung-thorax system, as well as inertia of some types of spirometers. It is disregarded for this reason. The average rate of airflow in the initial part of a forced expiration for a healthy young man is 6 to 7 L/sec (400 L/min). The $FEF_{200-1200}$ is a good index of airflow characteristics of the larger airways, but since it is calculated from the first segment of the forced expiration, airflow slowing caused by disease of the small (< 2 mm) airways may be overlooked. Decreased values for $FEF_{200-1200}$ indicate a mechanical problem; obstructive disease causes a decrease in $FEF_{200-1200}$, whereas restrictive disease may display a normal or sometimes increased $FEF_{200-1200}$. Flow rates as low as 1 L/sec (60 L/min) are not uncommon in obstructive patterns. $FEF_{200-1200}$ decreases significantly with age and is normally lower in women than in men (see Appendix). Low values for $FEF_{200-1200}$ are often seen in conjunction with decreased peak expiratory flow rates (see below). Similarly, large airway obstruction patterns seen on the expiratory limb of flow volume curves (see also below) also accompany a decreased $FEF_{200-1200}$. The nature of the mechanical problem in decreased flow rates is sometimes clarified by measuring the $FIF_{200-1200}$ (forced inspiratory flow) for the same interval from a forced inspiratory volume (FIV) maneuver. Healthy young men can normally attain rates of 5 L/sec (300 L/min) on inspiration. The validity of the test depends on subject cooperation and effort; low values are often a result of poor start-of-test because of inadequate explanation of the maneuver.

FORCED EXPIRATORY FLOW$_{25\%-75\%}$ (FEF$_{25\%-75\%}$)
Description

The $FEF_{25\%-75\%}$ is the average rate of flow during the middle half of an FEV maneuver. It is recorded in liters per second or liters per minute. The same test was formerly designated the maximum midexpiratory flow rate (MMFR).

Technique

The $FEF_{25\%-75\%}$ determination requires the same apparatus as an FEV maneuver. The length of time required for the subject to expire 50% of the FVC after exhaling the initial 25% of the FVC is divided into 50% of the FVC. Normally a volume-time spirogram is used, with 25% and 75% points marked on the curve

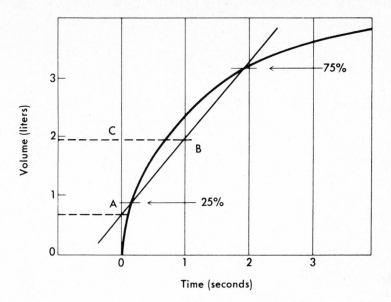

Fig. 3-4. FEF$_{25\%-75\%}$—FEV spirogram on which the 25% and 75% points of the expiration have been marked; these points are determined by multiplying the FVC by 0.25 and 0.75, respectively. A line connecting these points is extended to intersect two time lines 1 second apart, points A and B. The flow rate in liters per second can be read as the vertical distance between the points of intersection (AC)—in this case a little over 1 L/sec. Alternatively, the slope of the line connecting the 25% and 75% points can be determined by dividing one half of the FVC by the time interval between the points, or by using a protractor-like device.

(Fig. 3-4). A straight line connecting these points is extended to intersect two time lines 1 second apart, and the flow rate can be read directly as the distance between the points of intersection. The FEF$_{25\%-75\%}$ can be computed electronically, but its accuracy depends on the accuracy of the device. The FEF$_{25\%-75\%}$ is largely dependent on the FVC; large values for FEF$_{25\%-75\%}$ may be derived from maneuvers with small FVC values because the "middle half" of the volume is actually gas expired early on in the expiration. This effect is particularly evident when the subject terminates the FEV maneuver prematurely. (i.e., before reaching the RV). The FEF$_{25\%-75\%}$ should be measured from the maneuver with the largest sum of FVC and FEV$_1$. Volumes must be corrected to BTPS.

Significance

The FEF$_{25\%-75\%}$, like the FEF$_{200-1200}$, measures the average flow rate over a given interval (volume) but is based on a segment of the FVC that includes more than the initial part of the breath. It is normally somewhat slower than the FEF$_{200-1200}$, the values for a healthy young man averaging 4 to 5 L/sec (240-300 L/min). The FEF$_{25\%-75\%}$ is indicative of the status of the medium- to small-sized airways. Decreased flow rates are common in the early stages of obstructive disease, more so than in restrictive disease. Flows as low as 0.3 L/sec (20 L/min) may occur in cases of severe obstruction, such as advanced emphysema. $FEF_{25\%-75\%}$ values decrease with age. The $FEF_{25\%-75\%}$ varies significantly in normal subjects, such that a value as low as 65% of the predicted value may be statistically within normal limits. This variability limits the usefulness of the $FEF_{25\%-75\%}$ somewhat. Low values for $FEF_{25\%-75\%}$ in combination with normal values for other parameters (FVC, FEV_1, etc.) are often indicative of early small airway abnormality. The test depends on subject effort, but less so than does the $FEF_{200-1200}$. There is little evidence that the $FEF_{25\%-75\%}$ is more reliable than other flow measurements commonly used in assessing obstructive ventilatory

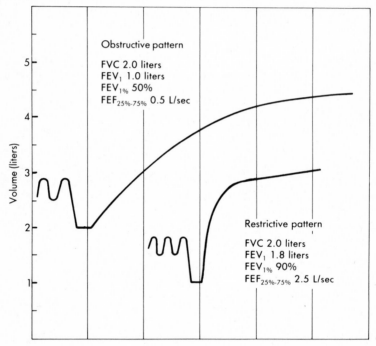

Obstructive pattern

FVC 2.0 liters
FEV_1 1.0 liters
$FEV_{1\%}$ 50%
$FEF_{25\%-75\%}$ 0.5 L/sec

Restrictive pattern

FVC 2.0 liters
FEV_1 1.8 liters
$FEV_{1\%}$ 90%
$FEF_{25\%-75\%}$ 2.5 L/sec

Volume (liters)

Time (seconds)

Fig. 3-5. Obstructive versus restrictive spirograms. The *obstructive pattern* shows a decreased FVC as well as expiratory airflow slowing; the volume expired in the first second (FEV_1) is only 50% of the FVC (FEV_1/FVC). The $FEF_{25\%-75\%}$ also shows a marked reduction. The *restrictive pattern* also shows a reduced FVC, equal to that observed in the obstructive defect, but the FEV_1FVC ratio is increased; almost all of the VC is expired in the first second. The $FEF_{25\%-75\%}$ is not decreased, as in the obstructive pattern. FVC alone cannot be used to distinguish obstructive from restrictive disease patterns; flow rates are typically decreased in obstructive patterns and are decreased significantly in restrictive disease only when the lung volumes are markedly reduced. The FEV_1/FVC ratio, used in conjunction with the actual measured values for FEV_1 and FVC, is helpful in ascertaining the type of defect (see text).

impairments, although it seems to be more commonly used. Reduced values for FEF$_{25\%-75\%}$ are sometimes seen in cases of severe restrictive patterns, when the restrictive lesion compresses the small airways. Fig. 3-5 shows typical abnormal spirograms for obstructive and restrictive patterns. Case study examples of spirometric measurements in both obstructive and restrictive disease patterns are included in Chapter 12. The general descriptions of FVC, FEV$_T$, and FEF measurements in this section may be used to help interpret the numerical data of the case studies.

PEAK EXPIRATORY FLOW RATE (PEFR)
Description

The PEFR is the maximum flow rate attained at any time during an FEV maneuver. It is recorded in liters per second or liters per minute.

Technique

PEFR can be measured by drawing a tangent to the *steepest* part of an FVC spirogram. The tracing should be made with the pen or paper moving at the

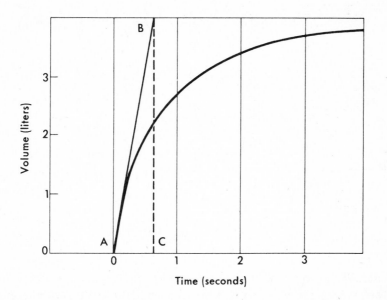

Fig. 3-6. Peak flow tangent—FEV spirogram on which a line has been drawn tangent to the steepest part of the curve, line *AB*. Normally the steepest part of the curve is near the very beginning. In this case the tangent has a slope such that it does not intersect the two closest time lines, 1 second apart. The flow rate can be computed by dividing the volume *(BC)* by the time interval *(AC)* of 4 L/0.67 sec. The peak flow in this instance is approximately 6 L/sec. This method is somewhat less than precise, especially in normal individuals, whose peak flows often exceed 10 L/sec. A pneumotachometer offers better results, especially at high flow rates. The PEFR can also be read easily from the MEFV curve (see text and Fig. 3-7).

fastest possible speed. The tangent may be extended to intersect two time lines and the flow read directly as the distance between the points of intersection for that interval (Fig. 3-6). This technique is difficult at best in subjects with normal peak flows. PEFR may be measured more accurately by means of a mechanical or electronic pneumotachometer; the latter uses a transducer to convert flow to an electrical output, which may be displayed either digitally or stored via computer (see Chapter 9). Temperature corrections must be made.

Significance

PEFR values as computed by the first method just given, are of doubtful accuracy, especially in normal subjects. The PEFR attainable by healthy young adults may exceed 10 L/sec (600 L/min). Even when measured by the pneumo-tachometer, PEFR measurements may be of limited value. Subjects with small airway obstructive disease may develop an initially high flow rate before airway closure occurs. A decreased PEFR is usually associated with upper or large air-way lesions but is largely nonspecific. A PEFR read from flow-volume loops (as well as peak inspiratory flow rate; PIFR) helps define the severity of large airway obstruction. The test, of course, depends on subject effort, and falsely low values may be obtained because of poor cooperation. However, reproducibility of the PEFR indicates validity, and comparison of peak flows obtained from maximum expiratory flow-volume (MEFV) curves is often helpful in quantifying subject effort.

Small, inexpensive devices that measure PEFR using some sort of flow gauge are available. The PEFR measured via such portable devices is most useful for following gross changes in airway function in outpatients. The PEFR measured thus should be correlated with spirometry done under laboratory conditions in order to be most meaningful. The primary application of the PEFR used in this way is to follow asthmatics on a continuous basis or during acute exacerbations, whether as outpatients or at the bedside.

FLOW-VOLUME CURVES
Description

The flow-volume curve is a graphic analysis of the flow generated during an FEV maneuver plotted against volume change, followed by an FIV maneuver plotted similarly (Fig. 3-7). Flow is usually recorded in liters per second, and the volume is recorded in liters. The MEFV curve or tracing delineates the expiratory portion of the curve in particular without reference to the maximum inspiratory flow-volume (MIFV) curve. When both the MEFV and MIFV curves are plotted together, the figure may be termed a flow-volume loop.

Technique

The subject performs an FEV maneuver followed by an FIV maneuver. Volume is plotted on the abscissa and the amount of flow generated on the ordinate. This type of spirogram must be done with a recorder capable of plotting flow and volume from their respective analog inputs (see Fig. 9-22), with a storage oscil-

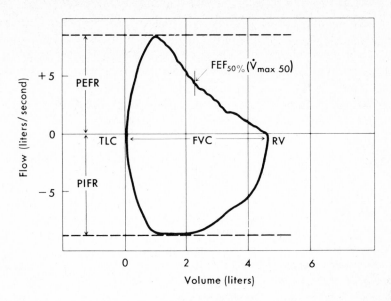

Fig. 3-7. Flow-volume loop—flow-volume spirogram in which an FEV and an FIV maneuver are recorded in succession. Flow rate is plotted on the vertical axis and volume on the horizontal axis. Peak flows for inspiration and expiration can be read directly, as can the FVC. The instantaneous flow rate at a particular point in the FVC can be measured directly. Recorders that are capable of interjecting time marks, or tics, in the tracing allow the FEVt to be read directly as well. Phenomena such as small or large airway obstruction show up as characteristic changes in the flow rate (see Fig. 3-8).

loscope, or by computer-generated graphics. From the loop the peak inspiratory and expiratory flows can be read, as well as the FVC. The instantaneous flow at any lung volume can be read directly from the MEFV tracing. Flows at 75%, 50%, and 25% of the VC are commonly reported as $\dot{V}_{max\ 75}$, $\dot{V}_{max\ 50}$, and $\dot{V}_{max\ 25}$, respectively. If automatic timing is available on the graphing device or via the computer, the FEVt% can be determined for whatever intervals are measured. Plotting of stored data points allows manipulation of the flow-volume tracings, which facilitates comparisons of individual maneuvers, bronchodilator studies, and challenge studies.

Significance

Predicted values for FEVt (if time marks are incorporated into the MEFV tracing) and for the FVC are the same as those for conventional volume-time curves. Significant decreases in either flow or volume (due to obstructive or restrictive processes) are available in a single graphic display to aid in differentiating specific abnormalities. The shape of the expiratory curve of the MEFV tracing from about 75% of TLC down to RV is largely independent of subject effort, flow being determined mainly by the elastic recoil properties of the lungs and the flow-resistive properties of the smaller airways. In normal subjects flow

$\dot{V}_{max}$) decreases linearly with volume over most of the VC range, so that the expiratory curve has a "straight line" appearance (Fig. 3-7). In subjects with small airway obstruction flow is decreased particularly at lower lung volumes and the independent segment of the flow-volume curve takes on a curvilinear or "scooped-out" appearance (Fig. 3-8). Values for $\dot{V}_{max\ 50}$ and $\dot{V}_{max\ 25}$ are characteristically decreased. Decreases in $\dot{V}_{max\ 50}$ correlate well with the $FEF_{25\%-75\%}$ in subjects with small airway obstructive lung disease. Because elastic recoil and

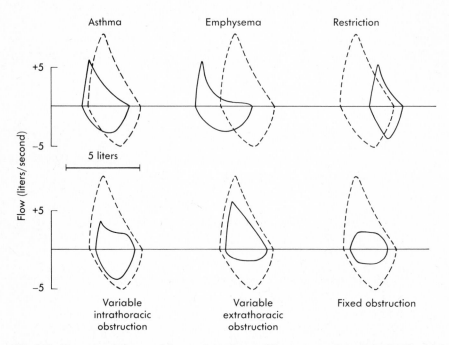

Fig. 3-8. Normal and abnormal flow-volume loops. Six curves are shown plotting flow in liters per second against the FVC. In each example the expected curve is shown by the dashed lines, and the curve typifying the particular lesion is superimposed. For asthma and emphysema, the latter portion of the expiratory curve is characteristically "scooped out" and the TLC and RV points are displaced toward higher lung volumes (hyperinflation and/or air trapping). In restrictive patterns the shape of the loop is preserved but the FVC is decreased, with the TLC and RV displaced toward lower lung volumes than might be expected. The bottom three examples depict types of large airway obstruction. Variable intrathoracic obstruction shows reduced flows on expiration with near normal flows on inspiration due to intrathoracic compression of the airways. Variable extrathoracic obstruction shows an opposite pattern, with inspiratory flow being reduced while expiratory flow is relatively well preserved. Fixed large airway obstruction is characterized by approximately equal inspiratory and expiratory flows. Comparison of the $FEF_{50\%}$ with the $FIF_{50\%}$ is often helpful in differentiating large airway obstructive processes. Since the magnitude of inspiratory flow is effort dependent, low inspiratory flows should be carefully evaluated.

resistance in the small airways determine the shape of the expiratory limb of the MEFV tracing, diseases that influence either of them result in decreased flows. Emphysema destroys terminal lung units, with a loss of elastic recoil; bronchitis, asthma, and similar inflammatory processes increase the resistance in the small airways; thus decreased flows (and the characteristic shape of the MEFV curve) occur despite somewhat distinct pathologic conditions.

Obstruction of the upper airway, trachea, and mainstream bronchi show characteristic limitations to expiratory flow, making the flow-volume curve useful in diagnosing these particular lesions (Fig. 3-8). Comparison of expiratory and inspiratory flows at the 50% point is helpful in distinguishing the site of the obstruction. Fixed large airway obstructions typically result in reduced, but approximately equal, flow at 50% of the VC for both inspiration and expiration (Fig. 3-9). Obstructive processes that vary with the phase of breathing also show

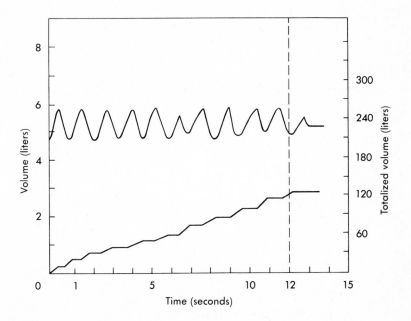

Fig. 3-9. Maximum voluntary ventilation (MVV)—composite MVV spirogram on which breath-by-breath volume change and totalized volume are plotted against time. The top tracing shows the actual volume moved on each breath over a 12-second interval; to calculate the MVV, the volumes of individual breaths are added and multiplied by a factor of 5 (60 sec/12 sec = 5). Since the MVV is stated as a flow rate in liters per minute, the values for 12 seconds must be extrapolated to 1 minute. The lower tracing is computer generated and depicts the totalized volume, in L/min, exhaled during the 12-second maneuver (in this example, approximately 120 L/min). Normal subjects will maintain the same MVV flow rate throughout the maneuver. Subjects with pulmonary disease will show decreased absolute values, and often the MVV will decrease significantly as the maneuver progresses, because of fatigue of the respiratory muscles, increased work of breathing, etc.

characteristic patterns. Variable extrathoracic obstruction usually shows normal expiratory flows with diminished inspiratory flows; the converse is true with variable intrathoracic obstruction.

Restrictive processes may show relatively normal peak expiratory flows and linear decreases in flow versus lung volume, but the lung volume itself is decreased. Moderate to severe restriction demonstrates equally reduced flows at all lung volumes and may appear as a *miniature* of the normal MEFV curve.

Before- and after-bronchodilator MEFV curves can be superimposed to facilitate measurement of relative increases in flow at each lung volume. Similarly, tidal breathing curves and maximum voluntary ventilation (MVV) curves can be superimposed on the flow-volume curve (inspiratory and expiratory curves) to evaluate ventilatory reserves by comparing the areas bounded by each of the curves. Subjects with severe chronic obstructive lung disease often generate flow-volume curves of only slightly greater dimensions than their tidal breathing curves. In general, the ability to assess both flow and volume in a single graphic representation is responsible for the widespread use of the flow-volume curve.

VOLUME OF ISOFLOW (Viso$\dot{V}$)
Description

The Viso$\dot{V}$ is the portion of the VC remaining in the lungs at which gas flow becomes independent of gas density and is determined by superimposing MEFV curves recorded with the subject breathing air and a mixture of 80% helium and 20% oxygen (Fig. 3-10). The Viso$\dot{V}$ is normally recorded as a percentage of the FVC.

Technique

MEFV curves are obtained as usual, with the subject breathing air. Then the MEFV maneuver is repeated with the subject breathing the He-O_2 mixture. The subject may either breathe the mixture for 10 minutes or take three slow VC breaths of the mixture before performing the maneuver; both techniques yield results that do not differ significantly. The He-O_2 mixture and air curves are then superimposed and matched at RV if the FVC values are different. The point at which the expiratory curves meet determines that part of the FVC that remains in the lungs when gas flow becomes identical after the subject has breathed the air and He-O_2 mixture (Fig. 3-10). This lung volume is known as the Viso$\dot{V}$ and is normally expressed as a percentage of the FVC. From the same tracing the increase in maximal flow at 50% of the VC ($\dot{V}_{max\ 50}$) can be determined. Since flow in larger airways depends on gas density, the amount of increase in $\dot{V}_{max\ 50}$ while the subject is breathing the He-O_2 mixture is relatively specific for changes in airway caliber. The increase in $\dot{V}_{max\ 50}$ while the subject is breathing the He-O_2 mixture is expressed as a percentage of the $\dot{V}_{max\ 50}$ while the subject is breathing air and is called the $\Delta\dot{V}_{max\ 50}$:

$$\Delta\dot{V}_{max\ 50} = \frac{\dot{V}_{max\ 50_{He}} - \dot{V}_{max\ 50_{air}}}{\dot{V}_{max\ 50_{air}}} \times 100$$

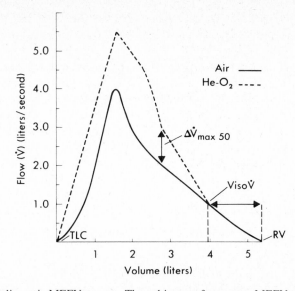

Fig. 3-10. Helium-air MEFV curves. The subject performs two MEFV maneuvers; the first is a simple MEFV maneuver of breathing air; the second MEFV maneuver is performed after the subject has breathed a mixture of 80% He and 20% O_2 for several minutes or for several VC breaths. The two curves are then superimposed by matching at RV. The $\dot{V}_{max\ 50}$ (or $\dot{V}_{max}$ at any other lung volume) can then be read directly from the tracing. Decreases in the $\dot{V}_{max\ 50}$ are consistent with diseases causing increased resistance in the small airways (< 2 mm), but there is apparently little change with loss of elastic recoil. The point at which both curves converge is the volume of isoflow (Viso$\dot{V}$). At this lung volume, maximum expiratory flow becomes independent of the gas density of the expirate. Diseases that compromise the small airways, either by increased resistance or loss of elastic recoil, tend to increase the Viso$\dot{V}$, so that the curves converge earlier during the expiratory maneuver.

Significance

Normal values for Viso$\dot{V}$ as a percentage of the FVC appear to be in the range of 10% to 20% for subjects 20 to 50 years of age.

An increase in Viso$\dot{V}$ above the normal level is consistent with obstruction of the small airways. During forced expiration in normal subjects, the site of flow limitation is in the large airways until low lung volumes are reached. Breathing a gas of low density improves flow in these larger airways, but as flow limitation shifts to the smaller airways (< 2 mm) toward the end of a forced expiration, resistance is determined by laminar airflow and is independent of gas density. At this point the He-O_2 mixture and air curves converge. Therefore in diseases of the small airways in which there is increased resistance (asthma) or in which there is a loss of elastic recoil (emphysema), the site of flow limitation is located in the smaller airways at a higher lung volume and the Viso$\dot{V}$ is increased.

The increase in $\Delta\dot{V}_{max\ 50}$ may be reduced in diseases that cause increased resistance, although loss of elastic recoil does not appear to influence $\dot{V}_{max\ 50}$. Thus $\Delta\dot{V}_{max\ 50}$ may be relatively specific for changes in the caliber of the small airways.

The Viso$\dot{V}$ is one of the most sensitive tests of small airway obstruction. It is relatively simple to perform and, in combination with measurement of the $\dot{V}_{max\ 50}$, may be helpful in differentiating large and small airway disease and determining whether the loss of elastic recoil or increased resistance is the causative factor.

MAXIMUM VOLUNTARY VENTILATION (MVV)
Description

The MVV is the largest volume that can be breathed over a 10- to 15-second interval (extrapolated to 1 minute) by voluntary effort. It is recorded in liters per minute.

Technique

The MVV is measured by having the subject breathe as deeply and rapidly as possible. The subject should set the rate and move more than the VT but less than the VC on each breath. The test is conducted for a specific interval (10,12, or 15 seconds). The volume expired (or inspired) may be measured by a suitable spirometer; it is important that the spirometer have an adequate frequency response (see Chapter 11). The volume may be read from an appropriate spirogram (Fig. 3-9) if the device is capable of recording accumulated volume. Most volume displacement spirometers produce simple volume-time tracings (Fig. 3-9), and manual calculation requires measurement and summing of each individual deflection, which can be quite time consuming. The actual values determined by either method are extrapolated from 10, 12, or 15 seconds to 1 minute and the result recorded as a flow rate, in liters per minute. The volumes must be corrected to BTPS.

Significance

The MVV is an overall test of the respiratory system, measuring the status of the respiratory muscles, the compliance of the lung-thorax system, and the resistance offered by the airways and tissues. Normal values vary by as much as 30% from the mean, so that only large reductions in MVV are considered significant. Healthy young men average 170 L/min. Values are lower in healthy women and decrease with age in both men and women. MVV is decreased greatly in subjects with moderate to severe obstructive disease. The maneuver exaggerates air trapping and exertion of the respiratory muscles. Assessment of the MVV may be useful in estimating the level of ventilation that can be expected during exercise testing. Subjects with moderate to severe obstruction who have MVV values much lower than 50 L/min usually exhibit ventilatory limitation during exercise. MVV may be within normal limits in some subjects with restrictive pulmonary disease, since limitation of lung or thoracic expansion may not interfere with flow. The MVV maneuver depends largely on subject effort, and low values should always be evaluated to ascertain whether the reduction is a result of obstruction, muscular weakness, inadequate ventilatory control, or poor subject effort.

An indirect index of subject effort on the MVV maneuver may be obtained by multiplying the FEV_1 by a factor of 35. For example, a subject with an FEV_1 of 2 liters might be expected to move about 70 L/min (35×2 liters) during the MVV test. If the measured MVV is much less than 70 L/min, then subject effort may be suspect. Criteria for acceptability of the MVV maneuver are outlined in Chapter 11.

COMPLIANCE
Description

Compliance is the volume change per unit of pressure change for the lungs (C_L), the thorax (C_T), or the lungs-thorax system (C_{LT}). The compliance for all three is recorded in liters or milliliters per centimeter of water. The elastic recoil pressure is the force generated by the lungs (or thorax) at a particular lung volume; it is recorded in cm H_2O and is usually reported for the measured value at TLC.

Technique

The C_{LT} may be measured as a unit; the C_L alone may be determined and the C_T calculated by subtraction if the C_{LT} was previously determined.

C_{LT} may be measured by having a subject in a sealed chamber inspire measured volumes by reducing the ''atmospheric'' pressure, as in an ''iron lung''; a volume-pressure curve is then plotted. The subject may likewise be intubated with an endotracheal tube, with pressure changes at various volumes above the end-expiratory level plotted to obtain a pressure-volume curve. This technique requires that the subject be anesthetized. Alternatively, a subject may be allowed to inspire known volumes from a spirometer, with pressure changes measured by means of a nasal plug in one nostril connected to a manometer. The subject must be instructed to relax all respiratory muscles so that the nasal pressure approximates alveolar pressure. Each of these techniques presents difficulties , which make them of limited usefulness for clinical studies.

Measurement of C_L is accomplished by passing a balloon catheter approximately 10 cm long into the esophagus at midthorax level and connecting it to a suitable pressure transducer. Serial pressure measurements are then recorded at various volumes and plotted (Fig. 3-11). Normally the subject inspires to TLC before the measurements, in order to standardize the lung volume history; lung compliance changes slightly after a full inspiration. Then the subject inspires again, and pressure and volume points are measured at points of zero airflow; the flow may be interrupted by means of a shutter. Similar measurements are recorded during the subsequent expiration. The compliance measurement (C_L) is usually taken from the slope of the pressure-volume curve over the interval from FRC to FRC plus 0.5 liters. Because of the effects of a previous deep inspiration on the measured compliance, measurements are usually recorded from the *defla-*

tion half of the curve. Maximum elastic recoil pressure is recorded as the most negative pressure recorded at the maximum lung volume attained, normally TLC. The optimal method of presenting compliance data is to plot the entire pressure curve (inflation and deflation) against either absolute lung volume or percent of TLC.

C_T can be derived if the total compliance and C_L are known:

$$\frac{1}{C_{LT}} - \frac{1}{C_L} = \frac{1}{C_T}$$

Significance

Measurements of compliance determine the elasticity of the lungs, the thorax, and the combination of the two. The average C_L in a normal adult is 0.2 L/cm H_2O. The C_T is also 0.2 L/cm H_2O. In series, the *total* compliance is:

$$\frac{1}{C_L} + \frac{1}{C_T} = \frac{1}{C_{LT}}$$

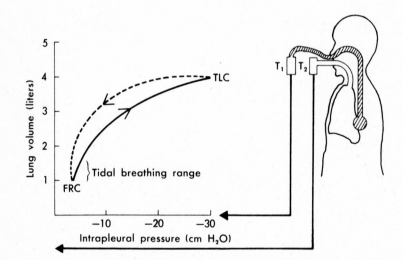

Fig. 3-11. Measurement of pulmonary compliance (C_L) (esophageal balloon technique). Determination of C_L requires measurement of intrapleural pressure at various lung volumes. Transducer T_1 is connected to an esophageal balloon containing a small amount of air and monitors changes in intrapleural pressure (ΔP). Transducer T_2 is actually a flow transducer (pneumotachometer) and is used to measure inspired or expired gas volumes (ΔV). Static C_L is the slope of the line defined by:

$$\frac{\Delta V \text{ (liters)}}{\Delta P \text{ (cm } H_2O)}$$

and is normally recorded from the tidal breathing range. C_L varies with the lung volume history, as illustrated by the steeper *expiratory* pressure-volume curve. Compliance measurements are often performed with the subject in the body plethysmograph to facilitate determination of absolute lung volumes.

or substituting the usual values:

$$\frac{1}{0.2} + \frac{1}{0.2} = 10$$

where the reciprocal of 10 is the compliance:

$$\frac{1}{10} \text{ or } 0.1 \text{ L/cm } H_2O$$

The total compliance is less than either of its two components because the forces act in series, resulting in the counterbalancing forces of the lung parenchyma and the thorax.

C_L varies with the volume of the lungs at the end-expiratory level (FRC). To compare the compliance of diseased lungs with that of normal lungs, the FRC in each case should be known. This is often stated as the compliance/FRC ratio. The C_{LT}/FRC ratio for adults ranges from 0.05 to 0.06. C_L is normally decreased in pulmonary edema or congestion, atelectasis, pneumonia, loss of surfactant, and restrictive diseases such as pulmonary fibrosis. These decreases, of course, may in many cases be caused by a reduction of the FRC. Emphysema is normally accompanied by an increase in compliance, since less pressure is required to maintain the FRC in the lungs. However, C_T may be decreased in obstructive

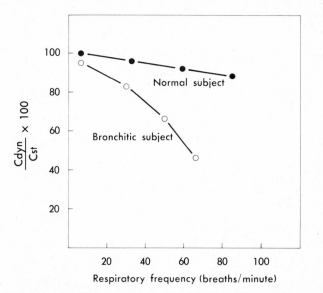

Fig. 3-12. Frequency dependence of compliance. Dynamic compliance (Cdyn) as a percentage of static compliance (Cst) for a normal subject *(solid circles)* and a bronchitic subject *(open circles)* is plotted at increasing respiratory frequencies. Increased resistance in small airways (< 2 mm) causes uneven distribution of gas, with most gas going to those lung units with normal resistance. At times of zero flow at the mouth, gas may still be moving within the lungs from one region to another (the Pendelluft phenomenon). Since some regions are out of phase with others, gas distribution becomes more uneven as breathing frequency increases and causes a fall in the ratio of Cdyn to Cst.

diseases because of chronic hyperinflation; hence total compliance may appear normal. CT may be decreased as a result of thoracic disease such as kyphoscoliosis or because of abdominal disorders such as obesity. CL normally decreases with age, presumably because of the changes in the connective tissues of the lung.

A special application of the determination of compliance is the measurement of CL at various breathing frequencies. Obstructive disease processes in airways smaller than 2 mm in diameter cause different regions of the lungs to ventilate asynchronously. This phenomenon can be detected by measurement of compliance at rapid breathing rates, usually 80 to 100/min. Compliance measured during breathing is called dynamic compliance (Cdyn). Normal subjects exhibit similar values for compliance under both static (Cst) and dynamic conditions. The frequency dependence of compliance is expressed as the ratio of Cdyn/Cst × 100. Values of less than 80% for this ratio are consistent with small airway obstruction. Frequency dependence is a very sensitive indicator of obstruction in smaller airways and may be present in persons with asthma and bronchitis in whom conventional tests such as FEV_1, $FEF_{25\%-75\%}$, and Raw are within normal limits (Fig. 3-12).

AIRWAY RESISTANCE (Raw) AND AIRWAY CONDUCTANCE (Gaw)
Description

Raw is the pressure difference developed per unit of flow change. Airway resistance is the difference in pressure between the mouth (atmospheric) and that in the alveoli, related to gas flow at the mouth. This pressure difference is created primarily by the friction of gas molecules coming in contact with the conducting airways. Raw is recorded in centimeters of water per liter per second. Gaw is the flow generated per unit of pressure drop in the airway. It is the reciprocal of Raw (1/Raw) and is recorded in liters per second per centimeter of water.

Technique

Raw is the ratio of alveolar pressure (PA) to airflow ($\dot{V}$). Gas flow can easily be measured with a pneumotachograph, and PA is measured with a body plethysmograph (Fig. 3-13). For gas to flow into the lungs (inspiration), PA must fall below atmospheric pressure; the opposite occurs during expiration. Since the total volume of gas in the lungs and plethysmograph remains constant, the changes in alveolar volume are reflected by reciprocal changes in the plethysmograph. (Pressures are monitored by sensitive pressure transducers at the mouth and in the plethysmograph, and flow is measured with a heated pneumotachometer.) Changes in $\dot{V}$ are plotted simultaneously against plethysmographic pressure changes (which are proportional to alveolar volume changes) on a storage oscilloscope.

The slope of this line is $\dot{V}/PP$, where $\dot{V}$ is airflow and PP is the plethysmographic pressure. Immediately after this measurement, an electronic shutter at the mouthpiece is closed and changes in plethysmographic pressure are plotted against airway pressure at the mouth, just as is done for measurement of the VTG.

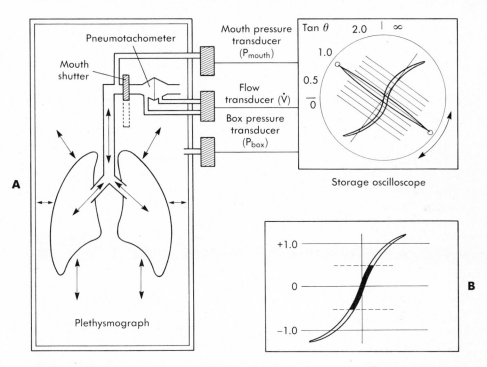

Fig. 3-13. Measurement of airway resistance (Raw). **A,** Diagrammatic representation of the measurement of airway resistance by the body plethysmograph method:

$$\text{Airway resistance} = \frac{\text{Atmospheric pressure} - \text{Alveolar pressure}}{\text{Flow}}$$

Flow ($\dot{V}$) is measured directly by means of the pneumotachometer. As the subject pants with the shutter open, flow is plotted against box pressure ($\dot{V}/P_{box}$) as an S-shaped curve on the oscilloscope. A shutter occludes the airway momentarily, usually at end-expiration, and a sloping line representing the ratio of mouth pressure (P_{mouth}/P_{box}) is recorded in a manner similar to that used for measurement of VTG. In this example the flow tracing (shutter open) and volume tracing (shutter closed) are superimposed. The P_{mouth}/P_{box} tangent is measured as for the VTG. **B,** The flow tangent is measured from the steep portion of the flow tracing, from about -0.5 L/sec to $+0.5$ L/sec. Airway resistance is then calculated as the ratio of these two tangents using appropriate calibration factors (see text and Appendix).

Since there is no airflow into or out of the lungs, the mouth pressure approximates P_A. The slope of this line is P_A/P_P, where P_A equals alveolar pressure. This step serves to calibrate changes in P_A to changes in P_P for each subject.

Raw is then calculated by taking the ratio of these two slopes:

$$Raw = \frac{P_A/P_P}{\dot{V}/P_P}$$

where

$\dot{V}$ = Airflow

P_A = Alveolar pressure

P_P = Plethysmographic pressure, which is measured with the shutter open and closed

The flow tangent is measured between the 0.5 L/sec points above and below the zero flow point (Fig. 3-13). Calibration factors for the flow and mouth pressure transducers are also included in the above equation. (See sample calculations in the Appendix.)

These measurements are made with the subject panting with an open glottis. Panting eliminates a number of artifacts from the tracing and allows measurements to be made at or near FRC. Corrections for the resistance of the mouthpiece and flowmeter are usually made. Conductance (Gaw) can be calculated as the reciprocal of Raw.

Lung volume determinations can easily be made at the same time, using the plethysmographic method (see Chapter 1). The Raw and Gaw may be expressed per liter of lung volume—specific resistance and specific conductance (SRaw and SGaw, respectively). Expressing Raw and Gaw in this way allows comparisons between subjects with different lung volumes and in the same subject when lung volume increases or decreases.

Significance

Normal values of Raw in adult subjects, panting and using a plethysmograph, range from 0.6 to 2.4 cm $H_2O/L/sec$. Gaw normally varies as the reciprocal between 0.42 and 1.67 L/sec/cm H_2O. Measurements are normally standardized at flow rates of 0.5 L/sec, as described above.

Airways resistance in the normal adult subject is divided thus:

Nose, mouth, upper airway $\simeq$ 50%

Trachea, bronchi $\simeq$ 30%

Small airways $\simeq$ 20%

Because the small airways contribute only about one fifth of the total resistance to flow, significant obstruction can occur in them with relatively little change in Raw. Lesions obstructing the larger airways may cause a significant increase in Raw and are often accompanied by increased work of breathing, as well as symptoms. Raw may be increased in asthma during an acute episode by as much as three times the normal values. Raw is increased in advanced emphysema because of airway narrowing and collapse in some of the larger airways as well as the more distal bronchioles. Other obstructive diseases, such as bronchitis, may cause increases in Raw proportionate to the degree of obstruction in medium and small airways.

Measurement of Raw may be useful in distinguishing between restrictive and obstructive diseases. The test is objective insofar as the subject cannot influence results by degree of effort. It should be noted, however, that acceptable performance of the panting maneuvers in the plethysmograph does require a certain degree of subject coordination, and not all subjects may be able to perform these maneuvers. Because Raw is decreased at increased lung volume, it is often advantageous to ascertain the FRC at the time of the Raw measurements. To use Gaw or Raw for comparative study, these values are often expressed per unit of lung volume.

In addition to resistance caused by $\dot{V}$ through the conducting tubes, some of the total pulmonary resistance results from the friction caused by the displacement of the lungs, rib cage, and diaphragm. Normally this "tissue" resistance is only about one fifth of the total resistance; therefore total pulmonary resistance is approximately 20% greater than the measured Raw.

MAXIMUM INSPIRATORY PRESSURE (MIP) and MAXIMUM EXPIRATORY PRESSURE (MEP)
Description

The MIP is the greatest subatmospheric pressure that can be developed by inspiring against an occluded airway. MIP is normally measured from the RV and is recorded in cm H_2O or mm Hg. The MEP is the greatest supraatmospheric pressure that can be developed during a forceful expiratory effort against an occluded airway. MEP is usually measured from the TLC and is also recorded in either cm H_2O or mm Hg.

Technique

The subject is connected to a three-way valve, or shutter apparatus, with a flanged mouthpiece and noseclip in place. The airway is occluded by switching the valve to one port, which is blocked, or by closing the shutter. In either method, a small leak is introduced between the occlusion and the mouth in order to negate any influence of the cheek muscles. The leak (usually a large-bore needle or similar opening) allows a small amount of gas to enter the oral cavity but does not significantly influence the lung volume or pressure measurement. For the MIP, the subject is instructed to expire maximally to the RV. It is sometimes helpful to monitor expiratory flow, or have the subject signal, to indicate when maximum expiration has been achieved. Then with the airway occluded, the subject inspires and maintains the inspiration for 1 to 3 seconds. The maximum subatmospheric pressure may be measured using a manometer, spring-type gauge, or pressure transducer. The pressure monitoring device should be linear and capable of recording pressures from -10 to approximately -200 cm H_2O. The greatest value from at least three efforts is reported, disregarding the first second of each maneuver, to eliminate transient pressures that occur initially with the maneuver. The MEP is recorded similarly, except that the subject inspires to TLC and then expires maximally against the occluded airway for 1 to 3 seconds.

Longer efforts should be avoided because of the possibility of reduction of cardiac output by the high thoracic pressures. Because MEP is typically larger than MIP, the pressure monitoring device should be able to accommodate the higher pressure developed. The best of three MEP efforts is reported, again disregarding any initial pressure transients. These tests require subject cooperation, and low values may reflect lack of understanding or insufficient effort.

Significance

The MIP primarily measures inspiratory muscle *strength*. The normal subject can generate inspiratory pressures in excess of -60 cm H_2O. (For prediction regressions, see the Appendix.) Decreased MIP is seen in subjects with neuromuscular disease, or diseases involving the diaphragm, intercostal muscles, and accessory muscles. MIP may also be decreased in patients with hyperinflation (such as emphysema), or in patients with chest wall or spinal deformities. The MIP is often used to assess subject response to training of the strength of the respiratory muscles. MIP, as a measure of respiratory muscle strength, may be measured in conjunction with MSVC (see Chapter 2), in the assessment of respiratory muscle function (see also Chapter 8, Bedside Testing).

The MEP measures the pressure generated during maximal expiration and depends on the function of the accessory muscles of respiration and the abdominal muscles, as well as the elastic recoil of the lungs and thorax. Normal adult subjects can generate MEP values of 80 to 100 cm H_2O. MEP may be decreased in neuromuscular disorders, particularly those that result in generalized muscle weakness. Reduced MEP may be related to an increased RV and may produce decreased expiratory flow rates on simple spirometry or flow-volume maneuvers. Decreased MEP is associated with inability to cough effectively and may complicate chronic bronchitis, cystic fibrosis, or other diseases that result in mucus hypersecretion.

SELF-ASSESSMENT QUESTIONS

1. A subject has an FVC of 2.1 liters; this value is only 49% of the predicted value for his age, height, and sex; this decrease may be caused by:
   a. Poor effort on the FVC maneuver
   b. Obstructive airway disease
   c. A restrictive disorder affecting the lung parenchyma
   d. Any of the above
   e. a or b
2. A subject has these results from simple spirometry:

	Measured	Predicted
FVC (L BTPS)	4.1	4.0
FEV$_1$ (L BTPS)	1.9	3.1

   These findings are consistent with:
   a. A restrictive disease process
   b. An obstructive disease process
   c. Normal lung function
   d. Cannot be determined without lung volumes

3. A subject has an $FEV_{1\%}$ of 82%; this is consistent with:
   a. Normal airway function
   b. Obstructive disease
   c. Restrictive disease
   d. a or c
4. A subject has flows measured using an acceptable spirometer; the following results are reported:

	Measured	Predicted
FVC (L BTPS)	4.4	4.6
FEV_1 (L BTPS)	3.4	3.5
$FEV_{1\%}$	77	76
$FEF_{25\%-75\%}$ (L/sec BTPS)	1.3	3.3

   These results are best described as consistent with:
   a. Normal pulmonary function
   b. Moderate obstructive airway disease
   c. Early small airway disease
   d. Moderate restrictive lung disease
5. A subject performs an MVV maneuver for 15 seconds; the total volume expired during this interval is 20 liters (BTPS). If the subject's predicted MVV is 100 L/min (BTPS), what percent of the predicted value did this subject perform?
   Percent of predicted MVV = _____%
6. A subject has her C_L measured using the esophageal balloon technique; a compliance of 0.410 L/cm H_2O is reported. This finding is consistent with which of the following disease entities?
   a. Emphysema
   b. Pulmonary fibrosis
   c. Atelectasis
   d. All of the above
   e. b and c
7. An asthmatic subject has his Raw measured according to the standard procedure using a body plethysmograph; an Raw of 1.71 cm H_2O/L/sec is obtained. This value is:
   a. Within normal limits
   b. Greater than normal, consistent with bronchospasm
   c. Lower than normal, indicating hyperinflation
   d. Physiologically impossible
8. The maximum static elastic recoil pressure of the lung is normally measured:
   a. At or near RV
   b. At or near FRC
   c. Over the interval from FRC to FRC plus 0.5 liters
   d. At or near TLC
9. The flow over the latter two thirds of the expiratory limb of the MEFV is:
   I. Determined by the elastic recoil properties of the lung
   II. Determined by the resistance to flow in the small airways (< 2 mm)
   III. Independent of subject effort
   IV. Termed the $\dot{V}_{max\ 75\%}$
   a. I, II, III, and IV
   b. I, II, and III
   c. II, III, and IV
   d. I and III

10. Large airway obstruction on an MEFV tracing is typically represented by
    a. Abnormally high peak flows
    b. A normal-shaped curve but with a low lung volume
    c. A "scooped-out" expiratory limb
    d. A "squared-off" expiratory limb
11. A subject performs MEFV maneuvers by breathing air and then breathing a mixture of 80% helium and 20% air. When the curves are superimposed, they coincide at approximately the same point as the $\dot{V}_{max\ 50}$. This finding is consistent with:
    a. Obstruction of small airways
    b. An improperly performed MEFV maneuver
    c. Large airway obstruction
    d. A restrictive disease process
12. A subject with myasthenia gravis performs MIP and MEP maneuvers to assess respiratory muscle function; the following values are reported:

	Measured
MIP (cm H_2O)	−94
MEP (cm H_2O)	+55

These findings are consistent with:
    a. Normal respiratory muscle function
    b. Normal inspiratory and abnormal expiratory muscle function
    c. Abnormal inspiratory and nomal expiratory muscle function
    d. Abnormal inspiratory and expiratory muscle function

SELECTED BIBLIOGRAPHY

General references
Bates, D.V., Macklem, P.T., and Christie, R.V.: Respiratory function in disease, ed. 2, Philadelphia, 1971, W.B. Saunders Co.
Comroe, J.H.: Physiology of respiration, Chicago, 1965, Year Book Medical Publishers, Inc.

Flow-volume curves
Acres, J., and Kryger, M.: Clinical significance of pulmonary function tests: upper airway obstruction, Chest **80**:207, 1981.
Bass, H.: The flow volume loop: normal standards and abnormalities in chronic obstructive pulmonary disease, Chest **63**:171, 1973.
Despas, P.J., Leroux, M., and Macklem, P.T.: Site of airway obstruction in asthma as determined by measuring flow breathing air and a helium-oxygen mixture, J. Clin. Invest. **51**:3235, 1972.
Gelb, A.F., and Klein, E.: The volume of isoflow and increase in maximal flow at 50 percent of forced vital capacity during helium-oxygen breathing as tests of small airway, Chest **71**:396, 1977.
Hyatt, R.E., and Black, L.F.: The flow volume curve, Am. Rev. Respir. Dis. **107**:191, 1973.
Knudson, R.J., et al.: The maximal expiratory flow-volume curve: normal standards, variability and effects of age, Am. Rev. Respir. Dis. **113**:587, 1976.
Knudson, R.J., et al.: Changes in the normal maximal expiratory flow-volume curve with growth and aging, Am. Rev. Respir. Dis. **127**:725, 1983.
Miller, R.D., and Hyatt, R.E.: Evaluation of obstructing lesions of the trachea and larynx by flow volume loops, Am. Rev. Respir. Dis. **108**:475, 1973.

Maximal respiratory pressures
Arora, N.S., and Rochester, D.F.: Respiratory muscle strength and maximal voluntary ventilation in undernourished patients, Am. Rev. Respir. Dis. **126**:5, 1982.
Block, L.F., and Hyatt, R.E.: Maximal static respiratory pressure in generalized neuromuscular disease, Am. Rev. Respir. Dis. **103**:641, 1971.
Gilbert, R., Auchincloss, J.H., Jr., and Bleb, S.: Measurement of maximum inspiratory pressures during routine spirometry, Lung **155**:23, 1978.

Compliance and airway resistance

Baydur, A., et al.: A simple method for assessing the validity of the esophageal balloon technique, Am. Rev. Respir. Dis. **126:**788, 1982.

Behrakis, P.K., et al.: Lung mechanics in sitting and horizontal body positions, Chest **83:**643, 1983.

Dubois, A.B., Bothello, S.V., and Comroe, J.H.: A new method for measuring airway resistance in man using a body plethysmograph: values in normal subjects and in patients with respiratory disease, J. Clin. Invest. **35:**327, 1956.

Gillespie, D.J.: Comparison of intraesophageal balloon pressure measurements with a nasogastric-esophageal balloon system in volunteers, Am. Rev. Respir. Dis. **126:**583, 1982.

Woolcock, A.J., Vincent, N.J., and Macklem, P.T.: Frequency dependence of compliance as a test for obstruction in the small airways, J. Clin. Invest. **48:**1099, 1969.

Spirometry

Knudson, R.J., and Lebowitz, M.D.: Maximal mid-expiratory flow ($FEF_{25\%-75\%}$): normal limits and assessment of sensitivity, Am. Rev. Respir. Dis. **117:**609, 1978.

Kuperman, A.S., and Riker, J.B.: The predicted normal maximal midexpiratory flow, Am. Rev. Respir. Dis. **107:**231, 1973.

Leuallen, E.C., and Fowler, W.S.: Maximal midexpiratory flow, Am. Rev. Tuberculosis **72:**783, 1955.

Morris, J.F., Koski, A., and Johnson, L.C.: Spirometric standards for healthy non-smoking adults, Am. Rev. Respir. Dis. **107:**57, 1971.

Sackner, M.A., et al. Assessment of time-volume and flow-volume components of forced vital capacity, Chest **82:**272, 1982.

Smith, A.A., and Gaensler, E.A.: Timing of forced expiratory volume in one second, Am. Rev. Respir. Dis. **112:**882, 1975.

Townsend, M.C., DuChene, A.G., and Fallat, R.J.: The effects of underrecording forces expirations on spirometric lung function indexes, Am. Rev. Respir. Dis. **126:**734, 1982.

CHAPTER FOUR

Gas distribution tests

SINGLE-BREATH NITROGEN ELIMINATION (SBN₂), CLOSING VOLUME (CV), AND CLOSING CAPACITY (CC)

Description

The SBN_2 test measures the distribution of ventilation by analyzing change in N_2 concentration during expiration of the VC after a single breath of 100% O_2. The evenness of distribution is assessed by two parameters: the $\Delta\%N_{2750-1250}$ and the slope of Phase III. Both of these parameters are recorded as percent change per unit of lung volume.

The CV is the lung volume at which airway closure begins and is expressed as a percentage of the VC. The CC is the sum of the CV and RV (see Chapter 1) and is expressed as a percentage of the TLC.

Technique

The subject expires to RV and then inhales a single breath of 100% O_2. Without holding the breath, the subject expires slowly and evenly (0.3 to 0.5 L/sec) into a spirometer through an N_2 analyzer that rapidly monitors the N_2 concentration of the expired gas. VE, as measured by the spirometer, is plotted against N_2 concentration on a suitable graph (Fig. 4-1). The curve can be divided into four phases: Phase I is extreme upper airway gas consisting of 100% O_2; Phase II is mixed VD gas in which the relative concentrations of O_2 and N_2 change abruptly as the VD volume is expired; Phase III is a plateau caused by the exhalation of alveolar gas, whose relative O_2 and N_2 concentrations change slowly and evenly; Phase IV is noted by an abrupt increase in the concentration of N_2 that continues until the RV is reached. The initial 750 ml of expired gas contains the VD volume of Phases I and II and is disregarded. The difference in N_2 concentration between the 750 ml and 1250 ml points is called the delta N_2 ($\Delta N_{2750-1250}$). The slope of Phase III is the change in N_2 concentration from the 30% point of the VC up to the onset of Phase IV and is recorded as $\Delta\%N_2$ per liter. The volume expired after the onset of Phase IV is called the CV. The CV may be added to the RV, if determined, and expressed as the CC. The CV is normally recorded as a percentage of the VC:

$$CV/VC \times 100$$

The CC is recorded as a percentage of the TLC:

$$CC/TLC \times 100$$

TLC can be determined from the SBN$_2$ test by measuring the area under the washout curve, either by electronic integration or planimetry, using a dilution equation to calculate the RV and then adding it to the measured VC. RV is calculated as follows:

$$RV = VC \times \frac{F\overline{E}_{N_2}}{F_{A_{N_2}} - F\overline{E}_{N_2}}$$

where

  $F\overline{E}_{N_2}$ = Mean expired N$_2$ concentration determined by a planimeter or electronic integration of the area under the curve

  $F_{A_{N_2}}$ = N$_2$ concentration in the lungs at the beginning of inspiration, approximately 0.75 to 0.79

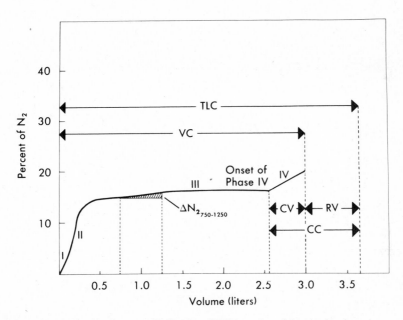

Fig. 4-1. Single-breath nitrogen elimination (SBN$_2$)—plot of the rise in nitrogen concentration on expiration following a single VC breath of pure O$_2$. The curve is divided into four parts or phases. Phase I is the extreme beginning of the expiration when only pure O$_2$ is being exhaled. Phase II shows an abrupt rise in N$_2$ concentration as mixed bronchial and alveolar air is expired. Phase III is the alveolar gas plateau, and nitrogen concentration changes only slightly as long as ventilation is uniformly distributed. Phase IV is an abrupt increase in N$_2$ concentration as basal airways close and a larger proportion of gas comes from the nitrogen-rich lung apices. Several useful parameters are derived from the SBN$_2$ tracing. Anatomic dead space can be calculated (see Chapter 2). The $\Delta N_{2_{750-1250}}$ and slope of Phase III are indices of the evenness of ventilation distribution. CV can be read directly from the onset of Phase IV until RV is reached; VC can also be read directly. RV, TLC, and CC can be calculated if the area under the curve is determined either by a planimeter or electronic integration (see text).

This method is accurate only in subjects without significant obstructive disease or dead space–producing disease.

Significance

$\Delta N_{2750\text{-}1250}$. The normal $\Delta N_{2750\text{-}1250}$ is 1.5% or less for healthy young adults and slightly higher for healthy older adults (approximately 3%). Increases in $\Delta N_{2750\text{-}1250}$ values are found in diseases characterized by uneven gas distribution during inspiration and unequal flow rates during expiration. In subjects with severe emphysema $\Delta N_{2750\text{-}1250}$ may exceed 10%. A best-fit line drawn through the Phase III segment of the tracing from about 30% of the VC to the onset of Phase IV is used to determine the slope of Phase III. This slope is used as an index of gas distribution, in a manner similar to the $\Delta N_{2750\text{-}1250}$. Very slow expiratory flow rates may cause oscillations in the tracing of Phase III, making the accurate measurement of $\Delta_{2750\text{-}1250}$ difficult. These oscillations are attributed to changes in alveolar N_2 concentrations as blood pulses through the pulmonary capillaries during cardiac systole. Increasing the expiratory flow rate slightly eliminates this common artifact. Subjects with small VC values may have difficulty exhaling enough gas to make the $\Delta\%N_{2750\text{-}1250}$ meaningful.

CV and CC. Phase IV of the SBN_2 test can be explained by the fact that after a maximal expiration there is proportionately more RV gas at the apices of the lungs than at the bases, and when a test gas is inspired, the apices receive the gas occupying the subject's dead space, with the test gas then going preferentially to the bases of the lungs. Gas concentrations in the lungs become widely different, since the apices contain RV gas plus V_D gas (largely nitrogen), whereas the bases contain predominantly test gas (oxygen in this case). Dynamic compression of the airways during the subsequent expiration causes airways to close as lung volume approaches RV. Dependent airways close first because of gravity and the weight of the lung in upright subjects. As the composition of gas switches from test gas to higher concentrations of N_2, Phase IV begins.

CV and CC indicate the lung volume at which airway closure begins and are thus indices of the status of the small airways. CV and CC may be increased (earlier onset of airway closure) with increases in age, in restrictive processes in which the FRC becomes less than the CV, in smokers and other subjects with early obstructive disease of the small airways, and in congestive heart failure when the caliber of the small airways is compromised by edema.

Subjects with moderate to severe obstructive disease may display no sharp demarcation between Phases III and IV of the SBN_2 because of grossly uneven distribution of gas in the lungs with little difference in gas composition between apices and bases.

CV and CC measurements may be in error if the subject does not perform a true VC maneuver. VC during the CV determination should not differ more than 5% from the subject's reproducible VC. Expiratory flow should be maintained between 0.3 and 0.5 L/sec.

To calculate normal values for CV and CC according to age and sex, see the Appendix.

NITROGEN WASHOUT TEST (7-MINUTE)
Description

The N_2 washout test measures the concentration of N_2 **in alveolar** gas at the end of 7 minutes of 100% O_2 breathing. The N_2 washout **test value is** recorded as a percentage of nitrogen.

Technique

The degree of N_2 washout in the lungs can be **calculated most** simply by having the subject breathe pure O_2 for 7 minutes and **then measuring the** N_2 concentration of a sample of alveolar gas collected at the end of a forced expiration. The evenness of ventilation determines whether practically all the N_2 has been washed out by O_2.

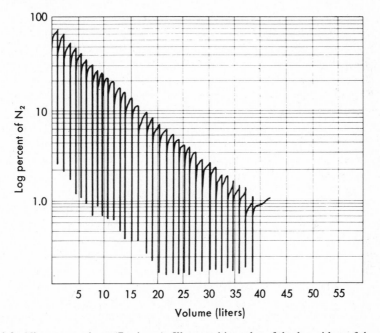

Fig. 4-2. Nitrogen washout (7-minute). Illustrated is a plot of the logarithm of the nitrogen concentration versus expired volume. The elimination of nitrogen from the lungs by O_2 breathing occurs exponentially. A single-chamber lung being washed out in this fashion would produce a J-shaped curve; however, since the percent of N_2 is usually plotted on semilog paper, the result is a straight line. Normal lungs produce an approximately straight line; lungs with deranged distribution tend to show a fast washout initially and progressive slowing as the test proceeds. This appears as a steep curve to begin, with more and more flattening toward the end. The slope of the washout curve is determined mainly by the rate, V_T, FRC, and V_D. The inspired gas distribution index (IDI) offers a more quantitative analysis of the distribution characteristics (see text). The test normally lasts 7 minutes, or until the alveolar N_2 concentration has been reduced to less than 1%, or until an expired volume limit has been reached (i.e., 60 liters). The log %N_2 may also be plotted against time or number of breaths.

A test of more quantitative value is that in which the dilution of N_2 by oxygen is graphed or displayed for each breath by means of rapid analysis of expired gas. Normally the percent of N_2 is plotted against the expired volume or number of breaths. The typical washout curve is an exponential or J-shaped curve, which becomes a straight line when the percent of N_2 is graphed on semilog paper (Fig. 4-2).

Significance

The normal value for the concentration of N_2 in alveolar gas after 7 minutes of O_2 breathing is less than 2.5%. The actual results of a 7-minute N_2 washout test are of little value without knowledge of the V_T, V_D, and FRC of the individual subject. Large increases in $\dot{V}_E$ can lower the percent of N_2 in the alveoli to near

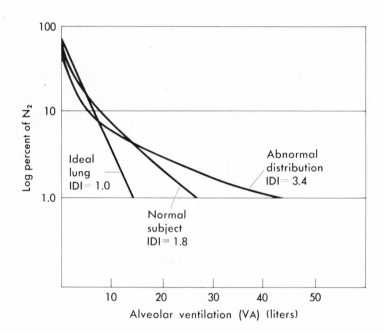

Fig. 4-3. Inspired gas distribution index (IDI). Illustrated is a plot of the logarithm of N_2 concentration versus the V_A. The IDI is derived thus:

$$IDI = \frac{V_A}{FRC\ (k)}$$

where

k = Constant equal to the natural log of 72 (see text)

By definition, the IDI for an ideal, single-chambered lung is 1.0. Plotting log $\%N_2$ concentration against V_A instead of total expired volume eliminates dependence on rate, V_T, and V_D as determinants of the shape of the washout curve and allows a quantitative measurement of the evenness of distribution. (From Application note AN729, San Diego, Hewlett-Packard Co.)

normal levels within the 7-minute limit even though there is marked unevenness of gas distribution.

The graphic method of displaying breath-by-breath washout yields somewhat more diagnostic results. The slope of the curve is determined by the FRC, V_T, V_D, and frequency of breathing. If the N_2 is washed out of the lungs evenly, the curve will appear as a straight line on semilog paper, no matter what the slope (Fig. 4-2). Because the lung is not a perfectly symmetric organ, the curve is seldom a straight line. The deviation from a straight line is indicative of the extent to which ventilation is uneven.

The data from the washout can be used to derive the inspired gas distribution index (IDI) (Fig. 4-3). The IDI is defined as being equal to the V_A (accumulated over the entire test) divided by the FRC and multiplied by a constant:

$$IDI = \frac{V_{A(tot)}}{FRC \ (k)}$$

where

k = Constant such that an ideal lung (single compartment) will have an IDI equal to 1.00

The technique eliminates the dependence on the V_T, f, and V_D as determinants of the slope of the washout curve. Total V_A can be calculated as follows:

$$V_{A(tot)} = V_{(tot)} - f(V_D)$$

where

$V_{(tot)}$ = Total volume expired during test
V_D = Respiratory dead space
f   = Number of breaths

In an ideal lung the IDI equals 1.00, and in normal subjects it is about 1.80 ± 0.2. Obstructive diseases show mean values of 3.40 ± 0.9. Thus the IDI is a quantitative expression of the gas distribution as analyzed by the multiple-breath N_2 technique.

Uneven distribution is characteristic of all obstructive disease patterns, with emphysema often showing the greatest degree of maldistribution; bronchitis and asthma show similar unevenness of ventilation during acute exacerbations. The effect of uneven distribution of ventilation is largely dependent on the matching of ventilation and perfusion (see Chapter 6). Some subjects with marked maldistribution, such as in emphysema, may have rather even matching of ventilation and perfusion if the disease process destroys capillaries along with the other alveolar structures. Pure restrictive patterns often show normal washout values, especially in subjects who hyperventilate as a result of restriction. However, tumors and other lesions that impinge on the airways may cause regional differences in ventilation. Both the simple multiple-breath N_2 test and the IDI are independent of subject effort, although the subject must maintain an adequate seal on the mouthpiece of the apparatus to prevent contamination of the test gas (O_2).

LUNG SCANS (^{133}Xe)
Description

The ^{133}Xe technique (as well as other techniques employing inhalation of radioactive gases) measures the regional distribution of ventilation.

Technique

1. The subjects, usually in a sitting position, inhale either a VT or a VC breath from a reservoir that contains a measured dose of ^{133}Xe (10 to 20 μCi). They then hold their breath for 10 to 20 seconds. During this time scintiphotos are made over the lung fields to demonstrate areas of poor ventilation (Fig. 4-4).
2. The subjects are allowed to rebreathe the gas mixture containing the ^{133}Xe for 3 to 5 minutes, during which time serial scintiphotos are made to demonstrate the rapidity and evenness of equilibration of the ^{133}Xe. Addition of O_2 and removal of CO_2 are required, since this is a closed circuit similar to that used in the He dilution FRC determination. Because the rebreathing period is usually short, the circuit may be flushed with pure O_2 to provide adequate oxygen during the maneuver.

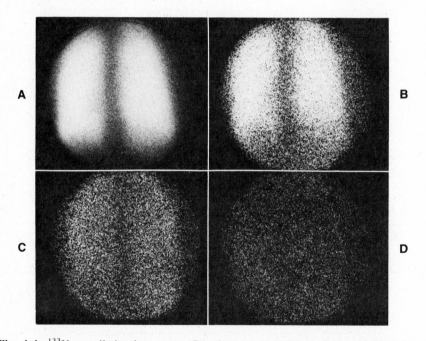

Fig. 4-4. ^{133}Xe ventilation lung scan—PA views of normal lung fields. **A,** Wash-in or equilibration after the subject has rebreathed radioactive Xe. **B,** Thirty seconds after washout begins; the subject is breathing room air. **C,** One minute after the subject has been breathing room air. **D,** Three minutes after the subject has been breathing air; only background radiation remains. (Courtesy Nuclear Medicine Department, St. Louis University Hospital, St. Louis, Mo.)

3. As a final step, the subjects return to breathing atmospheric gas to cause the ^{133}Xe to be washed out. Serial scintiphotos indicate those areas that have trapped the ^{133}Xe during the equilibration phase. Changing-count ratios in various lung zones can be used to determine the relative extent of ventilation by comparisons of the counting rates for each zone. This normally requires discrete counters or computerized segregation of counts from the various zones.

Significance

^{133}Xe is ideal for identifying regional ventilation disorders. It has a half-life of 5.27 days and requires sophisticated monitoring equipment, but it is not metabolized by the body and tends to remain in the gas phase. The three types of ^{133}Xe studies just outlined can be done individually or as a series and are helpful diagnostically in cases of pronounced regional differences in ventilation. Regional distribution of inspired gas is dependent on the volume of air in the lungs before the breath and the volume of the breath itself. Differences in regional ventilation can be quantified by calculating the concentration of ^{133}Xe in each lung zone by means of external counters placed over the chest. By comparing radiation counts

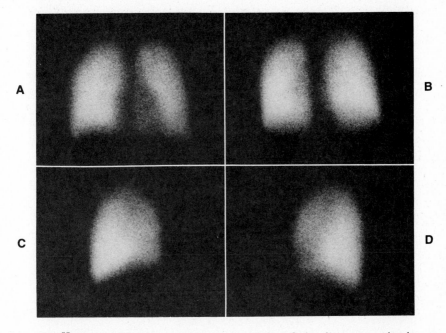

Fig. 4-5. ^{99m}Tc-HAM perfusion lung scan—normal perfusion lung scan using human albumin microspheres tagged with radioactive technetium. **A,** Anterior. **B,** Posterior. **C,** Right lateral. **D,** Left lateral. (Courtesy Nuclear Medicine Department, St. Louis University Hospital, St. Louis, Mo.)

during an initial breath of ^{133}Xe with counts at the same lung volume after rebreathing, when the concentration of ^{133}Xe is equal in both the lung and the breathing circuit, the fractional concentration of ^{133}Xe during the initial breath can be derived. This fractional concentration can then be stated as a ventilation index, expressed as a percentage of the simultaneous mean concentration of ^{133}Xe in the lungs. The concentration of ^{133}Xe is thus expressed per unit of lung volume, and similar data from different subjects can be compared. Typical values in normal upright subjects show proportionately greater ventilation in the bases than in the apices. This is important, since gravity causes most perfusion to be directed to the lower two thirds of the lungs. In spite of the smaller alveolar size in the lower lung zones (due to gravity and hydrostatic pressure) tidal ventilation is directed to those areas of gravity-dependent blood flow, so that a major portion of lung units have $\dot{V}/\dot{Q}$ ratios of 0.8 to 1.0.

The distribution of pulmonary blood flow may be demonstrated by intravenous injection of radioactive particles. Macroaggregated albumin labeled with ^{131}I (^{131}I-MAA), or human albumin microspheres labeled with ^{99m}Tc (^{99m}Tc-HAM) are commonly used. The particles, which measure 30 to 40 μm, are injected by a venous route; they then mix with blood passing through the right heart and lodge in the pulmonary arterioles. Their distribution matches the pulmonary blood flow at the time of injection. Scintiphotos are normally made of four views: anterior, posterior, left lateral, and right lateral (Fig. 4-5). These particles normally break up, pass through the pulmonary capillaries, and are removed in the liver and spleen. With the usual dosage, only 1 of every 1000 arterioles is occluded, and no functional abnormalities can be demonstrated following injection. Perfusion lung scanning may be contraindicated in subjects with severe pulmonary hypertension because of their reduced vascular bed, as well as in individuals with anatomic right-to-left shunts, because the particles pass unchanged through the lungs for embolization in the brain, kidney, heart, or other organs. Perfusion scanning is routinely combined with ventilation scans of the lung to evaluate subjects with obstructive airway disease or with suspected pulmonary emboli and may be computer enhanced to provide projection of the ventilation/perfusion characteristics of various lung segments.

SELF-ASSESSMENT QUESTIONS

1. Which of the following statements accurately describes Phase III of the SBN$_2$ test?
    I. The slope is dependent on the distribution of ventilation.
    II. It represents mixed dead space gas.
    III. The $\Delta N_{2750-150}$ is measured from this phase.
    IV. The closing volume is measured from this phase.
      a. I, II, III, and IV
      b. I, II, and IV
      c. I and III
      d. II and III
2. A subject performs an SBN$_2$ maneuver that is interpreted as "early onset of Phase IV"; this interpretation is consistent with:

a. Small airway obstruction
b. Mild restrictive pattern, such as found in fibrosis
c. Large airway obstruction (tumor, stenosis, etc.)
d. Normal airway function

3. A subject performs simple spirometry and an SBN_2:

	Measured	Predicted
FVC (L BTPS)	3.1	4.0
FEV_1 (L BTPS)	1.5	3.1
$FEV_{1\%}$ (%)	48	78
CV/VC (%)	27	13

These findings are consistent with:
a. Normal function in older healthy adults
b. Early small airway disease
c. Moderately advanced obstructive lung disease
d. a and b

4. A subject performs the 7-minute N_2 washout procedure; after 7 minutes the $\%N_2$ displayed on the graph of the washout is 0.7%. This is consistent with:
a. Severe obstructive lung disease
b. Early small airway obstruction
c. Increased intrapulmonary shunting
d. Normal distribution of ventilation

5. Radioactive xenon is well suited for assessing regional ventilation because:
a. It is not metabolized by the body
b. It has a half-life of 5.27 days
c. It is relatively insoluble, so that it remains in the gas phase
d. All of the above
e. a and c

6. In subjects with obstructive lung disease, breathing air after rebreathing ^{133}Xe will show:
a. ^{133}Xe trapped in poorly ventilated regions
b. A rapid washout of ^{133}Xe from poorly ventilated regions
c. Better ventilation at the bases of the lungs
d. b and c

7. Perfusion lung scanning may be contraindicated in subjects with:
a. Severe obstructive lung disease
b. Severe pulmonary hypertension
c. Right-to-left anatomic shunt
d. All of the above
e. b and c

8. Ventilation scans of normal upright subjects show:
a. Most ventilation goes to the bases of the lungs
b. Most ventilation goes to the apices of the lungs
c. Ventilation is almost evenly distributed throughout the lungs
d. Most ventilation occurs in the anatomic dead space

9. The inspired gas distribution index (IDI), if measured from a perfectly symmetric, single-chambered lung, would yield a value of:
a. Less than 2.5%
b. Less than 1.5%
c. 1.8
d. 1.0

10. Which of the following might be abnormal in a subject with early small airway obstruction?
    I. CV/VC ratio
    II. Slope of Phase III
    III. CC/TLC ratio
    IV. VisoV̇ (volume of isoflow)
    a. I, II, III, and IV
    b. I, III, and IV
    c. II, III, and IV
    d. II and IV

SELECTED BIBLIOGRAPHY

General references

Bouhuys, A.: Distribution of inspired gas in the lungs. In Fenn, W.O., and Rahn, H., editors: Handbook of physiology—respiration I, Washington, D.C., 1964, American Physiological Society.

Comroe, J.H., and Fowler, W.S.: Lung function studies. VI. Detection of uneven alveolar ventilation during a single breath of oxygen, Am. J. Med. **10**:408, 1951.

Darling, R.C., Cournand, A., and Richards, D.W.: Studies of intrapulmonary mixture of gases. V. Forms of inadequate ventilation in normal and emphysematous lungs analyzed by means of breathing pure oxygen, J. Clin. Invest. **23**:55, 1944.

Fowler, W.S.: Lung function studies. III. Uneven pulmonary ventilation in normal subjects and in patients with pulmonary disease, J. Appl. Physiol. **2**:283, 1949.

Hathirat, S., Renzetti, A.D., and Mitchell, M.: Intrapulmonary gas distribution: a comparison of the helium mixing time and nitrogen single breath test in normal and diseased subjects, Am. Rev. Respir. Dis. **102**:750, 1970.

Shinokazi, T., et al.: Theory of a digital nitrogen washout computer, J. Appl. Physiol. **21**:202, 1966.

Closing volume

Abboud, R., and Morton, J.: Comparison of maximal mid-expiratory flow, flow-volume curves, and nitrogen closing volumes in patients with mild airway obstruction, Am. Rev. Respir. Dis. **111**:405, 1975.

Buist, A.S., and Ross, B.B.: Predicted values for closing volumes using a modified single breath nitrogen test, Am. Rev. Respir. Dis. **107**:744, 1973.

Cormier, Y., and Belanger, J.: The role of gas exchange in phase IV of the single breath nitrogen test, Am. Rev. Respir. Dis. **125**:396, 1982.

MacFadden, E.R., Holmes, B., and Kiker, R.: Variability of closing volume measurements in normal man, Am. Rev. Respir. Dis. **111**:135, 1975.

Make, B., and Lapp, N.L.: Factors influencing the measurement of closing volume, Am. Rev. Respir. Dis. **111**:749, 1975.

Martin, R., and Macklem, P.T.: Suggested standardization procedures for closing volume determinations (nitrogen method), DHD-NHLBI, 1973.

McCarthy, D.S., et al.: Measurement of closing volume as a simple and sensitive test for early detection of small airway disease, Am. J. Med. **52**:747, 1972.

Lung scans

Bernier, D.R., Zangman, J.K., and Wells, L.D.: Nuclear medicine technology and techniques, St. Louis, 1981, The C.V. Mosby Co.

Dolfuss, R.E., Milic-Emili, J., and Bates, D.V.: Regional ventilation of the lung studied with boluses of [133]xenon, Respir. Physiol. **2**:234, 1967.

Secker-Walker, R.H., and Siegal, B.A.: The use of nuclear medicine in the diagnosis of lung disease, Radiol. Clin. North Am. **11**:215, 1973.

CHAPTER FIVE

Diffusion tests

CARBON MONOXIDE DIFFUSING CAPACITY (DL_{CO})
Description

DL_{CO} measures the factors that affect the movement of a diffusion-limited gas across the alveolocapillary membrane. The DL_{CO} is recorded as milliliters of CO per minute per millimeter of mercury at $0°C$, 760 mm Hg, dry (standard temperature, standard pressure, dry; STPD).

Technique

Carbon monoxide combines with hemoglobin about 210 times more readily than does O_2 but otherwise acts similar to oxygen. In the presence of normal amounts of hemoglobin and normal ventilatory function, the main limiting factor to diffusion is the status of the alveolocapillary membrane. Small amounts of CO in inspired gas produce measurable changes in the concentration of inspired versus expired gas. There are several methods for determining the DL_{CO} (Table 5-1). All of the methods measure diffusing capacity according to the general equation:

$$DL_{CO} = \frac{ml\ CO\ transferred/min}{P_{A_{CO}} - Pc_{CO}}$$

where

$P_{A_{CO}}$ = Mean alveolar partial pressure of CO
Pc_{CO} = Mean capillary partial pressure of CO

An additional method of quantifying diffusing capacity simply relates the inspired and expired CO concentrations during normal breathing.

Modified Krogh technique—single breath ($DL_{CO}SB$). The subject inspires a VC breath from a spirometer or reservoir (Fig. 5-1) containing a gas mixture of 0.3% CO, 10% He, and the remainder air, and then holds the breath for approximately 10 seconds. The subject then expires, and a sample of alveolar gas is taken with an end-tidal sampler after a suitable washout volume (usually 1000 ml) is discarded (Fig. 5-2). The sample is analyzed to obtain final fractional CO and He concentrations: $F_{A_{CO_{t2}}}$ and $F_{E_{He}}$, respectively. The concentration of CO in the alveolar gas at the beginning of the breath-hold ($F_{A_{CO_{t1}}}$) is computed thus:

$$F_{A_{CO_{t1}}} = 0.003 \times \frac{F_{E_{He}}}{F_{I_{He}}}$$

where

$FA_{CO_{t1}}$ = Fraction of CO at the beginning of the breath-hold

0.003 = CO fraction in the reservoir

FE_{He} = Exhaled fractional He concentration from the end-tidal sample

FI_{He} = Inspired He concentration (known)

The $DL_{CO}SB$ is then calculated as follows:

$$DL_{CO}SB = \frac{V_A \times 60}{(P_B - 47)(t2 - t1)} \times Ln \frac{FA_{CO_{t1}}}{FA_{CO_{t2}}}$$

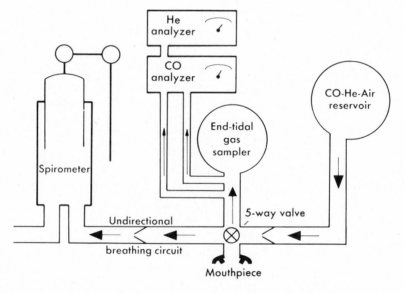

Fig. 5-1. DL_{CO} apparatus. The basic equipment for performing the DL_{CO} test (specifically the $DL_{CO}SB$) is illustrated. Included is a CO-He-air reservoir, which may be a large-volume bag, a sealed spirometer, or a demand valve–type system connected directly to a tank of special gas mixture. A five-way valve, which may be automatic, allows rapid switching of the breathing gases and directs exhaled gas to the end-tidal sampler or spirometer, or both. Some method of measuring the inspired volume is also required, and this is usually accomplished by using a bag-in-box or similar apparatus for the diffusion mixture reservoir. He and CO analyzers are used to analyze the end-tidal sample, as well as to determine inspired gas concentrations from the CO-He-air reservoir. Most automated systems include electronic timing of the manuever, automatic switching of the valve, and direct sampling of the end-tidal gas.

where

V_A = Alveolar volume (STPD)

60   = Correction from seconds to minutes

P_B = Barometric pressure

47   = Water vapor pressure (P_{H_2O})

$t2 - t1$ = Breath-hold interval (usually 10 seconds)

Ln   = Natural logarithm

$F_{ACO_{t1}}$ = Fraction of CO in alveolar gas before diffusion

$F_{ACO_{t2}}$ = Fraction of CO in alveolar gas at the end of diffusion

V_A may be calculated from the single-breath dilution of He:

$$V_A = \frac{VC}{F_{E_{He}}/F_{I_{He}}}$$

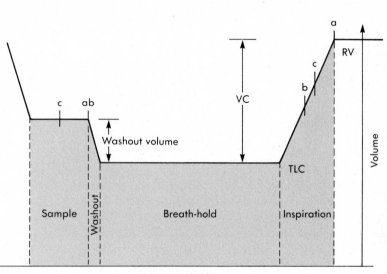

Fig. 5-2. Typical $D_{L_{CO}}SB$ maneuver tracing—tracing of the single-breath $D_{L_{CO}}$ maneuver proceeding from right to left: the subject starts from RV and inspires a VC breath rapidly to TLC, and then breath-holds for approximately 10 seconds. At the end of the breath-hold, the subject exhales a fixed washout volume (usually about 1 liter), and a sample of alveolar gas is taken; any remaining volume is exhaled. Various methods of timing are employed and are illustrated. Method *a* considers diffusion to be occurring from the beginning of inspiration to the beginning of alveolar sampling; method *b* considers diffusion to be occurring from the midpoint of inspiration to the beginning of alveolar sampling; method *c* measures diffusion from two thirds of the inspired VC to the midpoint of the alveolar sample (see text for further discussion).

where

VA = Alveolar volume

VC = Volume of test gas inspired (vital capacity) (Fig. 5-2)

FE_{He} = Exhaled fractional concentration of He

FI_{He} = Inspired fractional concentration of He

A simplification of the above single-breath method is widely employed. By calibrating both the He and CO analyzers to read full scale (100% or 1.000) when sampling the diffusion mixture and zeroing the analyzers appropriately, the FE_{He} obtained from the alveolar sample equals the $FA_{CO_{t_1}}$. The assumption here is that both He and CO are diluted equally during inspiration. The logarithmic ratio of CO disappearance from the alveoli can then be expressed:

$$Ln = \frac{FE_{He}}{FE_{CO}}$$

where

FE_{He} = Fraction of He in the alveolar sample (usually expressed as a percentage)

FE_{CO} = Fraction of CO in the alveolar sample (also expressed as a percentage)

This technique avoids the necessity of analyzing the absolute concentrations of the two gases but requires that both analyzers be linear. Because analysis of CO is often done using infrared analyzers (see Chapter 9), and because their output is nonlinear, care must be taken that corrected CO readings are used in the computation. This correction is easily accomplished via software in automated systems. Correction must be made for V_D and all lung volumes corrected from ATPS to STPD.

Filey technique—steady state ($DL_{CO}SS_1$). The subject breathes a gas mixture of 0.1% to 0.2% CO in air for 5 to 6 minutes. During the final 2 minutes, expired gas is collected in a Douglas bag and an arterial blood sample is drawn. The exhaled volume is measured, and the expired gas is analyzed for CO, CO_2, and O_2. The arterial blood is analyzed for PCO_2. Steady-state diffusing capacity is calculated by the equation:

$$DL_{CO}SS_1 = \frac{\dot{V}CO\ (STPD)}{PA_{CO}}$$

where

$\dot{V}CO$ = ml of CO transferred/min (STPD)

PA_{CO} = Partial pressure of CO in the alveoli

$\dot{V}CO$ is determined from an analysis of the fractional inspired and expired CO (FI_{CO} and FE_{CO} respectively), the $\dot{V}E$, and the inspired and expired N_2 fractions (FI_{N_2}, which is known, and FE_{N_2}, which is determined indirectly from the fractions of O_2, CO_2, and H_2O vapor in the exhaled gas):

$$\dot{V}CO = \dot{V}E\left(FICO\frac{FEN_2}{FIN_2} - FECO\right)$$

$PACO$ is determined by using a form of the Bohr equation:

$$PACO = PB - 47\left(\frac{FECO - rFICO}{1 - r}\right)$$

where

$$r = \frac{PACO_2 - PECO_2}{PECO_2}$$

Estimating $PACO$ in this way avoids the necessity of obtaining a direct alveolar sample.

End-tidal CO determination ($DLCOSS_2$). The $DLCOSS_2$ method is basically the same as the $DLCOSS_1$ in that the volume of CO transferred ($\dot{V}CO$) is derived similarly. $PACO$, however, is determined by taking the average end-tidal CO tension ($PETCO$) from instantaneous analysis of multiple breaths. The end-tidal value is assumed to be equal to the mean $PACO$.

Assumed VD technique ($DLCOSS_3$). Again, the $DLCOSS_3$ method resembles the $DLCOSS_1$. $\dot{V}CO$ is determined as in $DLCOSS_1$, but $PACO$ is measured differently. The fractional alveolar concentration ($FACO$), which can be used to derive $PACO$ when PB is known, is measured as follows:

$$FACO = \frac{VTFECO - VDFICO}{VT - VD}$$

where

VT   = Tidal volume
VD   = Dead space volume
FECO = Fraction of expired CO
FICO = Fraction of inspired CO

VT is measured by averaging multiple breaths. VD is often assumed to be equal to 1 ml/lb of body weight. The mechanical VD of the breathing circuit is subtracted.

Mixed venous PCO_2 technique ($DLCOSS_4$). $\dot{V}CO$ is obtained as in $DLCOSS_1$. $PACO$ is calculated by estimating the mixed venous PCO_2 ($P\bar{v}CO_2$) from an equilibration technique and then determining the $PACO_2$ from the $P\bar{v}CO_2$ and the normal gradient. Once the $PACO_2$ is derived, an equation similar to that used to determine $PACO$ in the $DLCOSS_1$ technique can be employed. Using mixed venous PCO_2 avoids the necessity of arterial puncture.

Rebreathing technique ($DLCORB$). The subject rebreathes from a reservoir containing a mixture of 0.3% CO, 10% He, and the remainder air for 30 to 60 seconds at a rate of about 30/min. After this interval, measurements of the final CO, He, and O_2 concentrations in the reservoir are made. An equation similar to that used for the single-breath technique is used (see p. 72):

$$DL_{CO}RB = \frac{Vs \times 60}{(PB - 47)\,(t2 - t1)} \times Ln\,\frac{FA_{CO_{t1}}}{FA_{CO_{t2}}}$$

where

Vs   = Volume of the lung reservoir system (initial volume $\times$ FI_{He}/FE_{He}

60   = Correction from seconds to minutes

PB   = Barometric pressure

47   = Water vapor pressure (PH_2O)

t2 − t1 = Rebreathing interval

Ln   = Natural logarithm

$FA_{CO_{t1}}$ = Fraction of CO in alveolar gas before diffusion

$FA_{CO_{t2}}$ = Fraction of CO in alveolar gas at the end of diffusion

Equilibration—washout method ($DL_{CO}SS_{He}$). The subject rebreathes from a reservoir containing 0.3% CO, 10% He, and the remainder air until equilibrium is reached. Then the subject again breathes room air, and the washouts of both CO and He are recorded by a rapid gas analyzer. During the washout, CO is removed at a rapid rate by diffusion as well as by ventilation, whereas He is removed more slowly by ventilation alone. The difference in washout rates is caused by the rate of CO diffusion. An equation similar to the $DL_{CO}SB$ equation is used to calculate $DL_{CO}SS_{He}$; a logarithmic expression of the ratio of final He concentration to initial He concentration is included as a factor, along with the CO concentration ratio. Representation of the washout curve in real time normally requires computerization.

Fractional CO uptake (FU_{CO}). The subject inspires a mixture of 0.1% CO in air from a reservoir to establish a steady-state breathing pattern. He or she expires into a spirometer or reservoir, from which an average expired CO sample is analyzed. The FU_{CO} is expressed as:

$$FU_{CO} = \frac{FI_{CO} - FE_{CO}}{FI_{CO}}$$

where

FI_{CO} = Fraction of inspired CO

FE_{CO} = Fraction of expired CO

The resultant fraction may be multiplied by 100 and expressed as a percentage. The level of VE is critical to valid determination of FU_{CO} and should be monitored closely.

Membrane diffusion coefficient (Dm) and capillary blood volume (Qc). The subject performs two $DL_{CO}SB$ tests, each at a different level of alveolar PO_2. The first $DL_{CO}SB$ is performed as outlined above. The subject then breathes a high concentration of O_2 (balance N_2) for approximately 5 minutes. He or she then immediately exhales to RV and performs the second $DL_{CO}SB$ maneuver. The DL_{CO} values are calculated for both the air and oxygen breathing maneuvers. The resistance caused by the alveolocapillary membrane (Dm) and the resistance caused by the rate of chemical combination with hemoglobin (Hb) and transfer into the red blood cell (θQc) are calculated according to the equation:

$$1/D_{L_{CO}} = 1/Dm + 1/\theta Qc$$

where

$1/D_{L_{CO}}$ = Reciprocal of diffusing capacity, or resistance

$1/Dm$ = Alveolocapillary membrane resistance

$1/\theta Qc$ = Resistance caused by the red blood cell membrane and rate of reaction with Hb

θ = Transfer rate of CO/ml of capillary blood

Qc = Capillary blood volume

Because CO and O_2 compete for binding sites on Hb, measurement of diffusion of CO at different levels of P_{O_2} can be used to distinguish resistance caused by the alveolocapillary membrane from resistance caused by the red blood cell membrane and Hb reaction rate. Qc is presumed to remain the same for both tests, but θ varies in response to changes in P_{O_2}. By plotting θ at two points against $1/D_{L_{CO}}$ and extrapolating back to zero (as if no O_2 were present), the resistance caused by the alveolocapillary membrane can be calculated.

Significance

The average value for resting subjects by the single-breath method is 25 ml CO/min/mm Hg (STPD). (Regression equations for calculation of normal values are included in the Appendix.) Values derived by steady-state methods are usually slightly less than those derived from the single-breath method in normal subjects but may vary by as much as 30%. Females show slightly lower normal values, presumably in correlation with smaller normal lung volumes. $D_{L_{CO}}$ values can increase two to three times in normal individuals during exercise.

Table 5-1 compares the advantages and disadvantages of the testing methods discussed in this chapter.

In general, the $D_{L_{CO}}SB$ is the most widely used method because of its simplicity and noninvasive nature. The rapidity with which several maneuvers can be performed also contributes to its popularity. Many automated systems use the $D_{L_{CO}}SB$, and this has contributed a certain degree of standardization to the methodology. However, because breath-holding at TLC is not a physiologic maneuver, and because the measured value of $D_{L_{CO}}$ varies with lung volume while holding the breath, the $D_{L_{CO}}SB$ may not be an entirely accurate description of diffusing capacity. It is not practical for use during exercise, and some subjects have difficulty expiring fully, inspiring fully, or breath-holding. (See Chapter 11 for criteria for acceptability for $D_{L_{CO}}$ maneuvers.)

The steady-state methods, $D_{L_{CO}}SS_{1-4}$, all use various methods of estimating the mean alveolar P_{CO}. $D_{L_{CO}}SS_1$ probably has the broadest application of the steady-state methods. The widespread availability of arterial blood gas analysis has enabled more common usage. The $D_{L_{CO}}SS_2$ is gaining in popularity because of the availability of fast-response CO analyzers (Chapter 9) and is often done in

Table 5-1. Advantages and disadvantages of testing methods

Method	Technique	Advantages	Disadvantages	Application
$DL_{CO}SB$ (breath-hold)	He and CO analysis relatively simple; 10-second breath-hold	Easy calculations, simple; fast; no COHb back pressure; can be automated	Sensitive to distribution of ventilation and $\dot{V}/\dot{Q}$; "nonphysiologic"; not practical for exercise	Screening and clinical application; good standardization
$DL_{CO}SS_1$ (Filey technique)	CO, CO_2, O_2 analysis; arterial blood sample; relatively simple	Most accurate steady-state method; good for exercise testing	Arterial puncture and blood gas analysis; sensitive to uneven $\dot{V}/\dot{Q}$	Clinical application; exercise studies
$DL_{CO}SS_2$ (end-tidal CO)	End-tidal sample, $F_{U_{CO}}$ simultaneously; CO analysis only	No arterial puncture or breath-hold; easy calculation	COHb back pressure; V_T must be maintained high; very sensitive to $\dot{V}/\dot{Q}$; sensitive to COHb	Fast, easy screening and clinical method; not used for exercise studies
$DL_{CO}SS_3$ (assumed V_D)	CO analysis (slow or fast); large V_T improves accuracy	Relatively simple calculations; good for exercise study	Large error if V_T is too small; sensitive to COHb	Screening and clinical applications; exercise studies

$DL_{CO}SS_4$ (mixed venous P_{CO_2})	CO, CO_2 analysis; rebreathing required	No arterial puncture; easy calculations; slow CO analyzer acceptable	Sensitive to COHb; rebreathing must be closely controlled	Not yet widely used clinically
$DL_{CO}RB$ (rebreathing)	He and CO analysis (rapid); rebreathing required	Less sensitive to V_A than $DL_{CO}SB$; less sensitive to $\dot{V}/\dot{Q}$ abnormalities	Complex calculations; rapid CO and He analyzers required; sensitive to COHb	Clinically applicable; provides most accurate DL_{CO}
$DL_{CO}SSHe$ (equilibration washout)	CO, He analysis rapid; sequencing required	Eliminates V_A, $\dot{V}/\dot{Q}$, and distribution problems	Complex calculations (computerized)	Research applications
$F_{U_{CO}}$ (fractional CO uptake)	CO analysis; may be done with $DL_{CO}SS_2$	Simple; CO analysis of inspired and expired gas only	Sensitive to $\dot{V}_E$, $\dot{V}/\dot{Q}$, and V_D/V_T	Screening or correlation to $DL_{CO}SS_2$
$1/Dm + 1/\theta Vc$ (membrane and red blood cell resistance)	$DL_{CO}SB$ repeated before and after O_2 breathing	Differentiates membrane from red blood cell components; calculates Vc	Complex calculations; estimates of alveolar Po_2 critical	Research with limited clinical applications

combination with the FU_{CO}. The $DL_{CO}SS_3$ is commonly used for measurement of diffusion capacity during exercise, since small differences in the assumed VD become less significant when the VT increases. All of the steady-state methods can be applied to exercise testing.

The rebreathing method is more complicated in terms of the calculations involved but offers the advantage of a normal breathing pattern without arterial puncture. The $DL_{CO}RB$ is less sensitive to $\dot{V}/\dot{Q}$ abnormalities and uneven ventilation distribution than either the $DL_{CO}SB$ or the steady-state methods. The rebreathing method and the steady-state methods may suffer some inaccuracy because of a buildup of COHb in the capillary blood and the resultant "back pressure." Capillary PCO is routinely assumed to be zero, but the actual alveolocapillary gradient at the time of testing can be estimated, though with some difficulty.

The $DL_{CO}SS_{He}$ is the most sophisticated technique. It is relatively insensitive to $\dot{V}/\dot{Q}$ and ventilation abnormalities but requires computerization and is probably limited to research applications.

Calculation of the membrane and red blood cell components of diffusion resistance has revealed that each component accounts for approximately half of the total resistance. Difficulty in quantifying the partial pressure of O_2 in the lungs (pulmonary capillaries) restricts the use of the membrane diffusing capacity determination.

The DL_{O_2} may be estimated from the DL_{CO} by multiplying the $DL_{CO} \times 1.23$, although the DL_{CO} is almost universally reported for clinical purposes.

Since DL_{CO} is directly related to VA, expression of this relationship is often useful in differentiating disease processes in which there may be decreased DL_{CO} as a direct result of loss of lung volume (restrictive) from those diseases in which decreased DL_{CO} is caused by uneven $\dot{V}/\dot{Q}$ or uneven distribution of inspired gas (obstructive). As an index, the measured DL_{CO} may be divided by the lung volume at which the measurement was made to obtain an expression of diffusing capacity per unit of lung volume. This is recorded as DL/VL or DL/VA and may be accomplished easily, since the VA must be calculated to derive the DL_{CO}.

Numerous other factors can influence the observed DL_{CO}:

1. Hematocrit and hemoglobin (decreased Hct and Hb decrease the DL_{CO}). The DL_{CO} may be corrected if the subject's Hb is known. CO uptake varies approximately 6.97% for each gram of Hb; the measured DL_{CO} may be "adjusted" so that the value reported is standardized to an Hb of approximately 14.4 g%. The adjustment factor may be calculated:

$$Hb\ correction = 1/(0.0697 \times Hb)$$

The DL_{CO} is corrected thus:

$$DL_{CO} = Hb\ correction \times DL_{CO}$$

It should be noted that when this correction is applied, the DL_{CO} will be reduced for hemoglobins greater than 14.4 and increased for hemoglobins less than 14.4. An alternate method corrects the *predicted* DL_{CO} rather than the observed value.

2. Alveolar P_{CO_2}. Increased P_{CO_2} raises DL_{CO}; significant increases in the alveolar P_{CO_2} lower the alveolar P_{O_2}.
3. COHb. Elevated carboxyhemoglobin levels, as found in smokers, reduce DL_{CO}; smokers may have COHb levels of 5% to 10% or even greater, causing significant CO "back pressure."
4. Pulmonary capillary blood volume. Increased Qc increases DL_{CO}.
5. Body position. Supine position increases DL_{CO}; changes in body position affect the volume of capillary blood flow.

In general, diffusing capacity is decreased in alveolar fibrosis associated with sarcoidosis, asbestosis, berylliosis, O_2 toxicity, or edema. These states are sometimes categorized as "diffusion defects," although they are probably more closely related to the loss of lung volume or capillary bed. DL_{CO} is decreased in emphysema because of the decrease in surface area, loss of capillary bed, increased distance from the terminal bronchiole to the alveolocapillary membrane, and mismatching of ventilation and blood flow. Diffusion capacity is decreased by parenchymal loss or replacement, space-occupying lesions, and lung resection.

Several technical considerations may affect the measurement of DL_{CO} (particularly $DL_{CO}SB$). Calculation of V_A from He dilution during the single-breath maneuver may result in an underestimation of the lung volume in subjects with moderate to severe obstruction. Low estimated V_A results in a low DL_{CO}. Some clinicians prefer to use a previously determined lung volume to estimate V_A. The RV, as measured by one of the foreign gas techniques, or by plethysmography, can be added to the inspired volume to derive the V_A. However, V_A calculated in this way is typically larger in subjects with obstruction than is V_A calculated from the single-breath dilution, resulting in a larger estimate of DL_{CO}. This approach may not be valid, since the single-breath He dilution value (FE_{He}) is also used to derive the logarithmic ratio that describes the disappearance of CO from the alveoli. Some laboratories report DL_{CO} calculated by both methods.

Various methods of measuring the breath-holding time may also lead to differing values for DL_{CO} (Fig. 5-2). Most systems measure breath-holding time by one of three methods: (1) from the beginning of inspiration (VC) to the beginning of alveolar sampling, (2) from the midpoint of inspiration (one half of the VC) to the beginning of alveolar sampling, or (3) from the two-thirds point of inspiration to the midpoint of the alveolar sample. Theoretically, the breath-holding time is considered the time during which diffusion occurs. However, because some gas transfer may take place early in inspiration, DL_{CO} may be greater if timing starts at the mid-VC point. Similarly, if the timing period is extended into the alveolar sampling phase, the actual time of breath-holding at TLC is reduced and DL_{CO} may be less. The exact timing method may become significant if the predicted values used for comparison were generated by one of the other methods.

Alveolar sampling technique also affects the measurement of DL_{CO}. Most automated systems allow variable washout volumes, with 1.0 liter being most commonly used. Washout volume may need to be reduced when the subject's VC is small (less than 1.5 liter). In subjects with obstruction, this may result in an increased volume of dead space gas being added to the alveolar sample. Since dead space gas resembles the diffusion mixture, D_{LCO} tends to be underestimated. A similar problem can arise if only a very small alveolar sample is taken. Continuous analysis of the expirate using a mass spectrometer allows better identification of ''alveolar'' gas, but this method is not yet practical for clinical use. Other procedural considerations affecting the $D_{LCO}SB$ are included in Chapter 11.

SELF-ASSESSMENT QUESTIONS

1. Carbon monoxide is ideal for measuring diffusing capacity because:
    a. The partial pressure in capillary blood is nearly zero
    b. It combines with Hb 210 times more readily than does O_2
    c. Only small amounts are required to compare inspired versus expired gas concentrations
    d. All of the above
    e. b and c
2. In the $D_{LCO}SB$ method, the alveolar volume is calculated from:
    a. The P_{ACO}
    b. The $P\bar{v}_{CO}$
    c. The expired CO
    d. A single-breath dilution of helium
3. Which of the following D_{LCO} methods is suitable for using during exercises?
    a. $D_{LCO}SB$
    b. $D_{LCO}SS_1$
    c. $D_{LCO}SS_2$
    d. All of the above
    e. b and c
4. The membrane diffusion coefficient (resistance to diffusion by the alveolocapillary membrane) is estimated by:
    a. The $D_{LCO}RB$ method
    b. The Fu_{CO} method
    c. Performing the $D_{LCO}SB$ test at two different levels of alveolar oxygen tension
    d. Subtracting the $F_{ACO_{t1}}$ from the $F_{ACO_{t1}}$ obtained from the $D_{LCO}SB$
5. The average D_{LCO} (by the single-breath method) for healthy adults is approximately 25 ml CO/min/mm Hg; the D_{LCO} by the steady-state methods is usually:
    a. Slightly less
    b. Slightly higher
    c. Two to three times that of the $D_{LCO}SB$
    d. Equal to the $D_{LCO}SB$
6. A subject with symptoms of shortness of breath has pulmonary function studies; his $D_{LCO}SB$ is 5 ml CO/min/mm Hg, and his TLC is 8 liters; these values are consistent with:
    a. A restrictive pattern
    b. An obstructive pattern
    c. Pulmonary fibrosis
    d. All of the above
    e. a and c

7. Which of the following factors might account for a decreased DL_{CO} in the absence of pulmonary disease?
   I. Increased alveolar carbon dioxide tension (PA_{CO_2})
   II. Decreased hemoglobin (anemia)
   III. Decreased capillary blood volume
   IV. Elevated carboxyhemoglobin (COHb)
   a. I, II, III, and IV
   b. I, III, and IV
   c. II, III, and IV
   d. I and IV

8. A subject with an Hb of 17.7 has a DL_{CO} of 24; if the observed value were adjusted for the increased hemoglobin, the "corrected" DL_{CO} would be:
   a. Higher
   b. Lower
   c. About the same
   d. Cannot be determined

9. If the VA is calculated from a multiple-breath lung volume technique and then used to compute the DL_{CO} in a subject with severe obstruction, the resulting DL_{CO} will be _____ _____ the DL_{CO} calculated from a single-breath dilution of He.
   a. Equal to
   b. Larger than
   c. Smaller than
   d. Either a or c

10. Breathholding time (in the $DL_{CO}SB$) is calculated from:
    I. The beginning of inspiration to the beginning of alveolar sampling
    II. Two thirds of the VC (volume inspired) on the midpoint of alveolar sampling
    III. One half of the VC (volume inspired) to the beginning of alveolar sampling
    IV. The end of inspiration to the end of alveolar sampling
    a. I, II, III, and IV
    b. I, II, and III
    c. II, III, and IV
    d. III only

SELECTED BIBLIOGRAPHY

General references
Bates, D.V., Macklem, P.T, and Christie, R.V.: Respiratory function in disease, Philadelphia, 1971, W.B. Saunders Co.
Dinakara, P., et al.: The effect of anemia on pulmonary diffusing capacity with derivation of a correction equation, Am. Rev. Respir. Dis. **102:**965, 1970.
Ferris, B.G.: Epidemiology standardization project: recommended standardized procedure for pulmonary function testing, Am. Rev. Respir. Dis. **118**(suppl. 2):**1,** 1978.
Forster, R.E.: Diffusion of gases. In Fenn, W.O., and Rahn, H., editors: Handbook of physiology—respiration I, Washington, D.C., 1964, American Physiological Society.
McNeill, R.S., Rankin, J., and Forster, R.E.: The diffusing capacity of the pulmonary membrane and the pulmonary capillary blood volume in cardiopulmonary disease, Clin. Sci. **17:**465, 1958.
Morris, A.H., et al.: Clinical pulmonary function testing, ed. 2, Salt Lake City, 1984, Intermountain Thoracic Society.
Symonds, G., Renzetti, A.D., Jr., and Mitchell, M.M.: The diffusing capacity in pulmonary emphysema, Am. Rev. Respir. Dis. **109:**391, 1974.
West, J.B.: Respiratory physiology: the essentials, Baltimore, 1974, Williams & Wilkins.
West, J.B.: Pulmonary pathophysiology: the essentials, Baltimore, 1977, Williams & Wilkins.

D$_{L_{CO}}$SB

Crapo, R.O., and Morris, A.H.: Standardized single breath normal values for carbon monoxide diffusing capacity, Am. Rev. Respir. Dis. **123:**185, 1981.

Gaensler, E.A., and Smith, A.A.: Attachment for automated single breath diffusing capacity measurement, Chest **63:**136, 1973.

Graham, B.L., Mink, J.T., and Cotton, D.J.: Overestimation of the single breath carbon monoxide diffusing capacity in patients with air-flow obstruction, Am. Rev. Respir. Dis. **129:** 403, 1984.

Mohsenifar, Z., and Tashkin, D.P.: Effect of carboxyhemoglobin on the single breath diffusing capacity: derivation of an empirical correction factor, Respiration **37:**185, 1979.

Ogilvie, C.M., et al.: A standardized breath-holding technique for the clinical measurement of the diffusing capacity of the lung for carbon monoxide, J. Clin. Invest. **36:**1, 1957.

D$_{L_{CO}}$SS

Filey, G.F., Macintosh, D.J., and Wright, G.W.: Carbon monoxide uptake and pulmonary diffusing capacity in normal subjects at rest and during exercise, J. Clin. Invest. **33:**530, 1954.

CHAPTER SIX

Blood gas analysis and related tests

BLOOD GAS ANALYSIS
ARTERIAL OXYGEN TENSION (Pa_{O_2})
Description

Pa_{O_2} is a measurement of the partial pressure exerted by O_2 dissolved in the serum portion of arterial blood. It is recorded in millimeters of mercury (mm Hg or torr) or in kilopascal units (Système International; 1 mm Hg = 0.133 kPa).

Technique

Pa_{O_2} is measured by submitting whole arterial blood, obtained by anaerobic arterial puncture, to a membrane-covered platinum electrode, which reacts with O_2 molecules (see Fig. 9-15). The blood is collected in a heparinized syringe and sealed from the atmosphere immediately. The sample should be stored in ice water if analysis is not to be done immediately. Mixed venous samples may be drawn from a pulmonary artery catheter and handled similarly. Venous samples are not useful for assessing oxygenation, since the blood reflects the metabolism of the area drained by that particular vein. Capillary samples are useful in infants when arterial puncture is impractical. The area for collection should be heated by a warm compress and lanced, and blood should be allowed to fill the required volume of heparinized capillary tube(s). Squeezing the tissue should be avoided, since predominately venous blood will be obtained. The capillary tubes should be carefully sealed to avoid bubbles. Guidelines for quality control for blood gas analysis are included in Chapter 11.

Significance

The Pa_{O_2} varies from 85 to 100 mm Hg in a healthy young adult and decreases slightly with age. The Pa_{O_2} can be increased with normal lungs by hyperventilation to values as high as 120 mm Hg. Normal subjects breathing 100% O_2 exhibit a Pa_{O_2} in excess of 600 mm Hg. Decreased Pa_{O_2} can result from (1) hypoventilation, (2) diffusion defects, (3) ventilation/blood flow imbalances, and (4) inadequate atmospheric O_2 (altitude). Since the Po_2 is the pressure of dissolved oxygen in blood, it is not influenced by the amount of hemoglobin present or by whether the Hb is capable of binding O_2. It is possible for the Pa_{O_2} to be normal or even elevated (as in O_2 breathing), and for hypoxemia to occur, if inadequate amounts or abnormal forms of Hb are present. Most automated blood gas analyzers allow *calculation* of the saturation (Sa_{O_2}) from the Pa_{O_2} and pH with the assumption that the normal hemoglobin reaction will occur. The actual ability of the Hb to bind O_2 at a particular pressure is quantified by the P_{50}, which specifies the partial pressure at which a specific hemoglobin is 50% saturated. Calculated saturations usually presume a value of 26 to 27 as the P_{50}, although this may be quite different depending on the types of hemoglobins and interfering substances present. A more accurate method is to measure Sa_{O_2} as described below.

The severity of arterial oxygenation impairment is indicated by the Pa_{O_2} at rest. The Pa_{O_2} describes the ability of the lungs to match pulmonary capillary blood flow with adequate ventilation. Because of the shape of the oxygen-hemoglobin dissociation curve, O_2 binding to hemoglobin is almost complete at Pa_{O_2} values greater than 60 mm Hg (90% saturation). As the Pa_{O_2} falls from 60 to 40, the saturation typically decreases from 90% to 75%, and symptoms of hypoxia (mental confusion, shortness of breath, etc.) increase. The delivery of O_2 to the tissues, however, depends on other factors in addition to the Pa_{O_2}. Since most O_2 transported is bound to Hb, there must be an adequate supply (12 to 15 g/dl) of functional hemoglobin. Adequate cardiac output (4 to 5 L/min) is necessary to deliver the oxygenated arterial blood to the tissues.

Severe obstructive or restrictive diseases may show decreased oxygen tension, occasionally as low as 40 mm Hg, in resting subjects. Less advanced pulmonary disease may show little decrease in Pa_{O_2} if hyperventilation is present or if the disease process affects both ventilation and perfusion in the same lung units. This is commonly observed in emphysema, wherein the destruction of alveolar septa removes pulmonary capillaries as well, resulting in poor ventilation and equally poor perfusion. Subjects with emphysema may have severe airway obstruction and relatively normal arterial oxygen tension. However, analysis of Pa_{O_2} during exercise often shows a decrease in Pa_{O_2} commensurate with the extent of the disease process. Pa_{O_2}, at rest and during exercise, correlates best with the subject's DL_{CO} and FEV_1, but a wide range of variability exists. Subjects with decreased DL_{CO} and FEV_1 typically show low Pa_{O_2} values at rest and during exercise, but the extent of arterial desaturation cannot be predicted from static pulmonary function measurements. Pa_{O_2} may be decreased for pulmonary reasons such as (1) anatomic shunts (intracardiac) or (2) neuromuscular hypoventilation. Pa_{O_2} is of greatest value when correlated with adequate spirometry (FEV_1, $FEF_{25\%-75\%}$), DL_{CO}, ventilation ($\dot{V}E$, VT, VD), and lung volume tests (VC, RV, TLC). The main disadvantage is the necessity of arterial puncture.

ARTERIAL OXYGEN SATURATION (Sa_{O_2})
Description

Sa_{O_2} measures the volume of oxygen in milliliters combined with hemoglobin as related to the maximum capacity of that same hemoglobin for binding O_2. This ratio of content to capacity is expressed as a percentage.

Technique

Oxygen saturation of hemoglobin is commonly measured in one of three ways:

1. The O_2 content of arterial blood is measured, and the blood is exposed to the atmosphere so that the Hb may combine with atmospheric O_2, after which the content is measured again. Saturation is determined after corrections for dissolved O_2 are made.
2. The O_2 saturation can also be measured spectrophotometrically by analyzing the ratio of oxyhemoglobin to total hemoglobin.
3. Saturation can also be obtained by ear or finger pulse oximetry.

Mixed venous oxygen saturation may be measured spectrophotometrically by an indwelling pulmonary artery catheter that includes fiberoptic bundles for in vivo measurements. Descriptions of the various types of oximeters are included in Chapter 9. Guidelines for quality control of blood gas analysis are included in Chapter 11.

Significance

The percent of saturation for a healthy young adult with a Pa_{O_2} of 95 mm Hg is approximately 97%. Because of the shape of the O_2-Hb dissociation curve, large changes in Pa_{O_2} effect small changes in saturation above partial pressures of 60 mm Hg. Therefore the Pa_{O_2} is a more sensitive indicator of oxygenation in lungs without gross abnormalities. As the partial pressure of O_2 falls below 60 mm Hg, the degree to which Hb binds to O_2 decreases rapidly. In essence, the percent of saturation is a measure of the relationship between O_2 and Hb.

Normal subjects have a small amount of other hemoglobins present that do not carry oxygen. Carboxyhemoglobin (COHb) is present in blood, usually in the range of 1% to 2% of the total Hb, as a result of metabolism and environmental exposure. In smokers the levels may be increased to between 3% and 15%, depending on the recent smoking history. Smoke inhalation or carbon monoxide poisoning from other sources may also result in elevated COHb levels. Methemoglobin (MetHb) results when the iron atoms of the hemoglobin molecule are oxidized from Fe^{++} to Fe^{+++}; normally the MetHb level is less than 1.5% of the total Hb. High levels of MetHb can result from ingestion of or exposure to strong oxidizing agents. Both COHb and MetHb reduce the oxygen-carrying capacity of the blood by reducing the available hemoglobin and shifting the O_2-Hb dissociation curve to the left.

The percent of saturation of mixed venous blood is 75% ($P\bar{v}_{O_2} = 40$ mm Hg). As the lungs fail to oxygenate mixed venous blood, arterial saturation falls from its normal 95% toward the mixed venous level of 75%. However, if the oxygen uptake and cardiac output remain constant, the mixed venous saturation also falls, so that about 5 vol% is removed. The percent of saturation does not indicate the O_2 content of either arterial or mixed venous blood (Ca_{O_2} and $C\bar{v}_{O_2}$, respectively), both of which are determined by the concentration of Hb as well as the Po_2. Ca_{O_2} is described by the equation:

$$Ca_{O_2} = (1.34 \times Hb \times Sa_{O_2}) + (0.0031 \times Pa_{O_2})$$

where

1.34 = O_2 binding capacity of Hb in ml/g (some clinicians prefer 1.36 or 1.39 ml/g)

Hb = Hemoglobin concentration, g/dl

Sa_{O_2} = Saturation expressed as a fraction ($Sa_{O_2}/100$)

0.0031 = Solubility coefficient for O_2 (ml/mm Hg)

Pa_{O_2} = Partial pressure of O_2 in the specimen

The two halves of the equation (terms in parentheses) define the volumes of O_2 transported bound to hemoglobin and in the dissolved form. The same calculation can be applied to a mixed venous sample by substituting the $S\bar{v}_{O_2}$ and $P\bar{v}_{O_2}$.

ARTERIAL CARBON DIOXIDE TENSION (Pa_{CO_2})
Description

Pa_{CO_2} is a measure of the partial pressure exerted by CO_2 in arterial blood. The measurement is expressed in millimeters of mercury (mm Hg or torr) or in kilopascal units (Système International; 1 mm Hg = 0.133 kPa).

Technique

Pa_{CO_2} is measured by submitting arterial blood to a special glass (pH) electrode behind a membrane in which the CO_2 combines with water to form carbonic acid (H_2CO_3). The dissociation of H_2CO_3 into H^+ and HCO_3^- is measured by the electrode and is proportional to the Pa_{CO_2} (see Fig. 9-15). The arterial blood must be kept in an anaerobic state, in an ice water bath, until analysis. P_{CO_2} may also be estimated using a transcutaneous electrode. Guidelines for quality control of blood gas analysis are included in Chapter 11.

Significance

The Pa_{CO_2} of a healthy adult is approximately 40 mm Hg (35 to 45 mm Hg). The Pa_{CO_2} is an index of the $\dot{V}A$ (see Chapter 2). A rise in Pa_{CO_2} is usually associated with hypoventilation; a fall in Pa_{CO_2} is associated with hyperventilation. Because CO_2 diffuses more readily than O_2, and because it is related to the *volume* of alveolar ventilation rather than matching of ventilation and perfusion, small changes in the ventilatory pattern or distribution of gas will show little or no change in Pa_{CO_2}. Subjects with localized lesions often hyperventilate functional alveoli and maintain a normal CO_2 tension. An increase in Pa_{CO_2} means that a significant number of lung units are being hypoventilated. Diffusion defects rarely raise the Pa_{CO_2}. The CO_2 tension may be normal or low even in moderately advanced pulmonary disease. The Pa_{CO_2} is most valuable as a diagnostic tool when correlated to the $\dot{V}E$, VT, f, Pa_{O_2}, and pH. The $\dot{V}E$ necessary to maintain a given Pa_{CO_2} is indicative of the number of functional lung units. A normal CO_2 tension accompanied by a large $\dot{V}E$ (15 to 20 liters) points to a large amount of wasted ventilation or VD, as might be seen with pulmonary embolization. The correlation of O_2 and CO_2 tensions often gives an indication of the extent of functional impairment. Subjects with high Pa_{CO_2} and low Pa_{O_2} values typically have the most severe derangements because a sufficiently large proportion of the pulmonary system is involved, so that even the fast-diffusing CO_2 cannot be eliminated efficiently. This is common in advanced emphysema, chronic bronchitis, and acute asthmatic episodes. A gas exchange system that cannot remove CO_2 can very rarely arterialize mixed venous blood, even in the presence of increased inspired O_2 concentrations. Similarly, a low Pa_{CO_2} coupled with a low Pa_{O_2} indicates that although enough mixed venous blood is passing through the pulmonary capillaries to cause an oxygenation defect, a sufficiently large portion of the gas exchange mechanism is working to remove an adequate amount of CO_2. In effect, hyperventilation caused by hypoxemia can often cause inappropriate removal of CO_2. Similarly, changes in the P_{CO_2} during breathing of supplementary O_2 must be carefully evaluated. Some subjects with chronic hypoxemia have a decreased ventilatory response to CO_2. Oxygen administered to such subjects may result in an elevation of the Pa_{CO_2}, so that O_2 therapy must be titrated to produce acceptable Pa_{O_2} values (usually 55 to 60 mm Hg) without hypercapnia or acidosis. The relationship of the Pa_{CO_2} to pH and HCO_3^- defines the acid-base status of the body (Table 6-1).

The only disadvantage of measuring Pa_{CO_2} is the required arterial sample. End-tidal P_{CO_2} is sometimes used to estimate Pa_{CO_2}.

ARTERIAL pH
Description

pH is the negative logarithm of the hydrogen ion (H^+) concentration used as a positive number. pH is recorded in pH units ranging from 1 to 14, 1 being most acid, 14 being most basic, and 7 being the pH of water, or neutral.

Table 6-1. Acid-base status

Status	pH	P_{CO_2}	HCO_3^-
Simple disorders			
Metabolic acidosis	Low	Normal	Low
Metabolic alkalosis	High	Normal	High
Respiratory acidosis	Low	High	Normal
Respiratory alkalosis	High	Low	Normal
Compensated disorders			
Compensated respiratory acidosis or metabolic alkalosis	Normal*	High	High
Compensated metabolic acidosis or respiratory alkalosis	Normal*	Low	Low
Combined disorders			
Metabolic/respiratory acidosis	Low	High	Low
Metabolic/respiratory alkalosis	High	Low	High

*Compensation cannot return values to within normal limits in severe acid-base disturbances. In addition, a normal pH may result in instances where there are respiratory and metabolic disturbances that occur together but are not compensatory.

Technique

Arterial pH is measured by submitting arterial blood to a glass electrode under anaerobic conditions (see Fig. 9-15). Normally pH measurements are made at 37° C. The pH can also be determined indirectly if the plasma HCO_3^- and Pa_{CO_2} are known, by application of the Henderson-Hasselbalch equation:

$$pH = pK + \log\frac{(HCO_3^-)}{(CO_2)}$$

where

pK   = Negative log of dissociation constant for carbonic acid (6.1)
(HCO_3^-) = Molar concentration of serum bicarbonate
(CO_2) = Molar concentration of CO_2

To simplify actual calculation, the Pa_{CO_2}, which can be measured directly, is substituted for (CO_2), and the total $CO_2 - Pa_{CO_2} \times (0.03)$ is substituted for (HCO_3); 0.03 is a solubility factor introduced to express the Pa_{CO_2} in milliequivalents per liter. The equation becomes:

$$pH = pK + \log\frac{(\text{Total } CO_2 - 0.03\,[Pa_{CO_2}])}{0.03\,(Pa_{CO_2})}$$

Guidelines for quality control of blood gas analysis are included in Chapter 11.

Significance

The pH of arterial blood of a healthy adult ranges from 7.35 to 7.45. As the pH falls below 7.35, the blood becomes acidotic; as it rises above 7.45, the blood becomes increasingly alkalotic.

One of the main functions of the lungs is to remove CO_2, and this ability is directly related to the acid-base status of the body. When CO_2 is retained, carbonic acid is formed and dissociates into HCO_3^- and H^+ ions, the pH falls, and the resulting acidosis is respiratory in origin. Similarly, if CO_2 is "blown off," respiratory alkalosis ensues (Table 6-1). Diagnostically, arterial pH is of greatest value when correlated to $\dot{V}E$ and Pa_{CO_2}. Increased Pa_{CO_2} normally causes acidosis, except in the presence of renal compensation (retention and production of bicarbonate). If the acidosis is of nonrespiratory origin (diabetes, etc.), hyperventilation and a fall in Pa_{CO_2} normally occur. Chronic obstructive pulmonary disease and chronic CO_2 retention often result in grossly exaggerated blood gas values and HCO_3^- levels with a resultant pH close to normal limits because of chronic compensation. Acute ventilatory impairment (pneumonia, etc.) often shows little or no renal compensation; when present, it is seldom as pronounced as in long-term compensation. Hence lung function and Pa_{CO_2} in particular often serve to define acid-base disorders.

Arterial blood is normally used for pH determinations because venous blood is slightly more acidic and reflects only local metabolism.

SINGLE-BREATH CARBON DIOXIDE ELIMINATION
Description

The single-breath CO_2 test measures the uniformity of both ventilation and pulmonary blood flow. The slope of the alveolar phase is recorded as a percentage.

Technique

The subject exhales into a CO_2 analyzer that continuously monitors the concentration of CO_2 in expired gas. The change in CO_2 concentration is recorded graphically, as is done in the SBN_2 test (Fig. 6-1). The change in percentage over a given interval after the V_D gas has been exhaled is measured to index the uniformity of ventilation to blood flow.

Significance

In normal individuals the concentration of CO_2 in expired gas rises to a plateau as alveolar gas is expired and remains more or less constant. The single-breath

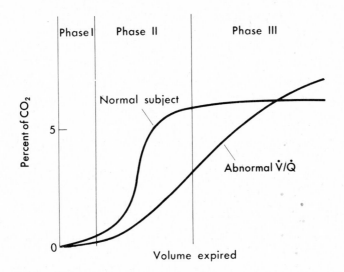

Fig. 6-1. Carbon dioxide elimination. A plot of expired CO_2 concentration against expired volume yields a curve distinctly similar to an SBN_2 curve. Three phases can be defined: *Phase I* includes the expiration of dead space gas containing little CO_2; *Phase II* shows an abrupt rise in the percent of CO_2 as mixed bronchial and alveolar air is expired; *Phase III* shows the typical plateau as alveolar gas is monitored. Also illustrated is an elimination curve typical of abnormal ventilation/blood flow ratios. When different parts of the lungs have different CO_2 concentrations and different parts empty at different rates, the CO_2 elimination curve will show a constant rise during the entire expiration. The SBN_2 test indicates abnormality of ventilation; the CO_2 elimination test indicates abnormal matching of blood flow and ventilation. If ventilation shifts to match uneven blood flow (or vice versa), the elimination curve will assure a more S shape.

CO_2 test will show a continuous rise with expired volume in lungs that exhibit uneven ventilation and at the same time determine if the blood flow matches the distribution of ventilation. If all parts of the lungs emptied CO_2 at exactly the same rate, there would be no rise in the concentration of carbon dioxide. But since lungs with ventilation and blood flow imbalances empty CO_2 at varying rates, the CO_2 concentration rises as more and more of the VC is expired. The slope of the CO_2 elimination curve (Fig. 6-1) is determined by the extent of variation in ventilation as compared with perfusion. The absolute concentrations of CO_2 expired depend on various factors (such as minute ventilation and $\dot{V}_{CO_2}$), but the quantitative value of the test is not influenced by the magnitude of the CO_2 concentration, only the amount of change.

The single-breath CO_2 test requires a CO_2 analyzer and a recording device for plotting CO_2 concentration against expired volume. Since it is not a strictly quantitative analysis, it is often replaced by a calculation of the physiologic V_D (see Chapter 2) or the percent of shunt. Rapid-responding CO_2 analyzers are often used at the bedside, and with appropriate recorders, can be employed to monitor the matching of ventilation to perfusion. With appropriate facilities the ^{133}Xe test and perfusion lung scan can be used to obtain similar qualitative judgments of ventilation/blood flow inequalities.

SHUNT CALCULATION ($\dot{Q}s/\dot{Q}T$)
Description

$\dot{Q}s/\dot{Q}T$ is a measurement of the fraction of blood that traverses the pulmonary system without participating in gas exchange. It is recorded as a percent of the total capillary flow, or sometimes as a fraction.

Technique

The shunt fraction is usually measured by one of two techniques:
1. Using O_2 content differences:

$$\frac{\dot{Q}s}{\dot{Q}T} = \frac{Cc_{O_2} - Ca_{O_2}}{Cc_{O_2} - C\bar{v}_{O_2}}$$

where

$\dot{Q}s/\dot{Q}T$ = Fraction of shunted blood to total perfusion

Cc_{O_2} = O_2 content of end-capillary blood, normally estimated from the saturation associated with the calculated $P_{A_{O_2}}$

Ca_{O_2} = Arterial O_2 content measured from an arterial sample (see Arterial Oxygen Saturation above)

$C\bar{v}_{O_2}$ = Mixed venous O_2 content measured from a sample obtained from an indwelling pulmonary artery catheter

The denominator in this equation reflects potential arterialization of mixed venous blood, whereas the numerator reflects the actual arterialization.

2. The subject is allowed to breathe 100% O_2 for at least 20 minutes at atmospheric pressure so that all N_2 is washed out of the lungs and the Hb can become completely saturated. The percent of shunt can then be calculated thus:

$$\frac{\dot{Q}s}{\dot{Q}T} = \frac{(P_{AO_2} - Pa_{O_2}) \times 0.0031}{C(a - v)o_2 + [(P_{AO_2} - Pa_{O_2}) \times 0.0031]}$$

where

$\dot{Q}s/\dot{Q}T$ = Ratio of shunted blood to total perfusion

P_{AO_2} = Alveolar O_2 tension

Pa_{O_2} = Arterial O_2 tension

$C(a - v)o_2$ = Arteriovenous oxygen content difference

0.0031 = Conversion factor to volume % for O_2

P_{AO_2}, with the subject breathing 100% O_2, can be estimated as follows:

$$P_{AO_2} = P_B - P_{AH_2O} - P_{ACO_2}/0.8$$

where

P_B = Barometric pressure

P_{AH_2O} = Partial pressure of water vapor at body temperature (47 mm Hg)

P_{ACO_2} = Alveolar CO_2 tension (estimated from arterial P_{CO_2})

0.8 = Correction based on respiratory exchange ratio

In both of these methods the shunt fraction or ratio may be multiplied by 100 and the result reported as a percentage (0.20 ratio × 100 equals a 20% shunt).

The second method of calculating the shunt is accurate only when the hemoglobin is completely saturated, and this normally requires a Pa_{O_2} of greater than 150 mm Hg. This is usually easily accomplished by breathing pure O_2. (See the Appendix for a more detailed description of the technique.) In situations where breathing 100% O_2 does not raise the Pa_{O_2} high enough to completely saturate the Hb, the content difference method (No. 1 above) should be used.

Significance

Normally less than 5% of the cardiac output is shunted. The accuracy of the shunt measurement using the second method above depends on the accuracy of the P_{O_2} determinations, since in small shunts the Hb still becomes 100% saturated, and the difference in P_{O_2} is a result of the amount of O_2 dissolved; in fact, it is the difference in the amount of dissolved oxygen that is the basis for the calculation. The actual value for the percent of shunt depends largely on the value of the O_2 content difference between arterial and mixed venous blood ($C[a-v]o_2$) used in the denominator of the equation. Since the a-v content difference is determined not only by the status of the pulmonary system, but also by the cardiac output and perfusion status, the value used in the equation should ideally be measured rather than estimated. Arterial content can be measured or calculated easily from a sample taken from a peripheral artery, but mixed venous content can only be measured accurately from a sample taken from the pulmonary artery. With subjects in whom the right side of the heart has not been catheterized, an estimated value must be used. Values from 4.5 to 5.0 vol% are reasonable a-v differences in subjects with good cardiac outputs and perfusion states. Values of

3.5 vol% are probably more realistic differences in individuals who are critically ill.

In instances where the a-v content difference cannot be reliably estimated or when the Hb cannot be maximally saturated by breathing 100% oxygen, the alveolar-arterial oxygen gradient (A-aDo$_2$) may be used as an index for matching of ventilation to blood flow. The $\dot{Q}s/\dot{Q}T$ does not derive any absolute values for $\dot{Q}s$, but if the cardiac output ($\dot{Q}T$) is known, the $\dot{Q}s$ can be determined simply. Increased shunting (percent) is indicative of low ventilation in relation to blood flow, as is often found in both obstructive and restrictive disease patterns. It should be noted, however, that even in advanced obstructive or severe restrictive diseases, blood flow to the areas of poor ventilation may be decreased by the lesions themselves or by compensatory mechanisms. In these cases there will be a minimal amount of shunting, even though severe ventilatory impairment may exist. Perhaps most common is increased shunting caused by acute disease patterns such as atelectasis or aspiration of a foreign body. Diseases such as pneumonia or the adult respiratory distress syndrome (ARDS) usually result in a shuntlike effect because of the reduction of ventilation in proportion to blood flow.

The shunt measurement's disadvantages are as follows: (1) method No. 1 requires placement of a pulmonary artery catheter to obtain mixed venous O$_2$ content, and (2) method No. 2 should also use measured a-v content differences; in addition, the second method requires inhalation of pure O$_2$ for 20 minutes, which may be contraindicated in subjects whose main respiratory drive is hypoxemia. Breathing pure O$_2$ washes N$_2$ out of the lungs completely. In subjects in whom certain lung units may be poorly ventilated, the washout of N$_2$ plus the removal of O$_2$ by the perfusing blood flow may reduce the size of alveoli to their critical limit and cause alveolar collapse. The net effect of the "nitrogen shunting" may be clinical shunt values that are falsely high, since a certain amount of shunting is induced by the testing procedure.

Measurement of the shunt fraction is often correlated with determination of the VD/VT ratio (see Chapter 2).

SELF-ASSESSMENT QUESTIONS

1. Arterial O$_2$ tension (Pa$_{O_2}$) may be decreased for which of the following reasons?
   I. Hypoventilation
   II. Inadequate hemoglobin
   III. Ventilation/blood flow imbalances
   IV. Inadequate atmospheric O$_2$
   a. I, II, III, and IV
   b. I, III, and IV
   c. II and III
   d. I and IV

2. In addition to a normal Pa$_{O_2}$, adequate delivery of oxygen to the tissues depends on:
   a. Adequate functional hemoglobin
   b. Normal amounts of dissolved oxygen

   c. Hb saturation greater than 97%

   d. Adequate cardiac output

   e. a and d

3. Calculate the oxygen content (ml O_2/100 ml blood) of a sample with the following blood gas measurements:

Hb	13.3 g/dl
Sa_{O_2}	89% (0.89)
Pa_{O_2}	60 mm Hg
Ca_{O_2} =	_____ml O_2/dl

4. Hyperventilation is defined as:

   a. Respiratory rate greater than 20/min

   b. Respiratory rate greater than 30/min

   c. Decreased Pa_{CO_2} and alkalosis (respiratory)

   d. Increased Pa_{CO_2} with a normal pH

5. The carboxyhemoglobin saturation (COHb) in smokers is often found in the range of:

   a. 1% to 3%

   b. 3% to 10%

   c. 20% to 40%

   d. Greater than 40%

6. Which of the following accurately describes the Pa_{CO_2}?

   I. It is often elevated in subjects with diffusion defects.

   II. It is inversely related to the alveolar ventilation.

   III. It may be low or normal in the presence of hypoxemia.

   IV. It may be elevated in the presence of hypoxemia.

   a. I, II, and III

   b. I, II, and IV

   c. II, III, and IV

   d. II and III

7. A subject has the following arterial blood gases:

pH	7.37
Pa_{CO_2}	62
Pa_{O_2}	55
HCO_3^-	35

These are best described as:

   a. Normal acid-base status, mild hypoxemia

   b. Compensated metabolic alkalosis, moderate hypoxemia

   c. Uncompensated respiratory acidosis with hypoxemia

   d. Compensated respiratory acidosis, moderate hypoxemia

8. The CO_2 elimination curve is particularly useful as an index for the matching of ventilation to blood flow because:

   a. The shape of the elimination curve is indicative of the extent of mismatching

   b. Only perfused and ventilated alveoli contribute CO_2 to the exhaled gas

   c. It is not influenced by the absolute concentration of the expired CO_2

   d. All of the above

9. Increased shunt values ($\dot{Q}s/\dot{Q}T$) are often found in subjects with:

   a. Acute restrictive disease patterns, such as pulmonary edema

   b. Obstructive disease patterns, such as COPD

   c. Atelectasis, as found in pneumonia or pneumonitis

   d. All of the above

10. Which of the following accurately describes the calculation of percent of shunt by the oxygen content difference method?
    I. The O_2 content of end-capillary blood must be estimated.
    II. The subject must breathe 100% O_2 for 20 minutes.
    III. A pulmonary artery catheter is required.
    IV. An arterial blood sample is required.
    a. I, II, III, and IV
    b. I, II, and IV
    c. I, III, and IV
    d. II and IV

SELECTED BIBLIOGRAPHY

General references

Comroe, J.H.: Physiology of respiration, Chicago, 1965, Year Book Medical Publishers, Inc.

Morris, A.H., et al.: Clinical pulmonary function testing, ed. 2, Salt Lake City, 1984, Intermountain Thoracic Society.

West, J.B.: Respiratory physiology: the essentials, Baltimore, 1974, Williams & Wilkins.

West, J.B.: Pulmonary pathophysiology: the essentials, Baltimore, 1977, Williams & Wilkins.

Blood gas analysis

Harris, E.A., et al.: The normal alveolar-arterial oxygen gradient in man, Clin. Sci. Molec. Med. **46:**89, 1974.

Harrison, R.A., et al.: Reassessment of the assumed a-v oxygen content difference in the shunt calculation, Anesth. Analg. **54:**198, 1975.

Severinghaus, J.W.: Blood gas calculator, J. Appl. Physiol. **21:**1108, 1966.

Severinghaus, J.W.: Simple, accurate equations for human blood O_2 dissociation computations, J. Appl. Physiol. **46:**599, 1979.

Shapiro, B.A., et al.: Clinical application of blood gases, ed. 2, Chicago, 1977, Year Book Medical Publishers, Inc.

Siggard-Anderson, O.: Acid-base and blood gas parameters—arterial or capillary blood? Scand. J. Clin. Lab. Invest. **21:**289, 1968.

Shunt and CO_2 elimination

Cane, R.D., et al.: Minimizing errors in intrapulmonary shunt calculations, Crit. Care Med. **8:**294, 1980.

Mellemgaard, K.: The alveolar-arterial oxygen difference: its size and components in normal man, Acta Physiol. Scand. **67:**10, 1966.

Rahn, H., and Farhi, L.E.: Ventilation, perfusion, and gas exchange—the VA/Q concept. In Fenn, W.O., and Rahn, H., editors: Handbook of physiology—respiration I, Washington, 1964, American Physiological Society.

CHAPTER SEVEN

Exercise testing

The efficiency of the cardiopulmonary system may be quite different during periods of increased metabolic demands from what it is at rest. For this reason, tests designed to assess ventilation, gas exchange, and cardiovascular function during exercise can provide information not obtainable with *static* tests of cardiopulmonary function. Exercise testing allows evaluation of the heart and lungs under conditions of increased metabolic demand, so that abnormalities not readily defined in terms of descreased flows, volumes, or diffusing capacities may be quantified. Limitations to work are not entirely predictable from any single static measurement of pulmonary function, although approximations may be made from multiple parameters (FEV_1, DL_{CO}, etc.). For quantification of the causes of work limitations, an exercise test under *stress* conditions is necessary. In all forms of exercise testing, measured parameters of cardiopulmonary function are assessed in relation to the level of exercise, or work load, performed. Indications for performing exercise testing in subjects whose chief complaint is dyspnea on exertion include (1) determining the presence and nature of ventilatory limitations to work, (2) determining the presence and nature of cardiac limitations to work, (3) assessing the extent of conditioning or deconditioning, (4) determining maximum tolerable work loads and safe levels of daily exercise, and (5) quantifying the extent of disability for rehabilitation purposes. Exercise testing may be indicated in apparently healthy individuals (particularly in adults over 40 years of age) for the sake of ascertaining fitness to engage in vigorous physical activities, such as running.

Chapter 12 includes examples of exercise studies (Cases 7, 8, and 9).

WORK LOAD DETERMINATION AND EXERCISE PROTOCOLS

Exercise tests can be divided into two categories in regard to the general protocol involved in performing the test: (1) progressive multistage tests and (2) steady-state tests.

Progressive multistage tests are designed to examine the effects of increasing work loads on various cardiopulmonary parameters without necessarily allowing a steady state to be achieved. Most often this protocol is used to determine a maximum tolerable work load and to establish trends for the various exercise parameters measured. In a typical progressive multistage test, the work load of the exercising subject is increased at predetermined intervals and all measurements are performed toward the end of each interval. Increments of work may be increased at intervals of 1 to 6 minutes, depending on the nature of the measurements being made. With a device that allows continuous adjustment of the work load in small intervals (see cycle ergometer below), a "ramp" test may be performed. During multistage tests using short intervals (1 to 3 minutes or a ramp protocol), a steady state of gas exchange, ventilation, and cardiovascular response may not be attained. Attainment of a steady state is not necessary if the primary objective of the evaluation is to determine the maximum tolerable work load. Incremental tests using intervals of 4 to 6 minutes at each work load may result in a steady state (relatively constant gas exchange, ventilation, and cardiovascular response), but these should not be confused with steady-state tests.

Steady-state tests are designed to assess parameters of cardiopulmonary function specifically under conditions of constant metabolic demand. This type of test is useful for assessing responses to a known work load and for evaluating the effectiveness of various therapies or pharmacologic agents on exercise ability. For example, a progressive multistage test may be performed initially to determine a subject's maximum tolerable work load; a steady-state test is then used to evaluate specific parameters at a submaximal level, such as 50% and 75% of the highest work load achieved. Work is performed for 5 to 8 minutes at the prede-

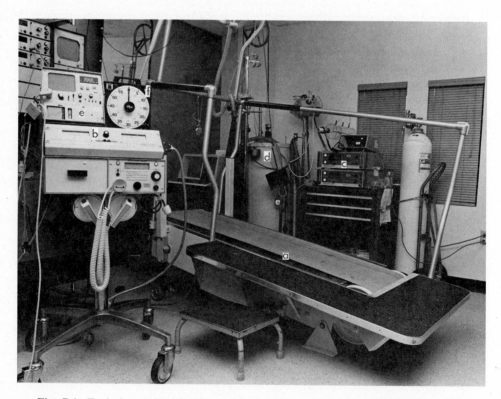

Fig. 7-1. Typical exercise laboratory setup. *a,* Motor-driven treadmill with adjustable slope and speed, side rails, and platform; *b,* treadmill controls with speed and slope indicators; *c,* gas analyzers (O_2 and CO_2); *d,* Tissot spirometer for ventilation measurements; *e,* cardiac monitor/recorder; *f,* electric timer.

termined level to allow a steady state to develop; measurements are performed during the last 1 or 2 minutes of the period. Successive steady-state determinations at higher power outputs may be made continuously or spaced with short periods of light exercise.

Two methods of varying exercise work load are commonly employed: the treadmill and the bicycle ergometer (Figs. 7-1 and 7-2). The work load on the treadmill is adjusted by changing the belt speed of the walking surface, the slope of the surface, or both. The speed of the treadmill may be calibrated in either miles per hour or in kilometers per hour; the slope is registered as "percent grade" on most devices. *Percent of grade* refers to the relationship between the length of the walking surface and the elevation of one end above level. The primary advantages of the treadmill are that it elicits walking, jogging, or running, which are familiar forms of exercise, and that maximal levels of exercise can be easily attained, even in conditioned healthy subjects. The actual work

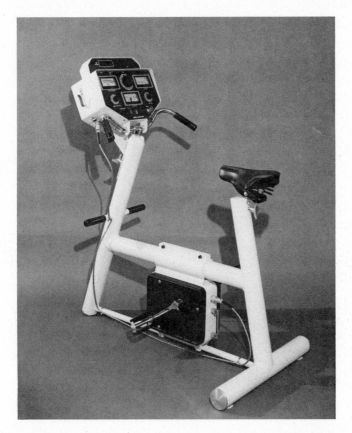

Fig. 7-2. Typical cycle ergometer with continuous adjustable electronic braking. Included are controls for adjusting the pedaling resistance, a timer, and analog meters for pedaling frequency (RPM) and external work load (watts). (Courtesy Warren E. Collins, Inc., Braintree, Mass.)

performed during treadmill walking is a function of the weight of the subject, as well as a function of the slope and speed of the device. Subjects of different weights walking at the same speed and slope perform different work loads; different walking patterns, stride length, and grip on the handrails may also affect the actual amount of work being done.

The bicycle ergometer allows the work load to be varied by adjustment of the resistance to pedaling. The flywheel of the ergometer turns against a belt or strap that has both ends connected to a weighted physical balance; the diameter of the wheel is known, the resistance can be measured easily, and when the pedaling speed is determined, the amount of work performed can be accurately calculated. On the cycle ergometer the work load can be changed rapidly and is independent of the weight of the subject. There are some differences in the work load performance between the treadmill and the cycle ergometer. In most subjects cycling does not produce as high a maximum O_2 consumption as does walking on the treadmill, but ventilation and lactate production are slightly greater, because of the different muscle groups used. These differences are not significant in most clinical situations. Electronically braked cycle ergometers (Fig. 7-2) provide a smooth, rapid, and somewhat more reproducible means of changing the exercise work load. Electronically braked ergometers allow the work load to be adjusted continuously, so that the exercise level can be "ramped." The ramp test allows the subject to advance from low to high work loads quickly and provides all the information normally sought during a progressive maximal exercise test.

Work load may be expressed quantitatively in several ways:

1. *Work*—normally may be expressed in kilopond-meters (KPM). One kilopond-meter equals the work of moving a 1 kg mass a vertical distance of 1 m against the force of gravity.
2. *Power*—expressed in kilopond-meters per minute (work per unit of time) or in *watts*. One watt equals 6.12 KPM/min (100 watts $\cong$ 600 KPM/min).
3. *Energy*—expressed by oxygen consumption ($\dot{V}O_2$), in liters or milliliters per minute (STPD), or in terms of multiples of the resting O_2 uptake (METS). Resting or baseline $\dot{V}O_2$ can be measured as described in the following paragraphs or estimated as 3.5 ml O_2/min/kg.

For purposes of exercise evaluation, it is particularly useful to relate the ventilatory and hemodynamic measurements to the $\dot{V}O_2$ as the independent variable. This requires measurement of ventilation and analysis of expired gas during exercise.

VENTILATION DURING EXERCISE

Collection and analysis of expired gas during graded exercise testing provides a noninvasive means of obtaining the following parameters:

$\dot{V}E$ (minute ventilation)
$\dot{V}T$ (tidal volume)
f (frequency of breathing; respiratory rate)
$\dot{V}O_2$ (oxygen uptake/consumption)
$\dot{V}CO_2$ (CO_2 production)

R (respiratory exchange ratio)

$\dot{V}E/\dot{V}O_2$ (ventilatory equivalent for oxygen)

$\dot{V}E/\dot{V}CO_2$ (ventilatory equivalent for CO_2)

Exhaled gas may be collected by using a one-way breathing circuit and either a collection system (Fig. 7-3) or a flow transducer (Fig. 7-4) with electronic integration for volumes (see Chapter 8), or by means of a breath-by-breath system (Fig. 7-5). The gas collection devices and analyzers should be routinely calibrated before each procedure (see Chapter 11). Tissot spirometers usually remain accurate for extended periods if leaks are not present in tubing or valves. Flow-sensing devices that are used to derive volumes should be checked by applying a known volume or flow signal (or both), or by being connected in a series with a spirometer of known accuracy. Gas analyzers should be calibrated and checked before each test procedure. Two-point calibrations using gases that approximate

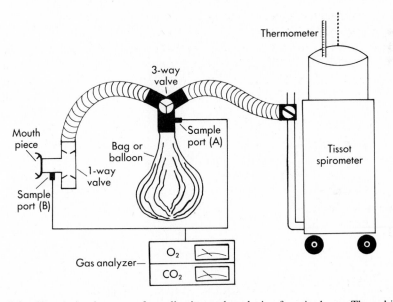

Fig. 7-3. Closed-circuit system for collection and analysis of expired gas. The subject inspires from a one-way valve and expires through large-bore tubing into a Douglas bag or a meteorologic balloon, or directly into a counterweighted Tissot spirometer. A three-way valve controls the breathing circuit. A sample may be collected over a timed interval into the bag or balloon; FE_{O_2} and FE_{CO_2} are determined by extracting a sample from port *A*. The volume in the bag/balloon may then be emptied into the Tissot spirometer for a volume measurement. The temperature of the gas in the spirometer is measured for conversion of gas volumes to BTPS and STPD. Alternatively, the volume may be collected directly into the Tissot spirometer, with a small sample collected in the bag/balloon for gas analysis; gas in the bag or balloon is then returned to the spirometer for the volume determination. Breath-by-breath measurements may be obtained by sampling gas at port *B*, allowing for determination of end-tidal CO_2 and O_2, as well as the respiratory rate. A valve or solenoid may be used to sample alternatively between ports *A* and *B*, so that breath-by-breath and mixed gas can be analyzed.

the physiologic range to be tested provide the best means of establishing the accuracy of the analyzers. Three-point calibration is necessary to check the linearity of the analyzers. For tests conducted without supplementary O_2, room air (20.93% O_2 and 0.03% CO_2) and a gas mixture containing 12% to 16% O_2 and 5% to 7% CO_2 provide suitable gases for a two-point calibration. The one-way valve of the breathing circuit should have a low resistance (1 to 2 cm H_2O at 100 L/min) and a small V_D. If a gas collection system (either a bag or Tissot spirometer) is being used, the subject should be allowed to breathe through the circuit with a noseclip in place long enough to wash out room air with expired gas. The exact washout volume (time) depends on the volume of the collection system and whether it can be emptied before gas is collected. If the exhaled gas is collected directly in a Tissot spirometer, it should be washed out thoroughly before gas sampling is performed. Circuits employing a mixing chamber and flow-sensing

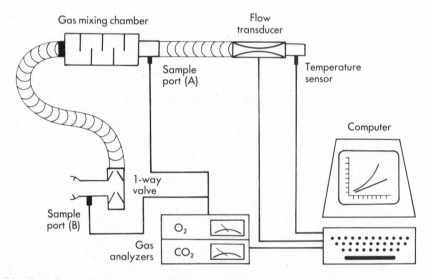

Fig. 7-4. Open-circuit gas system for analyzing expired gas concentrations and ventilation. The subject inspires room air through a one-way valve and expires through large-bore tubing into a mixing chamber that has a volume of about 5 liters. Baffles in the chamber cause the gas to be thoroughly mixed so that it is representative of mixed expired gas. A small volume is extracted at sample port A and directed to the O_2 and CO_2 analyzers for determination of F_{EO_2} and F_{ECO_2}. The expired gas then passes through a flow-sensing device from which volumes can be derived by integration. A temperature probe at the flow transducer provides data for conversion of the gas volume from ambient temperature to BTPS and STPD. Signals from the gas analyzers, flow transducer, and temperature sensor may be recorded directly on an analog recorder or converted to digital signals for processing by computer. Breath-by-breath analysis of expired gas can be obtained by sampling at port B. This technique allows end-tidal CO_2 and O_2 concentrations, as well as the respiratory rate, to be determined conveniently. A valve or solenoid can be used to sample alternatively between ports A and B, so that breath-by-breath and mixed expired samples can be analyzed.

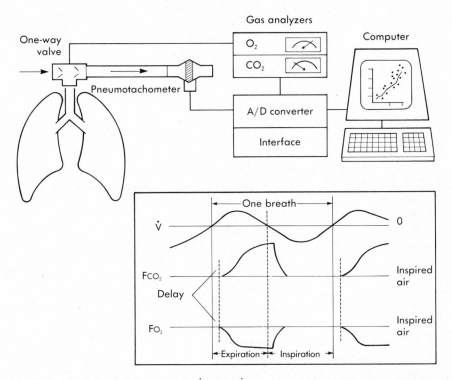

Fig. 7-5. Breath-by-breath system for $\dot{V}O_2$ and $\dot{V}CO_2$. The subject inspires room air from a one-way valve and expires through a pneumotachometer or similar flow-sensing device. Gas is continuously sampled at the subject's mouth for O_2 and CO_2. The flow signal and the signals from the gas analyzers are all integrated to derive the volume, FE_{O_2}, and FE_{CO_2}, and to calculate the $\dot{V}E$, $\dot{V}O_2$, $\dot{V}CO_2$, rate, and VT. To perform the necessary calculations and corrections, computerization is required. The insert shows the simultaneous recording of flow ($\dot{V}$) and fractional concentrations of O_2 and CO_2. During expiration, FCO_2 rises and FO_2 falls. Because of the lag time required to transport gas from the mouthpiece to the analyzers, and because of the response time of the analyzers themselves, gas concentrations and flow are out of phase. By storing appropriate delay corrections (determined from calibrations) in the computer, the necessary signals can be matched up so that ventilatory and gas exchange parameters can be monitored and displayed on a breath-by-breath basis. In many applications the breath-by-breath values are averaged over a short interval (10 to 60 seconds).

device for volume measurements can usually be washed out quickly. Breath-by-breath systems (Fig. 7-5) normally require no washout, since fractional gas concentrations are sampled directly at the mouth.

Depending on the protocol and equipment used, gas collection and analysis are performed over a specified interval toward the end of each exercise level. For steady-state protocols, collection is usually performed after 4 to 6 minutes at a constant work load. In progressive multistage protocols, the appropriate sampling may be performed during the last minute of each stage. In breath-by-breath systems, sampling is normally done continuously, with data being displayed for each breath; average values over a short interval or several breaths are usually reported. Six raw data parameters are measured for each sample collected:

1. *Volume* expired (liters)
2. *Temperature* of the gas at the measuring device (° C)
3. *Time* of the collection (seconds or minutes)
4. *Respiratory rate* during the collection interval
5. FE_{O_2}
6. FE_{CO_2}

These values can be recorded manually or by a multichannel recorder with appropriate analog signals. Similarly, the data may be entered into a computer either manually or *on line* by means of an analog-to-digital (A/D) converter (see Chapter 10). On-line data reduction offers the advantage of immediate feedback of all measurements, as well as greater flexibility for using different exercise protocols. Breath-by-breath analysis requires that signals from the flow-sensing or volume-measuring transducer be integrated with the gas analyzer signals for FE_{O_2} and FE_{CO_2} and that any lag time between the volume and gas analyzer signals be corrected. This can be done by computer if the appropriate delay times are measured.

Minute ventilation ($\dot{V}E$)

$\dot{V}E$ is the total volume of gas expired per minute by the exercising subject and is expressed in liters, corrected to BTPS. The normal adult at rest respires 5 to 10 L/min. During exercise this value may increase to more than 200 L/min in trained subjects and commonly exceeds 100 L/min in normal individuals (Figs. 7-6 and 7-7). The tremendous increase in ventilation provides adequate removal of CO_2, the primary product of exercising muscles, even at high work loads.

$\dot{V}E$ is calculated according to the following equation:

$$\dot{V}E = \frac{V \text{ expired} \times 60}{\text{Collection time (seconds)}} \times \text{BTPS factor}$$

(Sample calculations and BTPS factors are contained in the Appendix.)

Ventilation increases linearly with an increasing work load ($\dot{V}O_2$) at low and moderate levels of exercise. In normal subjects this increase in ventilation during exercise follows the rise in $\dot{V}CO_2$. As higher levels of work are achieved (greater than about 60% of the $\dot{V}O_{2_{max}}$), metabolic demand exceeds the threshold for anaerobic energy production. As the blood lactic acid rises, hydrogen ions (H^+)

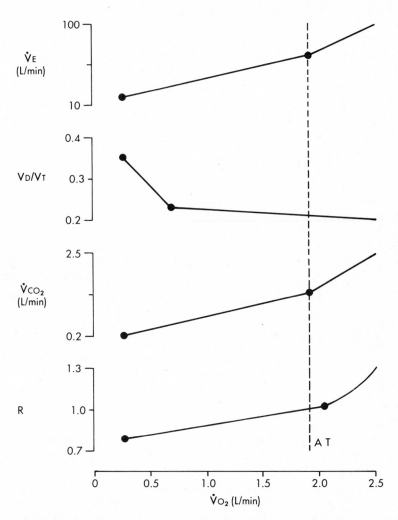

Fig. 7-6. Normal ventilation/gas exchange responses during exercise. Four parameters are plotted against $\dot{V}o_2$ as a measure of work rate, as they might appear in a healthy young adult. The dotted vertical line represents the anaerobic threshold (AT). $\dot{V}E$ increases linearly with work rate at low and moderate work loads up to the point of AT, as does $\dot{V}co_2$. At higher levels, both $\dot{V}E$ and $\dot{V}co_2$ increase at a faster rate as anaerobic metabolism (lactic acidosis) is buffered by HCO_3^- and CO_2 is produced. The ratio of $\dot{V}co_2$ to $\dot{V}o_2$ (R) follows a similar pattern. VD/VT, however, initially decreases rapidly as VT increases; it then continues to fall, but at a slower rate (see text).

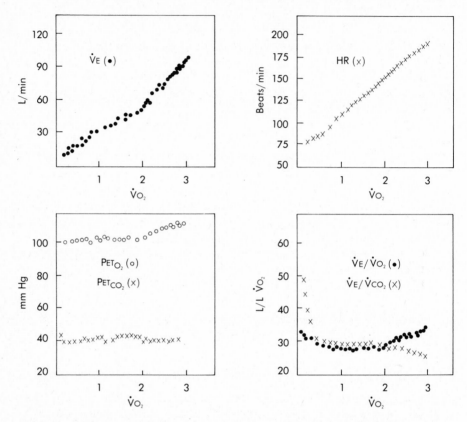

Fig. 7-7. Breath-by-breath exercise data—four plots of data obtained using a breath-by-breath technique, as in Fig. 7-5. Although values are recorded for each breath, the plots represent 30-second averages. All parameters are plotted against $\dot{V}_{O_2}$ as the measure of work being performed. $\dot{V}_E$ increases linearly up to about 2 L/min $\dot{V}_{O_2}$; HR increases linearly throughout the test. $P_{ET_{O_2}}$ and $P_{ET_{CO_2}}$ (end-tidal partial pressures of O_2 and CO_2, respectively) stay fairly constant up to approximately 2 L/min $\dot{V}_{O_2}$, where the O_2 begins to increase and the CO_2 begins to fall. A similar pattern is in evidence on the plot of ventilatory equivalents for oxygen and carbon dioxide ($\dot{V}_E/\dot{V}_{O_2}$ and $\dot{V}_E/\dot{V}_{CO_2}$, respectively). A primary advantage of breath-by-breath analysis is that these plots may be viewed in "real time" as they occur, thus allowing modification of the testing protocol as required. The data plots in this example indicate the occurrence of the anaerobic threshold at approximately 2 L/min of $\dot{V}_{O_2}$.

are buffered by HCO_3^-, and the result is an increase in the total $\dot{V}CO_2$. In healthy subjects ventilation also increases in order to remove the additional CO_2 generated by the buffering of lactic acid and to maintain the pH as close to normal as possible. Relating the $\dot{V}E_{max}$ achieved to static measures of ventilatory function may provide indices of the role of ventilatory limitations to exercise. The dyspnea index is an example of a commonly used technique of quantifying ventilation during exercise with a routine pulmonary function measurement, the maximum voluntary ventilation (see Chapter 3). This index relates the $\dot{V}E$ achieved during a submaximal exercise level, usually 6 minutes at 0% grade and 2 MPH, to the MVV and is calculated by this equation:

$$\text{Dyspnea index} = \frac{\dot{V}E \text{ (during the last minute)}}{MVV} \times 100$$

Values greater than 50% for this calculation are consistent with severe dyspnea. A valid MVV maneuver is essential, or the dyspnea index may be overestimated. The MVV can be similarly related to the $\dot{V}E$ achieved at the highest work load attained ($\dot{V}E_{max}$). The $\dot{V}E_{max}$ may approach the MVV if there is a primary ventilatory limitation to exercise. Since the MVV is extrapolated from a 10- to 15-second maneuver (see Chapter 3), the $\dot{V}E_{max}$ may also be compared with the FEV_1 multiplied by 35, because of the correlation between the MVV and the $FEV_1 \times 35$. The $FEV_1 \times 35$ provides a satisfactory estimate of the ventilation that can be maintained for 1 to 4 minutes in both normal subjects and those with moderate ventilatory impairment. In normal healthy subjects maximal exercise will produce a $\dot{V}E$ that approaches 70% of the MVV, or 70% of the $FEV_1 \times 35$. Subjects with airway obstruction may actually achieve a $\dot{V}E$ during exercise that equals the MVV, indicating a ventilatory limitation. Individuals with severe airway obstruction may actually achieve a $\dot{V}E$ that exceeds the $FEV_1 \times 35$ during maximal exercise. At high levels of ventilation (greater than 120 L/min in normal subjects), increases in O_2 uptake gained by further increases in ventilation serve mainly to supply O_2 to the respiratory muscles. The same phenomenon may occur at much lower levels of ventilation in subjects with abnormal lung parenchyma or airways and increased work of breathing. Because of the enormous ventilatory reserve in the normal subject, exercise is seldom limited by ventilation, but rather by inability to further increase cardiac output or inability to extract more O_2 at the tissue level in the exercising muscles.

Tidal volume (V_T) and respiratory rate (f)

V_T is derived by dividing the $\dot{V}E$ by f. In healthy subjects V_T increases to account for the increase in ventilation during exercise, with only a small initial increase in f. This pattern continues until the V_T approaches 60% of VC. Further increases in total ventilation are accomplished by increasing f. Subjects with airway obstruction may be able to increase their V_E, but not to predicted values, because of either a decreased VC or increased flow resistance. Obstruction occurring because of emphysematous changes (decreased elasticity) may be met by a marked increase in VT and a relatively low f during exercise to minimize the work of breathing. This pattern is not as pronounced if the obstruction is caused by bronchitis or bronchospasm. When the metabolic demands of exercise cannot be met by this type of ventilatory pattern, VT may decrease, and the sensation of dyspnea may occur. Unlike the pattern in obstruction, VT may remain relatively fixed in restrictive disease states, with increases in $\dot{V}E$ during exercise accomplished primarily by rapid respiratory rates. It is mechanically more efficient for subjects with reduced volumes and "stiff" lungs to move small VTs at fast rates to increase ventilation; in restrictive patterns flow limitation may be close to normal, whereas the work of distending the lung is increased.

OXYGEN CONSUMPTION ($\dot{V}o_2$), CO_2 PRODUCTION ($\dot{V}co_2$), AND RESPIRATORY EXCHANGE RATIO (R) IN EXERCISE

$\dot{V}O_2$ is the volume of O_2 taken up by the exercising (or resting) subject and is expressed in liters or milliliters per minute, (corrected to STPD). Its measurement is a result of the ventilation per minute and the rate of extraction from the gas breathed (the difference between the F_{IO_2} and the F_{EO_2} as seen in the next equation). Normal subjects at rest have a $\dot{V}o_2$ of approximately 0.25 L/min (STPD), or about 3.5 ml O_2/min/kg of body weight in the average adult. During exercise, $\dot{V}o_2$ may increase to over 4 L/min (STPD) in trained subjects. $\dot{V}o_2$ serves as the best single measure of the work load being performed; hence exercise limitations caused by abnormalities of gas exchange or inappropriate cardiovascular responses are quantified by relating specific measurements to the $\dot{V}o_2$. Figs. 7-6 to 7-8 provide examples of ventilatory and cardiovascular parameters as they relate to the $\dot{V}o_2$ in normal subjects. By analyzing the trends that these parameters take as the $\dot{V}o_2$ increases in the exercising subject, the causes of work limitations may be defined in terms of pulmonary disease, cardiac disease, deconditioning, or a combination of these.

To calculate $\dot{V}o_2$ (and $\dot{V}co_2$), the fractional concentrations of O_2 and CO_2 in expired gas must be analyzed, either from a collection device (Fig. 7-3), from an appropriate mixing chamber (Fig. 7-4), or by means of a breath-by-breath analysis (Fig. 7-5). In systems that accumulate a volume of gas (bag, balloon, Tissot, or mixing chamber), the water vapor is removed from the sample to be analyzed by means of a calcium chloride drying tube. If the sample for analysis is removed before the volume determination is made, the $\dot{V}E$ should be corrected for the volume withdrawn, or the sample itself returned to the volume measuring device.

$\dot{V}o_2$ is calculated from an accumulated gas volume using this equation:

$$\dot{V}O_2 = \left(\left[\left(\frac{1 - F_{EO_2} - F_{ECO_2}}{1 - F_{IO_2}} \right) \times F_{IO_2} \right] - F_{EO_2} \right) \times \dot{V}E \text{ (STPD)}$$

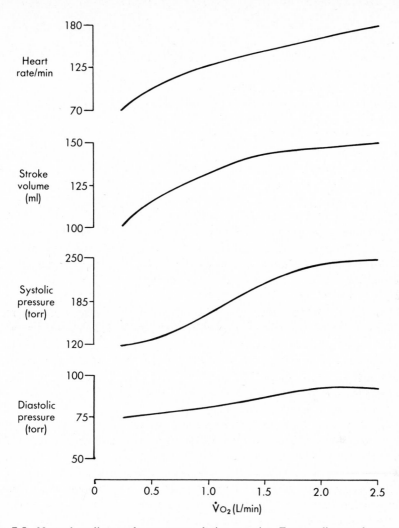

Fig. 7-8. Normal cardiovascular responses during exercise. Four cardiovascular parameters are plotted against $\dot{V}_{O_2}$ as a measure of work rate, as they might appear in a normal healthy adult. Heart rate (HR) increases linearly with work, with the maximum value attained declining with advancing age. Stroke volume (SV) increases initially at low to moderate work loads but then becomes fairly constant. Cardiac output, which equals HR × SV, is thus increased at low and moderate work loads by both HR and SV, but predominantly by HR at higher levels. Systolic blood pressure (BP) increases by about 100 mm Hg (torr) in a linear fashion, whereas diastolic BP increases only slightly (see test).

where

$F_{E_{O_2}}$ = Fraction of O_2 in the expired sample

$F_{E_{CO_2}}$ = Fraction of CO_2 in the expired sample

$F_{I_{O_2}}$ = Fraction of O_2 in inspired gas (room air = 0.2093)

$\dot{V}_E \text{ (STPD)}$ = $\dot{V}_E \text{ (BTPS)} \times \left(\dfrac{P_B - 47}{760}\right) \times 0.881$

$\left(\dfrac{1 - F_{E_{O_2}} - F_{E_{CO_2}}}{1 - F_{I_{O_2}}}\right)$ = Factor to correct for the small difference between inspired and expired volumes

$\dot{V}_{O_2}$ at the highest level of work attainable by a subject is termed $\dot{V}_{O_{2max}}$ and is useful for quantifying the work load for purposes of comparisons between subjects, or for comparison with an age-related predicted value of $\dot{V}_{O_{2max}}$. (Equations for deriving predicted $\dot{V}_{O_{2max}}$ are included in the Appendix.)

Several indices for relating a subject's $\dot{V}_{O_{2max}}$ to an expected value are commonly used. One such index is the functional aerobic impairment (FAI) index, originally used for subjects with heart disease, but useful for describing work limitations in general. The FAI is calculated using the predicted $\dot{V}_{O_{2max}}$:

$$FAI = \frac{\dot{V}_{O_{2max}} \text{ predicted} - \dot{V}_{O_{2max}} \text{ attained}}{\dot{V}_{O_{2max}} \text{ predicted}} \times 100$$

This index is generally interpreted:

$< 20\%$ Normal

20% to 30%   Mild impairment

30% to 40%   Moderate impairment

$> 40\%$ Marked or severe impairment

Indices such as the FAI allow comparisons between subjects and in the same subject before and after training or therapy. Several studies have attempted to estimate $\dot{V}_{O_2}$ based on the height and weight of the subject, and the speed and slope of a treadmill or the length of time spent walking. For the most part, $\dot{V}_{O_2}$ values estimated from treadmill walking are sufficiently variable to make their use somewhat limited in value. $\dot{V}_{O_2}$ values estimated by cycle ergometry are more accurate, because the values obtained are typically less influenced by weight or stride, but the actual $\dot{V}_{O_2}$ may differ significantly from the estimate.

$\dot{V}_{CO_2}$ is a direct reflection of the state of metabolism and is expressed in liters or milliliters per minute, corrected to STPD. Pulmonary ventilation, consisting of $\dot{V}_A$ and $\dot{V}_D$, may be expressed in terms of the $\dot{V}_{CO_2}$. $F_{A_{CO_2}}$ is directly proportional to the $\dot{V}_{CO_2}$ and inversely proportional to the $\dot{V}_A$. This relationship may be expressed:

$$F_{A_{CO_2}} = \frac{\dot{V}_{CO_2}}{\dot{V}_A}$$

$\dot{V}_{CO_2}$ in the normal subject at rest is about 0.2 L/min (STPD) and may increase to more than 4.0 L/min (STPD) during maximal exercise in trained individuals. The adequacy of $\dot{V}_A$ in response to the increase in $\dot{V}_{CO_2}$ is determined by the maintenance of the Pa_{CO_2} (in equilibrium with alveolar gas as determined by the FA_{CO_2}) at low and moderate work loads and the reduction of the Pa_{CO_2} at high work loads (see Pa_{CO_2} in the next equation).

$\dot{V}_{CO_2}$ may be calculated using this equation:

$$\dot{V}_{CO_2} = (F_{E_{CO_2}} - 0.0003) \times \dot{V}_E \text{ (STPD)}$$

where

$F_{E_{CO_2}}$ = Fraction of CO_2 in expired gas

0.0003   = Fraction of CO_2 in room air (may vary)

$\dot{V}_E$ (STPD) = Calculated as in the equation for $\dot{V}_{O_2}$

R, the respiratory exchange ratio, as defined by $\dot{V}_{O_2}$ and $\dot{V}_{CO_2}$ at the alveolar level, is calculated as the $\dot{V}_{CO_2}$ divided by the $\dot{V}_{O_2}$ expressed as a fraction. In some circumstances R is assumed to be equal to 0.8, but for exercise evaluation, particularly in metabolic studies, the actual value is reported. R typically increases from a resting level of between 0.75 and 0.85 as work increases. When anaerobic metabolism begins to produce CO_2 from the buffering of lactic acid, $\dot{V}_{CO_2}$ approaches $\dot{V}_{O_2}$ and, as exercise continues, exceeds it. R may be increased at submaximal work loads, or even at rest if hyperventilation is present, because R represents the exchange ratio between CO_2 and O_2 in the lungs, but not necessarily at the cellular level. In exercise tests in which a steady state is allowed to develop (4 to 6 minutes at a constant work load), R approaches or equals the respiratory quotient (RQ) and the ratio of $\dot{V}_{CO_2}/\dot{V}_{O_2}$ at the cellular level. Under steady-state conditions the $\dot{V}_{CO_2}$ reflects the CO_2 produced metabolically at the cellular level.

Sample calculations of $\dot{V}_E$, $\dot{V}_{O_2}$, $\dot{V}_{CO_2}$, and R (as used with one of the gas accumulation methods) are included in the Appendix.

VENTILATORY EQUIVALENT FOR OXYGEN AND O_2 PULSE IN EXERCISE

The minute ventilation (required to remove CO_2) may be related to the amount of work being performed (expressed as the $\dot{V}_{O_2}$). This ratio is termed the ventilatory equivalent for O_2, or $\dot{V}_E/\dot{V}_{O_2}$. Because ventilation is one of the determinants of the actual volume of O_2 that can be transported per minute, it is often useful to evaluate the level of total ventilation required for a particular work load to assess the role of the lungs in exercise limitations. The $\dot{V}_E/\dot{V}_{O_2}$ is calculated simply by dividing the $\dot{V}_E$ (BTPS) by the $\dot{V}_{O_2}$ (STPD) and expressing the ratio in liters of ventilation per liter of O_2 consumed per minute. In the presence of pulmonary disease the ratio may increase from the normal value of approximately 25 L/L $\dot{V}_{O_2}$ to as high as 50 L/L $\dot{V}_{O_2}$. In some pulmonary disease patterns the $\dot{V}_E/\dot{V}_{O_2}$ may be normal at rest but increase as the work load increases; subjects who hyperventilate at rest may show an increased $\dot{V}_E/\dot{V}_{O_2}$ that usually falls during exercise. The $\dot{V}_E/\dot{V}_{CO_2}$, similarly calculated, may be useful for estimating the maximum tolerable work load in subjects with moderate to severe ventilatory limitations. The ventilatory equivalents for O_2 and CO_2, measured by a breath-by-breath technique, are also useful in identifying the onset of the anaerobic threshold. Anaerobic metabolism is usually accompanied by a steady increase in the $\dot{V}E/\dot{V}o_2$ while the $\dot{V}E/\dot{V}co_2$ remains constant or falls slightly. This same pattern may also be seen on a breath-by-breath display of end-tidal O_2 and CO_2 (Fig. 7-7).

The heart rate (HR) may be related to the amount of work being done (the $\dot{V}o_2$) and expressed as the O_2 pulse. The O_2 pulse is defined as the amount of O_2 consumed per heartbeat and is easily derived, since the electrocardiogram (ECG) is always recorded during the exercise evaluation; the HR may be read manually or by an analog signal. The $\dot{V}o_2$ (STPD) in milliliters is divided by the HR, and the quotient is expressed as milliliters of $\dot{V}o_2$ per heartbeat. In normal subjects the O_2 pulse varies from 2.54 to 4.0 ml O_2/beat at rest to 10 to 15 ml O_2/beat during strenuous exercise. In subjects with cardiac disease the O_2 pulse may be normal or low at rest but does not rise to expected levels during exercise, consistent with an inappropriately high HR for a particular level of work. Since cardiac output, which normally increases with exercise, is the product of HR and stroke volume (HR $\times$ SV), a low O_2 pulse is generally consistent with an inability to increase the stroke volume. This pattern of low O_2 pulse with increasing work rate may be seen in subjects with coronary artery disease or valvular insufficiency but is most pronounced in those with cardiomyopathy. Tachycardia (tachyarrythmia) tends to lower the O_2 pulse because of the abnormal elevation of the HR. On the other hand, beta-blocking agents (which tend to reduce the HR) may falsely elevate the O_2 pulse. The O_2 pulse is often considered an index of fitness; at similar work rates a fit subject will have a higher O_2 pulse than one who is deconditioned. This is evidenced by the lowered HR, both at rest and at increasing work loads, and occurs because conditioning exercises increase stroke volume so that the heart beats less frequently to produce the same cardiac output.

GAS EXCHANGE AND EXERCISE BLOOD GASES

Pa_{O_2} tends to remain constant in normal subjects even up to relatively high work loads. A decrease in Pa_{O_2} with increasing exercise can result from increased right to left shunting, inequality of $\dot{V}A$ in relation to pulmonary capillary perfusion, potential diffusion limitations at the alveolocapillary interface, or a combination of these. Because exercise normally reduces the mixed venous oxygen tension ($P\bar{v}_{O_2}$), the presence of a shunt, or $\dot{V}/\dot{Q}$ inequality, may result in a decrease in Pa_{O_2} or a widening of the A-ao_2 gradient without an absolute change in the magnitude of the shunt. This is a direct result of the mixed venous blood with a lowered O_2 tension passing through the abnormal lung unit and then being mixed with normally arterialized blood. In some subjects with a decreased Pa_{O_2} at rest, or increased P(A-a)o_2, increased cardiac output or increased ventilation during exercise may increase the Pa_{O_2}. This may occur as a result of an increased PA_{O_2} caused by a reduction in PA_{CO_2} at moderate to high work rates, or because of improved $\dot{V}/\dot{Q}$ relationships resulting directly from the changes in ventilation or cardiac output, or both. Because of these types of changes, measuring Pa_{O_2}

during exercise may be particularly valuable in subjects with known or suspected pulmonary disorders.

An indwelling arterial catheter permits analysis of blood gas tensions (Pa_{O_2}, Pa_{CO_2}), saturation (Sa_{O_2}), O_2 content (Ca_{O_2}), pH, and lactate levels at various work loads. The indwelling catheter, in conjunction with a suitable pressure transducer (Fig. 7-9), allows continuous monitoring of systemic blood pressures (BPs) as well. Partial pressures of O_2 (and CO_2) may also be monitored via transcutaneous electrodes; Sa_{O_2} may be monitored via an ear (or finger pulse) oximeter (see Chapter 9). Transcutaneous Po_2 measurements offer a reasonable alternative to blood sampling for conventional measurements during exercise. Similarly, ear oximetry provides information as to the subject's ability to arterialize mixed venous blood. An obvious advantage of each of these methods is that they provide continuous measurements, in distinction to the conventional means of arterial sampling. Such "in vivo" measurements are extremely valuable in evaluating subjects with pulmonary disease in whom rapid changes in Pa_{O_2} and Sa_{O_2} frequently occur during exercise. A Pa_{O_2} falling to less than 50 to 55 mm Hg or an Sa_{O_2} decreasing to less than 85% is sufficient reason for terminating the exercise evaluation. Subjects with hypoxemia at rest, or at very low work rates, should be tested with supplementary O_2 via a controlled delivery system. It should be noted that ear oximetry may overestimate the true saturation if a significant concentration of COHb is present. A single arterial sample may be used to correlate the ear oximetry reading with true saturation, provided the specimen is analyzed with a cooximeter (see Chapter 6). Inadequate perfusion of the ear or finger may also confound oximetry during exercise testing.

Pa_{CO_2} normally remains constant as the work rate is progressively increased but, unlike Pa_{O_2}, not up to maximal work levels. At work loads in excess of 50% to 60% of the $\dot{V}o_{2_{max}}$, the metabolic acidosis resulting from anaerobic metabolism stimulates $\dot{V}E$ to increase curvilinearly with $\dot{V}o_2$ and $\dot{V}co_2$. Ventilation thus increases in excess of that required to keep the Pa_{CO_2} constant, causing a progressive decrease in Pa_{CO_2} and effecting a respiratory compensation for the lactic acidosis (Figs. 7-6 and 7-7). In subjects with airflow obstruction, this ventilatory compensation may be compromised, resulting in the development of acidosis. In some individuals with obstruction the $\dot{V}A$ may be adequate to maintain a normal Pa_{CO_2}, but not to reduce the Pa_{CO_2} to compensate for lactic acidosis; hence acidosis may occur even though ventilation appears appropriate. In a small number of subjects with airflow obstruction, the $\dot{V}A$ may not match the increase in $\dot{V}co_2$, resulting in hypercapnia and respiratory acidosis. If the obstruction is severe, the ventilatory limitation may occur at levels of work well below the anaerobic threshold.

The pH, like the Pa_{CO_2}, is regulated by the $\dot{V}A$ at low work rates. The $\dot{V}A$ increases in proportion to the $\dot{V}co_2$ up to the anaerobic threshold. At work rates above the anaerobic threshold, proportional increases in ventilation maintain the pH at normal levels, with most of the buffering of lactic acid provided by HCO_3^- and a decrease in Pa_{CO_2}. At the highest work rates (above 80% of the $\dot{V}o_{2_{max}}$), the pH decreases despite hyperventilation, and the compensation for lactic aci-

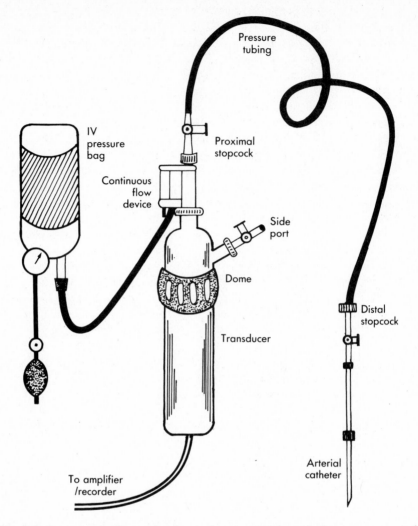

Fig. 7-9. Pressure transducer setup for continuous arterial monitoring—components for continuous monitoring of systemic BP via an arterial catheter. The catheter is normally inserted into the radial or brachial artery. Pressure tubing connects the catheter to a continuous flow device that maintains a constant pressure (and a small flow of solution) against the arterial line to prevent back flow of blood into the system. The continuous flow device also allows flushing of the system. Connected in line with the tubing is the transducer assembly. Pressure changes in the system are transmitted via a thin membrane at the base of the dome to a pressure transducer. Blood samples may be drawn by inserting a heparinized syringe at the distal stopcock, closing the proximal stopcock to block the continuous flow device, and withdrawing (the BP signal is temporarily lost during sampling). A similar assembly can be used for connection to a Swan-Ganz catheter for pulmonary artery monitoring during exercise.

dosis is incomplete. In the presence of airflow obstruction, ventilatory limitations may prevent compensation above the anaerobic threshold, resulting in the development of significant acidosis; however, subjects with moderate or severe obstruction generally cannot exercise up to a level that elicits anaerobic metabolism, and acidosis occurring in these subjects is usually a result of increased CO_2.

Arterial blood gases drawn during exercise allow several other parameters of gas exchange to be determined, namely V_D, $\dot{V}_A$, and V_D/V_T.

V_D (see Chapter 2) comprises anatomic and alveolar V_D and makes up that part of the $\dot{V}_E$ that does not participate in gas exchange. The V_D/V_T ratio expresses the relationship between "wasted" and tidal ventilation for the average breath. The normal adult subject at rest has a $\dot{V}_A$ of 4 to 7 L/min (BTPS) and a V_D/V_T ratio of approximately 0.25 to 0.35. V_D normally increases during exercise in conjunction with an increased $\dot{V}_E$. Because of increases in V_T and increased perfusion of well-ventilated segments of the lungs, such as the apices, the V_D/V_T ratio falls. This pattern is expected in normal healthy subjects (Fig. 7-6). Mild to moderate pulmonary disease may show a fall in the V_D/V_T ratio, whereas in severe airway obstruction or in pulmonary vascular disease the V_D/V_T may remain fixed or even rise. An increase in the V_D/V_T ratio is indicative of increased ventilation in relation to perfusion. During exercise, the $\dot{V}_A$ normally increases proportionately more than the $\dot{V}_E$ because the V_D/V_T falls. With subjects in whom the V_D/V_T ratio remains fixed or rises, the adequacy of $\dot{V}_A$ must be assessed in terms of the Pa_{CO_2}, not simply by the magnitude of the $\dot{V}_E$.

Calculation of V_D, $\dot{V}_A$, and V_D/V_T requires measurement of the Pa_{CO_2}. V_D is calculated using the following equation:

$$V_D \text{ (BTPS)} = V_T \text{ (BTPS)} \times \left(1 - \frac{F_{E_{CO_2}} \times (P_B - 47)}{Pa_{CO_2}} \right) - V_{D_{sys}}$$

where

V_T	= Tidal volume (liters)
$F_{E_{CO_2}}$	= Fraction of expired CO_2
$P_B - 47$	= Dry barometric pressure
Pa_{CO_2}	= Arterial CO_2 tension
$V_{D_{sys}}$	= Dead space of the one-way breathing valve (liters)

Once the V_D is determined, $\dot{V}_A$ can be calculated using this equation:

$$\dot{V}_A \text{ (BTPS)} = \dot{V}_E \text{ (BTPS)} - (f \times V_D \text{ (BTPS)})$$

where

$\dot{V}_E$ = Minute ventilation
f   = Respiratory rate

The dead space/tidal volume ratio is simply:

$$V_D/V_T$$

CARDIOVASCULAR MONITORS DURING EXERCISE

Continuous monitoring of the HR and ECG, and intermittent or continuous monitoring of the BP during exercise are essential to safe performance of the test. Assessment of HR, ECG, and BP allows work limitations caused by cardiac or vascular disease to be identified and quantitated.

Heart rate and electrocardiogram

The HR and rhythm are monitored continuously using one or more modified chest leads. Standard chest lead configurations allow comparison with resting 12-lead tracings. Twelve-lead monitoring during exercise is practical when devices are used that incorporate adequate filters (digital or analog) to eliminate movement artifact. Limb leads normally must be moved to the torso for ergometer or treadmill testing, and resting ECGs should be performed to record differences between the standard and modified leads. Single-lead monitoring allows only for gross arrhythmia detection and rate determination, and may not be adequate for testing subjects with known or suspected cardiac disease. The monitoring device should be able to provide tracings sufficiently free of artifact to allow assessment of intervals and segments up to the subject's predicted maximum HR. Computerized arrhythmia recording or manual ''freeze-frame'' storage is invaluable for careful evaluation of abnormalities, while allowing the testing protocol to be continued smoothly. The HR should be analyzed by visual inspection of a tracing with manual measurement of the rate, rather than by an automatic sensor, in order to detect subtle changes, such as occur with atrial arrhythmias. Accurate measurement of the HR is necessary to determine commonly used endpoints, such as 100% or 85% of the age-related predicted maximum. Significant S-T segment changes should be easily identifiable from the tracing up to the predicted maximum HR. Because artifacts caused by movement are the most common cause of unacceptable recordings during exercise, it is useful to allow the subject to ''practice'' the exercise (ergometer or treadmill), not only to familiarize the subject, but also to check for adequacy of the ECG signal. Carefully applied electrodes and secured lead wires greatly minimize movement artifact.

The HR normally increases linearly with the work load, up to an age-related maximum. Although several formulas are available for predicting the maximum HR, it should be noted that a variability of ±10 to 15 beats/min exists in healthy adult subjects. Two commonly used equations for predicting the maximum HR are:

(1) $$HR_{max} = 220 - Age_{years}$$
(2) $$HR_{max} = 210 - (0.65 \times Age_{years})$$

Equation 1 yields slightly higher predicted values in young adults, whereas equation 2 produces higher values in older adults. Other methods of predicting HR_{max} vary depending on the type of exercise protocol used in deriving the regression data. Specific criteria for terminating an exercise test should include factors based on symptom limitation as well as HR and blood pressure changes (see discussion of safety).

Blood pressure

The BP may be monitored intermittently by the standard cuff method or continuously by connection of a pressure transducer to an indwelling arterial catheter (Fig. 7-8). An indwelling line allows continuous display and recording of systolic and diastolic pressures. In addition, the catheter provides ready access for arterial blood sampling. Arterial catheterization can normally be easily accomplished using either the radial or brachial site. The catheter must be adequately secured to prevent loss of patency during vigorous exercise. Automated blood pressure monitors using a self-inflating cuff may also be used during exercise testing; these, however, suffer the same disadvantages as the manual cuff method, particularly the loss of adequate monitoring during vigorous exercise.

Systolic BP increases in healthy subjects by about 100 mm Hg during exercise up to approximately 200 to 250 mm Hg, whereas diastolic pressure rises only slightly (10 to 15 mm Hg) or not at all. The increase in systolic pressure is caused almost completely by the increase in the cardiac output; even though the cardiac output may increase fivefold (from 5 to 25 L/min), the systolic pressure increases only twofold because of a tremendous decrease in peripheral vascular resistance. Most of the decrease in resistance is assumed to result from vasodilatation in exercising muscles. Increases in the systolic pressure to greater than 250 mm Hg or increases in the diastolic pressure of more than 15 to 20 mm Hg should be considered indications for terminating the exercise evaluation. Similarly, if the systolic pressure fails to rise with an increasing work load, or if the diastolic pressure falls, the cardiac output is not increasing appropriately, and the procedure should be terminated and the subject's condition stabilized. In maximal tests, in which the subject is taken to his or her HR_{max}, it may be impossible to obtain a reliable BP at maximal exercise, even with an arterial catheter; additionally, the systolic pressure may transiently drop and the diastolic pressure fall to zero at the termination of exercise. To minimize the degree of hypotension resulting from the abrupt cessation of heavy exercise, the subject should "cool down" (i.e., continue working at a low work rate until the BP and HR have stabilized slightly above baseline levels).

Safety

Safe and effective exercise testing for cardiopulmonary disorders requires careful pretest evaluation to identify contraindications to the test procedure. Such contraindications include the following:
1. Pa_{O_2} less than 45 mm Hg with the subject breathing room air
2. Pa_{CO_2} greater than 70 mm Hg
3. FEV_1 less than 30% of the predicted value
4. Recent myocardial infarction
5. Unstable angina pectoris
6. Second- or third-degree heart block
7. Rapid ventricular/atrial arrhythmias
8. Orthopedic impairment
9. Severe aortic stenosis

   10. Congestive heart failure
   11. Uncontrolled hypertension
   12. Limiting neurologic disorders
   13. Dissecting/ventricular aneurysms
   14. Severe pulmonary hypertension

A preliminary workup should include a complete history and physical examination, a 12-lead ECG, a chest x-ray film, baseline pulmonary function studies before and after bronchodilator administration, and routine laboratory examinations (complete blood count and serum electrolyte counts). Subjects taking methylxanthines should have a recent theophylline level evaluation, particularly if the primary indication for exercise testing is ventilatory limitation or exercise-induced bronchospasm.

The entire procedure, including the risks involved, should be explained or demonstrated to the subject and appropriate informed consent forms signed. Criteria for terminating the exercise evaluation before the specified endpoint or symptom limitation occurs include the following:

   1. Dizziness or confusion
   2. Sweating and pallor, or systolic BP greater than 250 mm HG
   3. Cyanosis
   4. Nausea or vomiting
   5. Headache
   6. Muscle cramping

Following termination of the exercise evaluation for whatever reason, the subject should be monitored until cardiac and vascular parameters return to pretest levels.

Personnel conducting exercise tests should be trained in handling cardiovascular emergencies. The laboratory should have available resuscitation equipment, including:

   1. Standard intravenous medications (epinephrine, atropine, lidocaine, isoproterenol, propranolol, procainamide, sodium bicarbonate, and calcium gluconate)
   2. Syringes, needles, IV infusion apparatus
   3. Portable O_2 and suction equipment
   4. Airway equipment, endotracheal tubes, and laryngoscope
   5. DC defibrillator

CARDIAC OUTPUT (FICK METHOD)

Cardiac output can be measured by thermal or dye dilution, or by the Fick method (direct or indirect). The Fick methods require exhaled gas analysis and are often used in conjunction with exercise testing.

   1. Direct Fick method:

$$\dot{Q}_T = \frac{\dot{V}_{O_2}}{C(a - \bar{v})_{O_2}} \times 100$$

where

$\dot{Q}_T$ = Cardiac output (L/min)

$\dot{V}_{O_2}$ = Oxygen consumption (L/min)

$C(a - \bar{v})_{O_2}$ = Arterial–mixed venous O_2 content difference

100 = Factor to correct $C(a - \bar{v})_{O_2}$ to liters (content differences are normally reported in vol%)

$\dot{V}_{O_2}$ is measured by one of the methods described above; the $a - v$ content difference for O_2 is obtained by measuring (or calculating; see Chapter 6) the oxygen content in an arterial and mixed venous sample.

2. The indirect Fick method, also termed the CO_2 rebreathing technique:

$$\dot{Q}_T = \frac{\dot{V}_{CO_2}}{C(\bar{v} - a)_{CO_2}} \times 100$$

where

$\dot{Q}_T$ = Cardiac output (L/min)

$\dot{V}_{CO_2}$ = CO_2 production (L/min)

$C(\bar{v} - a)_{CO_2}$ = Mixed venous–arterial CO_2 content difference

100 = Factor to correct $C(\bar{v} - a)_{CO_2}$ to liters (content differences are normally reported in vol%)

$\dot{V}_{CO_2}$ is measured as described above. The content difference for CO_2 can be obtained completely noninvasively or in conjunction with arterial blood gas analysis. To estimate the $P\bar{v}CO_2$, a rebreathing technique is used. The subject, either at rest or during exercise, is switched to a rebreathing bag containing a mixture of CO_2 in air that is slightly higher than the P_{ACO_2} and that has a volume of one to two times the V_T. In general, bag F_{CO_2} must be adjusted between 7% and 15%, and the volume between 1 and 3 liters. The subject rebreathes rapidly from the bag until an equilibrium between the CO_2 in the bag and the CO_2 in the alveoli occurs (Fig. 7-10). Since there is no CO_2 removed during the rebreathing (because of the slightly higher CO_2 concentration in the bag), the fractional concentration at equilibrium closely resembles that in the pulmonary capillaries. From the fractional concentration the partial pressure, and hence the content, can be determined. The CO_2 content may be calculated or read from a standard nomogram. (The reader is referred to the excellent text by Jones et al. in the Selected Bibliography at the end of the chapter). The CO_2 content of arterial blood can be estimated similarly using either a measured Pa_{CO_2} or an estimated value derived from the end-tidal and mixed-expired CO_2 values, the V_T, and the respiratory rate:

$$Pa_{CO_2} = P_{ET_{CO_2}} + 4.4 - 0.0023V_T + 0.03f_b - 0.09P_{E_{CO_2}}$$

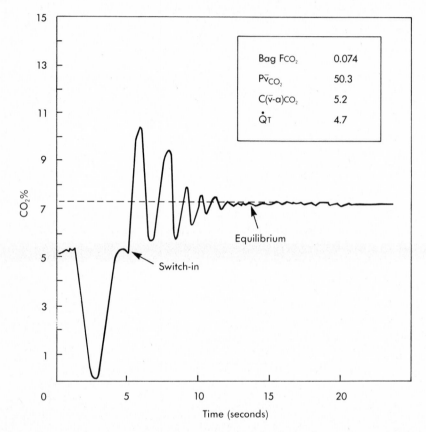

Fig. 7-10. Cardiac output determination by CO_2 rebreathing. Expired CO_2 (sampled at the mouth with a breath-by-breath system) is plotted against time as the subject is switched from breathing room air to rebreathing from a bag containing 7% to 15% CO_2. After switch-in, the subject takes several fast deep breaths until an equilibrium is established, as identified by a flat CO_2 tracing. For the maneuver to work correctly, the CO_2 concentration in the bag must be slightly higher than the subject's alveolar CO_2. The fractional concentration of CO_2 in the bag (bag Fco_2) is then used to estimate the mixed venous CO_2. A modified form of the Fick equation, using CO_2 content in arterial and mixed venous blood instead of O_2 content, is then used along with the $\dot{V}co_2$ to determine the cardiac output (see text).

where

PET_{CO_2} = End-tidal CO_2

V_T = Tidal volume

f_b = Frequency of breathing (respiratory rate)

PE_{CO_2} = Mixed expired CO_2

Similarly, Pa_{CO_2} can be estimated:

$$Pa_{CO_2} = PE_{CO_2} \div \left(1 - \frac{V_D + V_{D_{sys}}}{V_T}\right)$$

where

PE_{CO_2} = Mixed expired CO_2

V_D = Subject's dead space (estimated)

$V_{D_{sys}}$ = Dead space of the breathing circuit

After the CO_2 contents of mixed venous and arterial blood are calculated, the difference is divided into the $\dot{V}CO_2$, as above. These calculations may be performed manually or, because of their complexity, by computer. Corrections to the calculated CO_2 contents must be made if the subject's Hb is less than 15 g%, or if the Sa_{O_2} is much less than 95%, because of the effects of Hb and O_2 saturation on CO_2 transport. Because equilibrium must be achieved quickly (before recirculation occurs), a rapid-responding CO_2 analyzer is necessary; thus the CO_2 rebreathing method lends itself well to breath-by-breath analysis. Attainment of a true equilibrium can also be complicated by having a CO_2 concentration in the rebreathing bag that is either too high or too low, as well as by an inadequate volume to match the subject's tidal breathing. To rapidly adjust the gas concentrations and bag volume during exercise, a computerized valving system is quite useful.

The cardiac output is approximately 4 to 6 L/min at rest and rises during exercise to between 25 and 35 L in normal healthy subjects. Cardiac output is related to the HR:

$$\dot{Q}_T = HR \times SV$$

where

HR = Heart rate in beats/min

SV = Stroke volume in liters or milliliters

The stroke volume (SV) is approximately 70 to 100 ml at rest and increases to 100 to 150 with low or moderate exercise. The HR increases almost linearly with increasing work rate as described above, so that at low work loads the increase in $\dot{Q}$ is caused by a combination of the HR and SV. At moderate and high work loads further increases in $\dot{Q}_T$ are due mainly to increases in HR. Derivation of the SV from the $\dot{Q}_T$ and HR is useful in quantifying poor cardiac performance in subjects with various types of abnormalities. Conversely, if the $\dot{Q}_T$ is not measured and the SV not determined, inappropriately high HRs are usually equated with inadequate SVs. Reduced cardiac output is typical in both atrial and ventricular arrythmias, in valvular insufficiency, and in cardiomyopathies.

In subjects who are fit, the SV may be increased both at rest and during exercise. These individuals typically have low resting HRs and exceed their predicted $\dot{V}o_{2max}$, since their cardiac output is greater when they reach their maximum HR.

The main disadvantage of the direct Fick method is that placement of a pulmonary artery catheter is required to obtain a mixed venous sample. The indirect Fick method (CO_2 rebreathing) is somewhat complicated and requires careful attention to the correct CO_2 concentration in the rebreathing bag. Additionally, if arterial Pco_2 is estimated rather than measured, the content difference may be in error. In subjects with obstructive pulmonary disease this may be a serious limitation, in spite of the fact that CO_2 rebreathing appears to work well with uneven distribution of ventilation.

SELF-ASSESSMENT QUESTIONS

1. Which of the following exercise protocols could be used to determine the maximum tolerable work load?
   - I. Steady state
   - II. Constant power output
   - III. Progressive multistage
   - IV. Ramp test
     - a. I, II, III, and IV
     - b. I and III
     - c. II and IV
     - d. III and IV

2. During treadmill exercise, the external work performed depends on:
   - a. The speed and slope of the treadmill
   - b. The weight of the subject
   - c. The walking style of the subject (gait and stride)
   - d. All of the above

3. A subject has his maximum oxygen consumption ($\dot{V}o_{2max}$) measured using a cycle ergometer; the reported value is 3.3 L/min (STPD). How many METS is this, if the subject weighs 60 kg?
   - a. 3.3 METS
   - b. 55 METS
   - c. 16 METS
   - d. 18 METS

4. Which of the following must be measured in order to calculate the oxygen consumption ($\dot{V}o_2$) during an exercise test using a gas accumulation method (bag or balloon):
   - I. Fe_{CO_2} and Fe_{O_2}
   - II. Temperature (at the volume measuring device)
   - III. Respiratory Rate
   - IV. $\dot{V}e$
     - a. I, II, III, and IV
     - b. I, II, and IV

    c. I and IV

    d. I only

5. A subject has an exercise evaluation using an incremental protocol (progressive mul-tistage); his $\dot{V}_{E_{max}}$ is 55 L/min with a maximum HR of 120 beats/min and no arryth-mias or ECG abnormalities noted. If this subject's MVV is 59 L/min and his FEV_1 is 1.71 L, then he could be described as:

    a. Having severe aerobic impairment

    b. Having a primary cardiac (HR) limitation to exercise

    c. Having a primary ventilatory limitation to exercise

    d. Being moderately deconditioned

    e. a and d

6. Which of the following describe breath-by-breath gas analysis for measurement of $\dot{V}_{O_2}$ and $\dot{V}_{CO_2}$?

    I. Rapid-response gas analyzers are required.

    II. Computerization is necessary to integrate flow (volume) and gas fractional con-centrations.

    III. The mixing device must be 5 liters or larger.

    IV. Delay times between flow (volume) and gas concentration signals must be mea-sured.

    a. I, II, III, and IV

    b. II, III, and IV

    c. I, II, and IV

    d. II only

7. The best measure of the actual energy expenditure during any type of exercise is the:

    a. Speed/slope of the treadmill

    b. Pa_{O_2}

    c. $\dot{V}_{O_2}$

    d. $\dot{V}_{CO_2}$

    e. HR_{max}

8. A subject at rest has a $\dot{V}_E/\dot{V}_{O_2}$ of 45 L/L O_2; this might be due to:

    a. Primary lung disease

    b. Hyperventilation (anxiety, etc.)

    c. Cardiomyopathy

    d. All of the above

    e. a and b

9. Subject A and subject B are given progressive multistage exercise tests to determine their fitness; subject A has an HR_{max} of 177 and an O_2 pulse of 17 ml/beat; subject B has an HR_{max} of 187 and an O_2 pulse of 9 ml/beat. Which subject is "most fit"?

    a. Subject A

    b. Subject B

    c. Both are equally fit

    d. Cannot be determined

10. A subject with a resting BP of 140/95 begins an exercise test; after 3 minutes of walking at 1.7 MPH and 10% grade, his BP is 110/60. This is:

    a. A normal response

    b. An abnormal response

    c. An indication to discontinue the test

    d. a and c

    e. b and c

11. In normal subjects during exercise, the V_D/V_T ratio:
    a. Decreases from 0.30 to about 0.15
    b. Decreases from 0.50 to about 0.40
    c. Increases from 0.25 to 0.35
    d. Remains constant even at high work loads
12. During exercise in normal subjects, which of the following parameters increases at the highest levels of work?
    a. Pa_{O_2}
    b. $\dot{V}_E/\dot{V}_{O_2}$
    c. Pa_{CO_2}
    d. pH
    e. a and b

SELECTED BIBLIOGRAPHY

General references
American College of Sports Medicine: Guidelines for graded exercise testing and exercise prescription, Philadelphia, 1975, Lea & Febiger.
Astrand, P.O., and Rodahl, K.: Textbook of work physiology, New York, 1970, McGraw-Hill Book Co.
Hansen, J.E.: Exercise instruments, schemes, and protocols for evaluating the dyspneic patient, Am. Rev. Respir. Dis. **129**(suppl.):S25, 1984.
Hansen, J.E., Sue, D.Y., and Wasserman, K.: Predicted values for clinical exercise testing, Am. Rev. Respir. Dis. **129**(suppl.):S49, 1984.
Hellerstein, H.K., Brock, L.L., and Bruce, R.A.: Exercise testing and training of apparently healthy individuals: a handbook for physicians, New York, 1972, Committee on Exercise, American Heart Association.
Jones, N.L., and Campbell, E.J.M.: Clinical exercise testing, ed. 2, Philadelphia, 1982, W.B. Saunders Co.
Lange-Anderson, K. et al.: Fundamentals of exercise testing, Geneva, 1971, World Health Organization.
Spiro, S.G.: Exercise testing in clinical medicine, Br. J. Dis. Chest **71**:145, 1977.

Ventilation, gas exchange, and blood gases
Jones, N.L.: Exercise testing in pulmonary evaluation: rationale, methods and the normal respiratory response to exercise, I and II, N. Engl. J. Med. **293**:541, 1975.
Jones, N.L.: Normal values for pulmonary gas exchange during exercise, Am. Rev. Respir. Dis. **129**(suppl.):S44, 1984.
Sue, D.Y., et al.: Measurement and analysis of gas exchange during exercise using a programmable calculator, J. Appl. Physiol. **49**:456, 1980.
Wasserman, K., and Whipp, B.J.: Exercise physiology in health and disease, Am. Rev. Respir. Dis. **112**:219, 1975.
Whipp, B.J., Ward, S.A., and Wasserman, K.: Ventilatory responses to exercise and their control in man, Am. Rev. Respir. Dis. **129**(suppl.):S17, 1984.

Cardiovascular monitoring during exercise
Bruce, R.A.: Value and limitations of the electrocardiogram in progressive exercise testing, Am. Rev. Respir. Dis. **129**(suppl.):S28, 1984.
Ellestad, M.H., et al.: Maximal treadmill stress testing for cardiovascular evaluation, Circulation **39**:517, 1969.
Pollack, M.L., et al.: A comparative analysis of four protocols for maximal stress testing, Am. Heart J. **92**:39, 1976.
Stone, H.L., and Liang, I.Y.S.: Cardiovascular response and control during exercise, Am. Rev. Respir. Dis. **129**(suppl.):S13, 1984.

CHAPTER EIGHT

Testing regimens

Most individual pulmonary function tests measure the functional relationships of various aspects of the pulmonary system. The diagnosis of specific pulmonary disorders requires the performance of an appropriate battery of tests. Too often, accurate diagnoses are lacking because of inappropriate testing or insufficient pulmonary history. It is seldom necessary to perform all of the various tests available; in many instances simple spirometry and blood gas analysis provide sufficient information to delineate a disease process or recommend a course of therapy. Some of the more specialized regimens described in this chapter, such as inhalation challenge testing, presuppose that the simpler tests have been performed and the patient's history and clinical presentation adequately studied.

PULMONARY HISTORY AND RESULTS REPORTING

Basic to accurate diagnosis on any level—from simple screening at the bedside to a cardiopulmonary laboratory—is a background of information pertinent to possible pulmonary disorders. An ordered array of questions that can easily be answered by the subject is the most useful type of history. It should be kept in mind that in many instances the interpreter of the pulmonary function studies will have little clinical information regarding the subject other than the history. For this reason, it is important that an appropriate history be taken as a routine part of pulmonary function testing. As a minimum, the following should be included in the pulmonary history:

1. **Age** _____ **Sex** _____ **Height** _____ **Weight** _____ **Race** _____
   Diagnosis _____
2. **Family history**—has anyone in your family (mother, father, brother, sister) ever had:
   Tuberculosis _____
   Emphysema _____
   Chronic bronchitis _____
   Asthma _____
   Hay fever or other allergies _____
   Cancer _____
   Other lung disorders _____
3. **Personal history**—have you ever had, or been told that you had:
   Tuberculosis _____
   Emphysema _____
   Chronic bronchitis _____

Asthma _____

Recurrent infections _____

Colds _____

Pneumonia or pleurisy _____

Hay fever or other allergies _____

Chest injury _____

Chest surgery _____

4. **Occupation**—have you ever worked:

In a mine, quarry, or foundry _____

In a mill _____

On a farm _____

Near gases or fumes _____

In a dusty place _____

5. **Smoking habits**—have you ever smoked:

Cigarettes   (_____/day)

Cigars   (_____/day)

Pipe   (_____/day)

How long?   (_____years)

Still smoke?   (Yes/No) _____

6. **Cough**—do you cough:

In the morning _____

At night _____

At a particular time of the year _____

Blood   (when   _____)

Phlegm   (when   _____)

(color   _____)

(volume _____/day)

7. **Dyspnea**—do you get short of breath:

At rest _____

On exertion   (when   _____)

At night _____

8. **Subject disposition at time of test**

Dyspneic _____

Wheezing _____

Coughing _____

Cyanotic _____

Apprehensive _____

Cooperative/uncooperative _____

Most of these questions can be answered by yes or no. In addition, space may be provided for comments either by the subject or history taker. A list of current medications, and the time last taken, is also helpful. An outline history of this type provides an intelligence base for evaluation of the various tests. In instances

NAME _____ SEX _____			
AGE _____ HEIGHT _____ WEIGHT _____			

Test	Subject	Predicted	% Normal
Lung Volumes			
VC i-e			
e-i			
FRC			
RV			
TLC			
RV/TLC x 100%			
Ventilation			
V_T			
$\dot{V}_E$			
f			
Pulmonary Mechanics			
FVC			
FEV 0.5			
FEV 1.0			
FEV 1.0%			
FEF 25-75%			
MVV			
Arterial Blood Gases			
Pa_{O_2}			
% Sat.			
Pa_{CO_2}			
pH			
Distribution			
SBN_2			
7 Minute N_2			
Miscellaneous			

INTERPRETATION:

DIAGNOSIS:

Interpreted by_____

Performed by_____

Fig. 8-1. Typical data record sheet.

in which the physician performs the test, such a history may be redundant if a medical history is available.

Standardized reporting helps simplify test interpretation; a common method of recording test results follows a format such as that outlined in Fig. 8-1. Test results are usually reported in conjunction with the appropriate predicted normal values and a corresponding percent of normal. Since many studies providing predicted normal values are available for the more common pulmonary function tests, it is important that the normal values chosen for a particular laboratory represent the methodology employed. For example, a laboratory using a water-sealed spirometer at or near sea level would use predicted values obtained under similar conditions. Because trying to match methodologies may not always be practical, predicted normal values that represent a large and diverse population should be used (see Appendix for a more detailed discussion on selecting normal values). In addition to the predicted value, the standard deviation (SD) or standard error of estimate (SEE) for any predicted normal value should be taken into consideration in the final evaluation of the extent of lung dysfunction. The SD or SEE is a measure of the ''variability'' that exists in the sample population that was tested in order to generate the predicted values. Using a statistical approach (SD or SEE) to define the difference between the subject's measured value and the predicted value is usually more sound than using simple percentages. Perhaps the best method to accomplish this is to calculate the confidence interval (CI) for each predicted value. The CI is:

$$CI = 1.65 \times SD$$

where

    SD = Standard deviation for the particular parameter in question
    1.65 = Number of SDs *below* the mean, which includes 95% of the normal population

This method accounts for the variability associated with each individual pulmonary function parameter. One drawback of reporting the relationship between measured and predicted values in this way is that some parameters ($FEF_{25\%-75\%}$, etc.) are so variable in the normal population that 1 CI may include extremely low or even negative values. This points out the importance of considering how variable a particular parameter is in the normal population when using the parameter to diagnose pulmonary abnormalities (see Appendix, Using Predicted Values).

Reporting of results should include any other information that is pertinent to the interpretation of the test. If predicted values are corrected, either to reflect racial adjustments or to standardize the predicted value, that fact should be included. If a computer-assisted interpretation is generated, it should be clearly marked as such. Questionable test results should not be reported, but in many instances it is impossible to differentiate between an abnormal finding and an erroneous one. In such an instance the questionable value should be noted as such. Following predefined criteria for acceptability for each test may be helpful in elucidating the causes for questionable results (see Chapter 11 for criteria for acceptability).

BEFORE AND AFTER BRONCHODILATOR STUDIES

Perhaps the most practical application of pulmonary function testing is the determination of a course of therapy over and above the delineation of the nature and extent of a lesion.

Pulmonary function tests, and spirometry in particular, can be performed before and after bronchodilator therapy to determine the reversibility of airway obstruction. A good indication for performing bronchodilator studies is an $FEV_{1\%}$ of less than 70%; except in older adults, low FEV_1/FVC ratios are associated with some degree of obstruction. Even subjects whose FEV_1 and FVC values are "within normal limits" compared with predicted values may display a low $FEV_{1\%}$. The value of 70% is relative; bronchodilator studies may be indicated any time there is clinical evidence of altered airway reactivity. The tests of pulmonary mechanics are the usual parameters examined. The subject is given a normal battery of tests. TLC determinations done by He dilution or the open-circuit nitrogen method should be performed before bronchodilator administration to provide an accurate baseline on which to judge any changes in the lung volume compartments that occur as a result of the dilator. Even though indices of flow such as the FEV_1 and $FEF_{25\%-75\%}$ change most dramatically, lung volumes and DL_{CO} may also respond to bronchodilator therapy.

A bronchodilator, usually a beta-adrenergic agent or a preparation of similar action, can be administered by an aerosol generator, intermittent positive pressure breathing (IPPB), or a metered-dosage device. A metered-dosage device provides a more reproducible (thus quantifiable) administration of bronchodilator when an inhalational method is used. The type of therapy may be determined by the subject's requirements. For example, known asthmatic individuals may be given their regular bronchodilator orally, by inhalation, or both, between tests to determine that particular drug regimen's effectiveness. Depending on the type of bronchodilator used and the means of administration, the therapy should last long enough to achieve the maximum effects. Most aerosolized bronchodilators begin taking effect on inhalation and continue for an indefinite period, usually at least an hour. If the bronchodilator is administered by IPPB, the "after" tests should be delayed for 5 to 10 minutes to allow for the return of the blood gases to their normal values.

Reversibility of airway obstruction and improvement in flow rates is considered significant for increases of greater than 15% to 20%. The percent of change may be calculated:

$$\% \text{ Change} = \frac{\text{Postdrug} - \text{Predrug}}{\text{Predrug}} \times 100$$

where

Postdrug = Test parameter after administration

Predrug = Test parameter before administration

It should be noted that a pulmonary function parameter that worsens following bronchodilator administration will produce a negative value using this scheme. In addition, parameters that have small absolute values (for example, an $FEF_{25\%-75\%}$

less than 0.5 L/sec) may show large-percentage changes even though the actual improvement in flow is minimal.

Disease patterns involving the bronchial (and bronchiolar) musculature show the most pronounced change from "before" to "after." Uncomplicated asthma often shows improvements of greater than 50% in parameters such as the FEV_1 and $FEF_{25\%-75\%}$. Moderate to severe chronic obstructive disease may fail to show any improvement and may even yield poorer results for the "after" tests because of the exertion of performing the forced expiratory tests several times. Since bronchodilators effect the greatest change in the pulmonary mechanics, repetition of the lung volume tests and $D_{L_{CO}}$ are usually unnecessary. An increase in VC is normally at the expense of the previously increased RV. However, if symptomatic improvement occurs with bronchodilator administration in the absence of increased flows, it may be a result of changes in the lung volume compartments, changes in $D_{L_{CO}}$, or changes in the matching of ventilation to perfusion. A common change is one in which the VC increases only slightly, but the $FEF_{25\%-75\%}$ or FEV_1 shows significant increase. This is caused by the opening of previously obstructed airways without notable increase in the actual volume of air moved by a forced expiratory maneuver. A related improvement is a significant increase in the FVC but little or no change in the FEV_1; this results in a decrease in the FEV_1/FVC ratio, despite increases in the absolute values. Failure of the FEV_1 to increase by more than 15% to 20% does not preclude the use of bronchodilator therapy, particularly if symptomatic improvement or increased exercise tolerance is demonstrated. A paradoxical fall in Pa_{O_2} may occur in some subjects following administration of an inhaled bronchodilator. This hypoxemia is thought to result from alterations that occur in the matching of ventilation and blood flow in the lungs when a beta-adrenergic drug enters the circulatory system via the lungs and is then distributed to poorly ventilated lung regions during recirculation. An increased blood flow to poorly ventilated lung units results in an increased venous admixture, with a fall in Pa_{O_2}. Blood gas analysis before and after bronchodilator administration may be required to document the paradoxical hypoxemia, particularly if flows improve but symptoms of hypoxemia worsen.

QUANTITATIVE METHACHOLINE CHALLENGE TEST

Bronchial provocation testing is useful in determining the extent of airway reactivity, particularly in subjects who may be symptomatic but who have normal pulmonary function studies or equivocal bronchodilator studies. Challenge testing may be performed in conjunction with before and after bronchodilator studies and is often done as a preliminary to an exercise-induced asthma evaluation. The objective of the test is to determine the minimum exposure of methacholine that can precipitate a 20% decrease in the FEV_1; this is usually referred to as the provocative dose, or $PD_{20\%}$. Methacholine increases parasympathetic tone in bronchial smooth muscle, resulting in bronchoconstriction. In the doses usually employed, normal subjects do not display decreases greater than 20% in the FEV_1; thus the methacholine challenge test is highly specific for airway hyperreactivity.

Subjects to be tested should be in an asymptomatic state and have a baseline FEV_1 equivalent to at least 80% of their highest previously observed value. If the subject is taking medication, the following steps are recommended:

1. Beta-adrenergic agents withheld for 8 hours
2. Sustained-action beta-adrenergic agents and methylxanthines withheld for 12 hours
3. Cromolyn sodium withheld for 24 hours
4. Antihistamines withheld for 48 hours and subjects receiving corticosteroids should be challenged while taking a stable dosage

Baseline spirometry is performed to establish that the subject's values are above 80% of the previously observed best values. The subject then inhales five breaths of nebulized diluent. A simple nebulizer may be used, but a dosimeter provides a true "quantitative" challenge test. After 10 minutes, spirometry is repeated. The diluent value then becomes the "control," and if the FEV_1 is not reduced 10% from the baseline, the quantitative challenge is performed. The following methacholine dilutions may be used:

0.075 mg/ml	2.50 mg/ml
0.15 mg/ml	5.00 mg/ml
0.31 mg/ml	10.00 mg/ml
0.60 mg/ml	25.00 mg/ml
1.25 mg/ml	

Each of these dilutions may be prepared from a 25 mg/ml stock. One-milliliter volumes are suitable for five inhalations in commonly used nebulization devices. The subject inhales five breaths from the nebulizer, beginning with the most dilute solution (0.075 mg/ml). Spirometry is repeated at 1.5 and 3.0 minutes, with the "best" test selected from duplicate or triplicate efforts. The percent of decrease is calculated as follows:

$$\% \text{ Fall} = \frac{X - Y}{X} \times 100$$

where

$X = \text{Control } FEV_1$

$Y = \text{Current } FEV_1 \text{ following methacholine inhalation}$

A 20% or greater fall in the FEV_1 is considered a positive test. If the test is negative, then five breaths of the next higher dilution are administered and the measurements repeated. If the test is borderline positive, less than five inhalations of the next dilution may be given.

At each dilution the subject should be observed and questioned for the perception of symptoms (chest tightness, wheezing), and auscultation performed. As soon as a 20% fall in the FEV_1 is observed, administration of the methacholine is terminated. The bronchospasm may be reversed by means of an appropriate bronchodilator, usually by inhalation.

Several methods of quantifying the results of the procedure are commonly used. The dilution that produced the 20% decrease FEV_1 is most often reported as the $PD_{20\%}$. A more precise method totals the amount of methacholine inhaled to produce the requisite decrease. This is done by multiplying the number of breaths times the dilution, times the volume per breath. This method requires a dosimeter or metered-dosage type of nebulizer, so that a constant volume of drug is given with each inhalation. Table 8-1 lists the cumulative amounts of methacholine delivered using the five breaths per 3-minute routine.

Methacholine challenge testing presents some risk to the subject, so a physician familiar with the procedure should be present. Medications for reversal of the bronchospasm, as well as for resuscitation, should be immediately available in the event of an untoward reaction.

The spirometer used should meet the minimal standards set by the American Thoracic Society (see Appendix) and should provide hard copy results for later evaluation.

Similar protocols may be employed for antigen and histamine challenge testing, both for testing and for expressing results. Antigen inhalation challenge requires intradermal (cutaneous) testing to establish a safe initial dosage for inhalation challenge.

TESTING FOR EXERCISE-INDUCED ASTHMA (EIA)

Exercise-induced asthma is typified by bronchospasm during or immediately following vigorous exercise. It is thought to be related to heat loss from the upper airway, which accompanies increased ventilation during exercise. Evaluation of exercise-induced bronchospasm is helpful in quantifying the extent of reversible airway obstruction in the following instances:

1. In subjects with shortness of breath on exertion, but normal resting pulmonary functions

Table 8-1. Units for methacholine challenge*

Methacholine concentration (mg/ml)	Cumulative No. of breaths	Cumulative units/five breaths	Cumulative No. of minutes
0.075	5	0.375	3
0.15	10	1.125	6
0.31	15	2.68	9
0.62	20	5.78	12
1.25	25	12.00	15
2.50	30	24.50	18
5.00	35	49.50	21
10.00	40	99.50	24
25.00	45	225.00	27

*One methacholine unit is arbitrarily defined as one inhalation of 1 mg/ml of methacholine in diluent. The quantity of drug required to provoke a 20% decrease in FEV_1 is expressed in X units/X min (e.g., 12 methacholine units/15 min).

2. In symptomatic subjects in whom bronchial provocation tests (methacholine) produce negative or equivocal results
3. In subjects with known EIA in whom therapy is being evaluated
4. In screening subjects where some risk to asthmatics might be involved (athletics, etc.)

Subjects for exercise challenge should receive an appropriate history, physical examination, and laboratory studies, including an ECG, to evaluate potential contraindications to exercise testing (see Chapter 7). Methylxanthine and beta-adrenergic bronchodilators should be withheld for 8 to 12 hours before testing, depending on the preparation. Cromolyn sodium should be excluded for 24 hours, but corticosteroids may be maintained for subjects receiving stable dosages. Before exercise, the subject's pulmonary functions should be greater than 80% of the previously determined "best" values and the FEV_1 not less than 65% of the predicted value.

Either a treadmill or cycle ergometer may be used, depending on the type of physiologic measurements being made. The subject's response to an increasing work load should be monitored via a continuous ECG. Ventilatory parameters may be helpful in assessing the extent of pulmonary limitation to exercise. A spirometer that meets the American Thoracic Society requirements (see Chapter 11) is necessary. The device should be simple enough for repeated measurements following the exercise and should allow for multiple recordings of either volume-time tracings or flow-volume curves, or both. Some automated systems provide software specifically for challenge testing (either by inhalation or exercise) with capability for superimposing MEFV curves, etc. Resuscitation equipment (as described in Chapter 7) must be available.

A progressive multistage protocol should be used initially to allow evaluation of ventilatory and cardiovascular responses to work. For subsequent testing, a 5- to 8-minute steady-state protocol may be used, with the work load determined by the subject's response to the initial multistage regimen. In either protocol the level of provocation should be determined by objective criteria, such as attainment of 85% of the predicted maximum HR, or $\dot{V}O_2$. In most instances, a short period of moderately heavy work is all that is required to trigger exercise-induced bronchospasm. Normally bronchospasm occurs immediately following the exercise, not during it, unless the test is extended over a longer interval.

Pulmonary function baseline values are established before testing and compared with the subject's usual values. Following exercise, measurements should be taken at 1 to 2 mintues, then every 5 minutes as the selected parameter (usually FEV_1 or SGaw) decreases to a minimum, and then until the parameter returns to baseline. The best value of duplicate measurements is recorded. Ambient temperature, relative humidity, and P_B should be recorded because of their influence on airway muscle tone. Several methods of reporting the response to exercise are in common use:

1. Maximum percent of decrease of baseline function:

$$\frac{X - Y}{X} \times 100$$

where

X = Baseline value (FEV$_1$, etc.)
Y = Lowest value after exercise

2. Maximum decrease as a percentage of the predicted value:

$$\frac{X - Y}{P} \times 100$$

where

X = Baseline value (FEV$_1$, etc.)
Y = Lowest value after exercise
P = Subject's predicted value

3. Lowest value as a percent of predicted value:

$$\frac{Y}{P} \times 100$$

where

Y = Lowest value after exercise
P = Subject's predicted value

The advantage of the first method is that the baseline parameter is included in both the numerator and denominator and provides a unit that is independent of the absolute values, making it useful for comparisons between subjects. The second method can be used similarly. Baseline values should always be reported, particularly if the third method is used.

Exercise-induced asthma (bronchospasm) has been demonstrated to be related to respiratory heat and/or water loss in the upper airway as a result of increased minute ventilation. Some individuals with EIA are protected from bronchospasm during exercise if warm moist air is inhaled. It is likely that the stimulus to bronchospasm during exercise testing is the level of ventilation achieved, as well as the ambient temperature and humidity. Recently, cold air inhalation has been suggested as a means of evaluating airway responsiveness. The difficulties associated with control of temperature and humidity in the testing context may limit the usefulness of this type of challenge. The exercise-induced asthma test, particularly if used to evaluate prophylactic therapy, is a quite practical means of quantifying airway reactivity.

PREOPERATIVE PULMONARY FUNCTION TESTING

Preoperative pulmonary function testing is one of several means available to clinicians to evaluate surgical candidates. Preoperative testing, in conjunction with a history and physical examination, ECG, and chest x-ray study, is indicated for one or more of the following reasons:

1. To determine the level of risk involved in the surgical procedure (morbidity and mortality)
2. To plan perioperative care, including preoperative preparation, type and duration of anesthetic during surgery, and postoperative care to minimize complications
3. To estimate postoperative lung function in candidates for pneumonectomy or lobectomy

The type of surgical candidate who needs preoperative pulmonary function testing is determined by the type of surgical procedure and the risk factors that the individual may have. Many investigations, both prospective and retrospective, have identified that the risk of postoperative pulmonary complications are highest in *thoracic procedures,* followed by *upper abdominal* and *lower abdominal* procedures. Increased incidence of complications appears in both normal subjects and those with pulmonary disorders, with the latter being at higher risk in proportion to the degree of pulmonary impairment.

Preoperative pulmonary function testing is definitely indicated in:

1. Subjects with a smoking history
2. Subjects with symptoms of pulmonary disease (i.e., cough, sputum production, shortness of breath)
3. Subjects with abnormal physical examination findings, particularly of the chest (i.e., abnormal breath sounds, ventilatory pattern, respiratory rate)
4. Subjects with abnormal chest x-ray films

Preoperative testing may also be indicated in:

1. Subjects with morbid obesity (greater than 30% above ideal body weight)
2. Subjects advanced in age, usually greater than 70 years
3. Subjects with current or recent respiratory infections, or a history or respiratory infections.
4. Subjects with marked debilitation or malnutrition

In each of these subjects the primary purpose of pulmonary function testing is to uncover preexisting pulmonary disease. Decreases in the VC of more than 50% of the preoperative value place individuals with compromised function at high risk of developing atelectasis and pneumonia. Decreases in the FRC and increases in the CV may lead to $\dot{V}/\dot{Q}$ abnormalities and hypoxemia. Abnormal ventilatory function, in terms of the central control of respiration and the status of the ventilatory muscles, may also play a role in postoperative complications.

Certain tests of pulmonary function appear to be better predictors of postoperative complications and hence should be used both for risk evaluation and to assist in planning the perioperative care of the individual. These include:

1. *Spirometry* (FVC, FEV_1, $FEF_{25\%-75\%}$, MVV). Because obstructive disease can be easily identified with simple spirometry, a significant percentage of subjects who might develop postoperative problems can be detected with minimal screening. Subjects with a reduced FVC, with or without airway

obstruction, typically have impaired ability to cough effectively when the VC decreases further during the immediate postoperative period. The MVV, although dependent on subject effort, appears to be uniquely suited to detecting postoperative risk. This may be due in part to the fact that the MVV tests lung parenchyma, airway function, ventilatory muscle function, and subject cooperation. The measured MVV correlates better with the incidence of postoperative problems than does the estimated MVV ($FEV_1 \times 35$ or 40); this may be attributable to measurement of both inspiratory and expiratory flow during the MVV, whereas the FEV_1 assesses just expiration. Since the ventilatory muscles may be involved in the development of postoperative complications, a test like the MVV may be a more sensitive predictor than forced expiratory flows.

2. *Bronchodilator studies.* Operative candidates with obstruction, either known or demonstrated via spirometry, should also be tested with bronchodilators. Postbronchodilator values for FVC, FEV_1, $FEF_{25\%-75\%}$, and MVV may be used in estimating the surgical risk and may make a significant difference in the degree of risk if there is substantial reversibility. Bronchodilator studies are similarly helpful in planning perioperative care; bronchodilator therapy may improve the subject's bronchial hygiene preoperatively as well as postoperatively.

3. *Blood gas analysis.* In subjects with documented lung disease arterial blood gases are helpful in assessing the subjects' overall response to the pulmonary changes known to occur postoperatively. The Pa_{O_2} itself is not a good prognosticator of postoperative problems, but individuals with hypoxemia at rest usually also have abnormal spirometric values and hence are at risk. The Pa_{O_2} may actually improve postoperatively in subjects undergoing thoractomy for lung resection if the resected portion was contributing to $\dot{V}/\dot{Q}$ abnormalities. The Pa_{CO_2} appears to be the most useful blood gas indicator of surgical risk. If the Pa_{CO_2} is above 45 mm Hg, there is a marked increase in postoperative morbidity and mortality. Again, elevated Pa_{CO_2} values are most commonly encountered in subjects with significant airway obstruction.

4. *Lung volumes.* Even though they may be reduced dramatically in the immediate postsurgical phase, lung volumes do not correlate well preoperatively with postoperative complications and do not enhance the estimate of complications.

5. *Diffusion studies* (DL_{CO}). Diffusion studies, like lung volume determinations, do not appear to improve the prediction of postoperative complications.

6. *Exercise testing.* Exercise studies can accurately predict subjects at risk in that those who fail to tolerate moderate work loads typically have airway obstruction or similar ventilatory limitations.

In addition to these tests for predicting postoperative problems, several other tests are employed specifically for predicting postoperative lung function in candidates for pneumonectomy or lobectomy. These procedures, normally used in conjunction with spirometry and blood gas analysis, include:

1. *Perfusion and $\dot{V}/\dot{Q}$ scans.* Lung scans (see Chapter 4) are particularly useful in estimating the remaining lung function in subjects who are likely to require removal of all or part of a lung. Split-function scans are performed; these allow partitioning of lungs into right and left halves or into multiple lung regions. Although ventilation/perfusion scans give the best estimate of overall function, simple perfusion scans yield quite similar information. Lung scan values, in the form of regional function percentages, are used in combination with simple spirometric indices to calculate the subject's postoperative capacity. For example:

$$\text{Postop } FEV_1 = \text{Preop } FEV_1 \times \% \text{ Perfusion to unaffected portions}$$

Subjects whose postoperative FEV_1 values are calculated to be less than 800 ml are typically not considered surgical candidates.

Table 8-2. Preoperative pulmonary functions

Test	Increased postoperative risk	High postoperative risk	Candidate for pneumonectomy*
FVC	Less than 50% of predicted value	Less than 1.5 L	—
FEV_1	Less than 2 L or 50% of predicted value	Less than 1 L	Greater than 2 L
$FEF_{25\%-75\%}$	Less than 50% of predicted value	—	—
MVV	—	Less than 50 L/min or 50% of predicted value	Greater than 50 L/min or 50% of predicted value
Pa_{CO_2}	—	Greater than 45 mm Hg	—
Predicted postoperative FEV_1	—	—	Greater than 0.8 L
Pulmonary artery occlusion	—	—	Less than 35 mm Hg

*Values in this column determine if the subject is to be considered a candidate for lung resection (see text).

2. *Pulmonary artery occlusion pressure*. In some candidates for pneumonectomy the development of postoperative pulmonary hypertension may be a limiting factor. To estimate the effect of redirecting the entire right ventricular output to the remaining lung, a catheter is inserted into the pulmonary artery of the affected lung and blood flow occluded by means of a balloon. The resulting pressure increase in the remaining lung is then measured. A pressure increasing to less than 35 mm Hg is usually considered consistent with acceptable postoperative pressures. The effect of redirected blood flow on oxygenation may also be a consideration, and this can also be examined during occlusion to estimate postoperative Pa_{O_2}.

These tests to predict the effects of resection on the remaining lung are normally used in series, with spirometry done first, followed by split-function lung scans if the spirometry is acceptable, and then pulmonary artery occlusion pressure if the development of cor pulmonale is a concern. Table 8-2 summarizes some general ranges of values used for preoperative pulmonary function testing.

PULMONARY FUNCTION TESTING FOR DISABILITY

Pulmonary function tests are one of several means of determining a subject's inability to perform certain tasks. Respiratory impairment and disability, however, are not synonymous. Respiratory impairment relates to the failure of one or more of the functions of the lungs; this is what most pulmonary function studies measure. Disability is the inability to perform tasks that are required either for employment or for everyday activities. Those pulmonary function tests used to determine impairment leading to disability should characterize the type, extent, and cause of the impairment. Pulmonary function testing may not completely describe all the factors involved in the disabling impairment; other factors involved may be the age, educational background, and motivation of the subject, and the energy requirements of the task in question.

Determination of the level of impairment usually consists of the following:
1. *Physical examination*—does not allow quantification of disabling symptoms but is useful in grading shortness of breath. Shortness of breath is the most prominent feature of respiratory impairment but, like pain, is subjective. Tachypnea, cyanosis, and abnormal respiratory patterns are not indicative of the extent of impairment but may be helpful in elucidating the findings from pulmonary function studies.
2. *Chest x-ray study*—does not correlate well with shortness of breath or pulmonary function studies, except in advanced cases of pneumoconioses. Absence of usual findings in the pneumoconioses may be helpful in excluding occupational exposure as part of the impairment.
3. *Pulmonary function studies*—should be objective, reproducible, and, most important, specific to the disorder being investigated.
   a. *FVC and FEV_1*. Spirometry is the most useful index for the assessment of impairment due to airway obstruction. A permanent record of the tracings must be kept. The volume-time tracing should have the time

sensitivity marked on the horizontal axis and the volume sensitivity marked on the vertical axis. The paper speed should be at least 20 mm /sec and the volume excursion at least 10 mm/L. The three largest FVC and FEV_1 values should be within 5%, and each maneuver should be continued for at least 10 seconds. The largest FVC and FEV_1 of three acceptable maneuvers is reported. FEV_1 calculated from a flow-volume curve is not acceptable. Spirometry is normally repeated following bronchodilator therapy.

b. *MVV*. The maximum voluntary ventilation has some drawbacks in that it is influenced by subject effort, which may be in question in disability determinations. The test is also affected by muscular coordination, heart disease, neurologic function, and chest wall compliance. One satisfactory MVV maneuver is required (see Chapter 11), but it should not be calculated from the FEV_1. The tracing should show both inspiratory and expiratory excursions, rather than just accumulated volume; the recording should be continued for 10 to 15 seconds.

c. *Lung volumes*. Lung volume determinations correlate poorly with shortness of breath and disability but may be necessary to assess the extent of restriction present. The VC may be required for disability determination, but other lung volumes are not.

d. DL_{CO}. The diffusing capacity is useful in determining impairment in restrictive disorders such as fibrosis. Either single-breath or steady-state methods may be used; the predicted normal value for the method should also be reported.

e. *Arterial blood gas analysis*. Although blood gas results are objective, they are largely nonspecific in determining impairment. The $A\text{-a}_{O_2}$ gradient is not reliable, since it may be affected by hyperventilation. Blood gas analysis may be required in diffuse pulmonary fibrosis and should include both the Pa_{O_2} and the Pa_{CO_2}. Blood gases (and the A-a gradient) are helpful if measured during exercise. The requirement for supplementary O_2 may also be quantified by exercise blood gas analysis.

f. *Exercise testing*. Exercise testing may be indicated if the results of simple spirometry, diffusing capacity, or blood gases are equivocal with regard to the extent of respiratory impairment. The $\dot{V}E_{max}$, compared with the MVV, helps to determine the ventilatory reserve, if any, that remains. Similarly, the HR_{max}, if much less than that predicted for the work load, indicates a ventilatory rather than cardiovascular limitation. Ventilatory equivalents for O_2 and CO_2 ($\dot{V}E/\dot{V}O_2$ and $\dot{V}E/\dot{V}CO_2$) are most useful if measured during sustained exercise. They may be used to estimate functional limits that can be compared with the job requirements of the individual. The dyspnea index (see Chapter 7) is considered normal if less than 12% of the MVV; values between 35% and 50% are equivocal, and values greater than 50% are almost always considered abnormal.

Limits for determining disability on the basis of respiratory impairment have been set by the U.S. Social Security Administration. Criteria are set according to the disease category:

COPD

FEV_1 less than 1.0 to 1.4 liters (heights of 57 to 73 inches, respectively)

MVV less than 32 to 48 L/min (heights of 57 to 73 inches, respectively)

Asthma

As for COPD *or*

Episodes of severe attacks in spite of treatment every 2 months *or*

Episodes six times a year with wheezing between attacks

Diffuse pulmonary fibrosis

VC less than 1.2 to 2.0 liters (heights of 57 to 73 inches, respectively) *or*

$DL_{CO}SS$ less than 6 ml CO/min/mm Hg; $DL_{CO}SB$ less than 9 ml CO/min/mm Hg *or*

Pa_{O_2} less than 65 mm Hg (at a Pa_{CO_2} of 30 mm Hg); Pa_{O_2} less than 55 mm Hg (at a Pa_{CO_2} of 40 mm Hg)

Other restrictive ventilatory disorders (kyphoscoliosis, thoracoplasty, lung resection)

VC less than 1.0 to 1.4 liters (heights of 59 to 70 inches, respectively)

Pneumoconioses (demonstrated by chest x-ray film)

Nodular focal fibrosis evaluated as for COPD *or*

Interstitial disseminated fibrosis evaluated as for pulmonary fibrosis

In reporting impairment for disability purposes, the remaining functional capacity is as important in determining the subject's ability to carry out a certain task as the percentage of lost function. Some statement of the subject's ability to understand and cooperate with the pulmonary function measurements should accompany the tabular and graphic data.

PULMONARY FUNCTION TESTING IN CHILDREN

Pulmonary function testing in children uses many of the same basic tests as are used in adults. Differences between adult and pediatric testing exist not only in the absolute dimensions of the developing pulmonary system, but also in two main areas concerned with the testing regimens themselves:

1. Newborns, infants, and very young children cannot strictly perform those tests that require and depend on subject cooperation.
2. Young children and adolescents may perform variably on those tests that are effort dependent or that require detailed instruction.

Tests of lung function in infants and very young children normally assess lung volumes and those mechanical factors that are not determined by the functional limits of the respiratory system. Inability to perform maximal efforts elminates such parameters as FVC, FEV_1, and FEF. Reasonable estimates of basic measurements, such as the VC, can be made by compromise techniques, but the details are beyond the scope of this text, and the reader is directed toward the Selected Bibliography at the end of this chapter.

Pulmonary function testing in children and adolescents is often directed toward diagnosis and evaluation of disease states most common in pediatric subjects. These are (1) asthma, (2) cystic fibrosis, and (3) chest deformities.

The presence and severity of asthma in children is evaluated using a method similar to that used for testing the extent of reversible obstructive lung disease in adults:

1. *Lung volume measurements* (VC, TLC, RV, FRC, RV/TLC) provide information concerning hyperinflation (air trapping), particularly in acute asthmatic episodes.
2. *Flow measurements* (FEFx, FEV_T, $FEV_T\%$, MEFV curves, PEFR) help to establish the extent of obstruction and determine the effectiveness of bronchodilators. The PEFR can be particularly useful, since it can be measured conveniently (at the bedside with a portable peak flow meter) and provides serial measurements for planning and evaluating therapy. The PEFR should be correlated with the FEV_1 or other flow measurements in order to detect changes that may be due to obstruction and not just effort.
3. *Exericse testing* may be used to determine the presence of exercise-induced bronchospasm and to evaluate the effectiveness of particular therapeutic regimens.

The deterioration of lung function in children with *cystic fibrosis* is measured in a manner similar to that used in adults with COPD:

1. *Lung volumes* (VC, FRC, RV, TLC, RV/TLC) provide data concerning air trapping.
2. *Flow measurements* (FEFx, FEV_T, $FEV_T\%$, MEFV curves) assess the extent of obstruction caused by mucus plugging, bronchospasm, and edema.
3. *Arterial blood gas studies* provide information concerning the degree of respiratory insufficiency.

Chest deformities that are commonly evaluated by pulmonary function studies include kyphoscoliosis and pectus excavatum. In both cases, measurements include those parameters that are useful in assessing restrictive ventilatory patterns, such as lung volumes and $D_{L_{CO}}$.

Normal values of lung function for children in all cases depend on height, sex, and age. Lung function predicted values in children vary mainly with height, and many parameters change dramatically at the onset of puberty. For spirometric variables (FVC, FEV_1, etc.) lung function increases up to about age 18 in boys and about age 16 in girls. After these ages volumes and flows plateau and then begin to decline. Nomograms for lung volumes and various flow measurements for common parameters are included in the Appendix.

BEDSIDE TESTING

The determination of a course of therapy is one of the most common indications for pulmonary function studies. In many situations these determinations must necessarily be performed at the bedside rather than under laboratory conditions. Bedside evaluation of subjects involves three main types of pulmonary function tests: (1) ventilation, (2) pulmonary mechanics, and (3) matching of ventilation and blood flow.

Ventilation tests ($\dot{V}E$, VT, f, VC, NIF)

Basic ventilatory measurements are fundamental to the treatment of subjects requiring continuous ventilatory assistance, those with impending ventilatory failure, or those in the early stages of recovery from ventilatory failure. Ventilation tests correlate well with arterial blood gas studies in determining the type and duration of ventilatory assistance required for individuals in acute ventilatory failure. Tests of ventilatory muscle function may also be important in planning therapy for subjects with neuromuscular disorders, or for subjects who are being weaned from mechanical ventilation (see Chapter 2). The negative inspiratory force (NIF) is similar to the maximum inspiratory pressure (MIP) and is measured by connecting a pressure manometer to an occluded airway and noting the maximum negative pressure that can be developed. The NIF (sometimes referred to as the maximum inspiratory force; MIF) is used in obtunded individuals in whom the VC cannot be obtained. Occlusion of the airway produces maximum values within 10 to 20 seconds but may not be tolerated well by subjects with unstable cardiovascular status. A VC of 15 ml/kg requires development of approximately -20 cm H_2O, and this value is considered the minimum below which a subject usually will not be able to maintain adequate spontaneous ventilation over an extended period. Values greater than -80 cm H_2O are observed in healthy individuals, but negative pressures greater than -20 cm H_2O in obtunded subjects have not been well correlated with specific VC values.

Pulmonary mechanics tests (FVC, FEV, FEF, PEFR)

Measurements of FVC and flow rates at the bedside provide a quantitative basis for therapy in obstructive airway processes, particularly asthma. Portable spirometers and pneumotachometers allow serial measurements, on a daily or even hourly basis, to assess the effectiveness of bronchodilators, respiratory therapy, or chest physical therapy.

PEFR values, though used often, do not by themselves quantify the reversibility of obstruction, since normal peak flows may be developed early in a forced expiration despite decreased FEV or FEF values. PEFR should be correlated with other flow measurements rather than used alone. Peak flows, as measured with a small portable device, may be beneficial in evaluating the control of asthma in subjects who use the device routinely and for whom conventional spirometric measurements are well documented. Serial measurements, daily or more often, can serve as an index for evaluation of therapeutic maneuvers to control bronchospasm.

Blood gases and related tests

Arterial blood gas analysis (see Chapter 6) is the most commonly used method of evaluating the adequacy of ventilation/blood flow matching.

Two techniques that have proved especially valuable in the clinical setting are the determinations of VD/VT ratio and $\dot{Q}s/\dot{Q}T$ (see Chapter 6). Shunt and VD/VT measurements may be performed on subjects requiring continuous ventilatory assistance without interruption of the therapy. Serial measurements of shunt and

V_D/V_T provide data concerning the progression of an individual's clinical status and allow for changes in the ventilator therapy appropriate for the subject's status. Simple measurement of the alveolar-arterial oxygen gradient ($P[A-a]o_2$) with the subject breathing 100% O_2 provides similar information in instances where the calculation of percent of shunt may be unreliable, such as when the true a-v content difference cannot be measured. $P(A-a)o_2$ values of less than 250 mm Hg while breathing 100% O_2 are consistent with adequate matching of ventilation and perfusion to allow weaning from mechanical ventilation to be considered. Normal healthy adults show a $P(A-a)o_2$ of 50 to 100 mm Hg while breathing O_2.

Measurement of end-tidal Pco_2 ($P_{ET_{CO_2}}$), either by manual or automatic sampling, provides information similar to that obtained from the V_D measurement. Averaged end-tidal values may be used to calculate the V_D/V_T ratio if the Pa_{CO_2} is known, but these values may be inaccurate in the presence of severe $\dot{V}/\dot{Q}$ abnormalties.

Mechanical spirometers, such as the Wright respirometer (see Chapter 8), provide the simplest and most portable means of measuring $\dot{V}E$, V_T, and VC. Measurement of FVC, FEV_T, and FEFx is most easily accomplished by means of a portable electronic spirometer, using one of several flow-sensing transducer principles and integrating circuitry. Many available portable spirometers provide digital output, including measured, predicted, and percent of predicted, and can be adapted to provide hard copy printout. PEFR can be measured by portable electronic spirometers or by mechanical flow-sensing devices such as the Wright peak flow meter. NIF is measured simply by connecting a manometer, calibrated in centimeters of water or millimeters of mercury, to either an anatomically fitting face mask or a standard artificial airway connector. A means for rapidly occluding and reopening the airway must be provided. For chart recording, a suitable transducer may be placed in line and coupled to a single- or multiple-channel recorder.

SELF-ASSESSMENT QUESTIONS

1. A pulmonary history for use in conjunction with pulmonary function testing should include:
   a. A smoking history
   b. A family history of lung disease
   c. A description of cough and sputum production
   d. A description of shortness of breath
   e. All of the above
2. A subject is given a before and after bronchodilator study (spirometry), and these values are recorded:

	Before drug	After drug
FVC (L)	2.30	3.30
FEV_1 (L)	1.38	1.73
$FEV_{1\%}$	60	52
$FEF_{25\%-75\%}$ (L)	0.60	0.90
MVV (L/min)	57.0	65.0

These results are consistent with:

a. Severe obstruction with no bronchodilator response

b. Moderate obstruction with significant bronchodilator response

c. Paradoxical response to bronchodilator administration

d. Erroneous postdrug data

3. A subject is given a methacholine challenge test, and the following results are recorded:

Dosage	FEV_1
Baseline	4.01
Control (saline)	3.77
0.075	3.71
0.150	3.65
0.310	3.66
0.625	3.30
1.25	3.15
2.50	2.99
5.00	2.66

These findings are consistent with:

a. Negative methacholine challenge study

b. Positive methacholine challenge; provocative dose is 1.25 units

c. Positive methacholine challenge; provocative dose is 2.50 units

d. Incomplete methacholine challenge study

4. Before testing for EIA, beta-adrenergic bronchodilators should be withheld for:

a. 1 hour

b. 8 to 12 hours

c. 24 to 48 hours

d. 48 to 72 hours

5. Spirometric measurements made to detect EIA should be made:

a. Every 1 to 2 minutes during the exercise

b. 1 to 2 minutes following the exercise

c. Every 5 minutes during the exercise

d. Every 5 minutes following the exercise

e. b and d

6. Which of the following tests may not produce reliable results in infants or very young children?

a. $\dot{V}_{max\ 50}$

b. FVC and FEV_1

c. Arterial blood gases

d. a and b only

7. A peak flow measurement, as determined with a portable peak flow meter, may be valuable:

a. When it has been correlated with the FEV_1

b. In asthmatics who use the device routinely

c. When used before and after bronchodilator administration

d. All of the above

8. A patient about to undergo upper abdominal surgery is referred for pulmonary function evaluation of postoperative risk; which of the following would best predict pulmonary complications?

a. Spirometry (FVC, FEV_1, etc.)

b. Shunt study

   c. Lung volumes (FRC, RV, TLC)

   d. $DL_{CO}SB$

   e. a, b, and d

9. A patient scheduled for lung resection has an FEV_1 of 1.2 liters; to estimate postoperative FEV_1, one could:

   a. Sum the FVC and FEV_1 and divide by two

   b. Multiply the preoperative FEV_1 by the percent of perfusion to the unaffected lung

   c. Multiply the preoperative FEV_1 by the shunt fraction

   d. Divide the FEV_1 by one half the FVC

10. In order for spirometric tracings to be acceptable for determining respiratory impairment for disability, which of the following must be met?

   I. The FEV_1 should be marked on the F-V loop.

   II. The recording device should have a volume excursion of at least 10 mm/L.

   III. The FEV_1 should be recorded at a paper speed of at least 20 mm/sec.

   IV. The FEV_1 should be the largest value from three acceptable maneuvers.

   a. I, II, III, and IV

   b. I, III, and IV

   c. II, III, and IV

   d. III and IV

11. A subject who is 54 years old and 65 inches tall has a diagnosis of COPD; his postbronchodilator FEV_1 is 0.95 liter, and his MVV is 32 L/min. These are consistent with:

   a. Severe obstruction meeting disability requirements

   b. Moderate obstruction but not meeting disability requirements

   c. Moderate restriction but not meeting disability requirements

   d. Obstruction, but blood gas analysis is required for disability determination

12. A subject is tested for exercise-induced asthma (EIA). Her pretest FEV_1 is 3.8 liters, and the lowest FEV_1 recorded following exercise to 85% of her predicted HR was 3.3 liters. This represents a maximum decrease of:

   a. 13%

   b. 15%

   c. 21%

   d. 41%

SELECTED BIBLIOGRAPHY

Testing regimens

Becklake, M.R., and Permutt, S.: Evaluation of tests of lung function for screening for early detection of chronic obstructive lung disease. In Macklem, P., et al., editors: The lung in transition between health and disease, New York, 1979, Marcel Dekker, Inc.

Cotes, J.E.: Lung function throughout life; determinants and reference values. In Cotes, J.E.: Lung function: assessment and application in medicine, Oxford, ed. 4, 1979, Blackwell Scientific Publications, Ltd.

Before and after bronchodilator studies

Girard, W.M., and Light, R.W.: Should the FVC be considered in evaluating response to bronchodilator? Chest **84:**87, 1983.

Light, R.W., Conrad, S.A., and George, R.B.: The one best test for evaluating the effects of bronchodilator therapy, Chest **72:**512, 1977.

Sourk, R.L., and Nugent, K.M.: Bronchodilator testing: confidence intervals derived from placebo inhalations, Am. Rev. Respir. Dis. **128:**153, 1983.

Bronchial challenge and exercise-induced asthma

Bhagat, R.G., and Grunstein, M.M.: Comparison of responsiveness to methacholine, histamine, and exercise in subgroups of asthmatic children, Am. Rev. Respir. Dis. **129:**221, 1984.

Chai, H., et al.: Standardization of bronchial inhalation challenge procedures, J. Allergy Clin. Immunol. **56:**323, 1975.

Cockroft, D.W., and Berscheid, B.A.: Standardization of inhalational provocation test: dose vs concentration of histamine, Chest **82:**572, 1982.

Cockcroft, D.W., et al.: Bronchial reactivity to inhaled histamine: a method and clinical survey, Clin. Allergy **7:**235, 1977.

Eggleston, P.A., and Rosenthal, R.R.: Guidelines for the methodology of exercise challenge testing of asthmatics, J. Allergy Clin. Immunol. **64:**642, 1979.

Fish, J.E., and Kelly, J.F.: Measurements of responsiveness in bronchoprovocation testing, J. Allergy Clin. Immunol. **64:**592, 1979.

McLaughlin, F.J., and Dozor, A.J.: Cold air inhalation challenge in the diagnosis of asthma in children, Pediatrics **72:**503, 1983.

Michoud, M.C., Ghezzo, H., and Amyot, R.: A comparison of pulmonary function tests used for bronchial challenges, Bull. Eur. Physiopathol. Respir. **18:**609, 1982.

Pepys, G., and Hutchcroft, B.J.: Bronchial provocation tests in etiologic diagnosis and analysis of asthma, Am. Rev. Respir. Dis. **112:**829, 1975.

Preoperative pulmonary function testing

Boysen, P.G.: Preoperative pulmonary function tests and complications after coronary artery by-pass, Anesthesiology **57:**A499, 1982.

Cain, H.D., Stevens, P.M., and Adaniya, R.: Preoperative pulmonary function and complications after cardiovascular surgery, Chest **76:**130, 1979.

Olsen, G.N., et al.: Pulmonary function evaluation of the lung resection candidate: prospective study, Am. Rev. Respir. Dis. **111:**379, 1975.

Reichel, J.: Assessment of operative risk of pneumonectomy, Chest **62:**570, 1972.

Tisi, G.M.: Preoperative evaluation of pulmonary function: validity, indications, and benefits, Am. Rev. Respir. Dis. **119:**293, 1979.

Respiratory impairment for disability

Gaensler, E.M., and Wright, G.W.: Evaluation of respiratory impairment, Arch. Environ. Health **12:**146, 1966.

Harber, P., et al.: Statistical "biases" in respiratory disability determinations, Am. Rev. Respir. Dis. **128:**413, 1983.

Morgan, W.K.C.: Pulmonary disability and impairment: can't work? won't work? Basics of RD, Am. Thoracic Soc. **10**(5), 1982.

Social Security Regulations: Rule for determining disability and blindness, U.S. Department of Health and Human Services, SSA Publ. No. 64-014, 1981.

Pulmonary function testing in children

Falliers, C.J.: Why test function in children routinely? J. Respir. Dis. **3**(1):37, 1982.

Hsu, K.H.K., et al.: Ventilatory functions of normal children and young adults—Mexican-American, white, and black. I. Spirometry, J. Pediatr. **95:**14, 1979.

Kanner, R.E., et al.: Spirometry in children: methodology for obtaining optimal results for clinical and epidemiologic studies, Am. Rev. Respir. Dis. **127:**720, 1983.

Polgar, G., and Promadhat, V.: Pulmonary function testing in children: techniques and standards, Philadelphia, 1971, W.B. Saunders Co.

Taussig, L.M.: Standardization of lung function testing in children, J. Pediatr. **97:**668, 1980.

Wall, M.A., Misley, M.C., and Dickerson, D.: Partial expiratory flow-volume curves in young children, Am. Rev. Respir. Dis. **129:**557, 1984.

CHAPTER NINE

Pulmonary function testing equipment

Although many of the principles of pulmonary function testing that date back over a hundred years are still in use, recent years have seen an astounding multiplication of devices for assessing the various parameters of pulmonary function. Testing by means of electronic as well as mechanical apparatus has proceeded toward a highly specialized technology. The use of small computers (see Chapter 10) has eliminated many time-consuming calculations, and complex testing procedures are common on a widespread basis.

Many of the common tests now in use developed as a result of technical advances in regard to their respective testing devices. This chapter enumerates and attempts to explain the principles of the more common pieces of hardware in terms of specific testing applications. Included are volume displacement spirometers, pneumotachometers, gas analyzers, plethysmographs, the respiratory inductive plethysmograph, and recording/output devices.

SPIROMETERS
Water-seal spirometers

For many years the basic tool in the determination of lung volumes and capacities and flow rates has been the water-seal spirometer. The water-seal spirometer consists of a large bell suspended in a container of water with the open end of the bell below the surface of the water (Fig. 9-1). A breathing system into and out of the interior of the bell allows for the addition or removal of accurate volumes of gas. Normally the subject breathes into and out of the spirometer and in so doing moves the bell a proportional distance. The movement of the bell can be used to mechanically manipulate a pen attached to a kymograph or to activate an electrical potentiometer to produce an analog output signal. For rebreathing studies, the breathing system necessarily includes a CO_2 absorber (soda lime) and separates inspiratory and expiratory circuits to eliminate dead space. For simple spirometry, a single hose carries both inspiratory and expiratory gases.

Water-seal spirometers may be used for the following tests:
1. Lung volumes and subdivisions, including RV and TLC, when used with appropriate gas analyzers
2. Ventilation ($\dot{V}E$ and VT)
3. Diffusing capacity (with appropriate gas analyzers)
4. Pulmonary mechanics, including FVC, FEV_T, $FEV_T\%$, inspiratory and expiratory flow rates, and MVV

The reliability of the water-seal spirometer depends on a number of factors. Primarily, the spirometer bell must be either precisely counterweighted or bal-

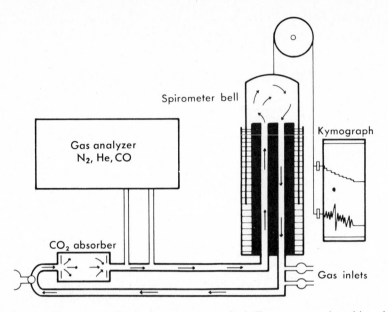

Spirometer bell

Gas analyzer
N₂, He, CO

Kymograph

CO₂ absorber

Gas inlets

Fig. 9-1. Typical water-seal spirometer apparatus, including a one-way breathing circuit, CO_2 absorber, and recording kymograph (see text). (From Clinical spirometry, Warren E. Collins, Inc., Braintree, Mass.)

anced so that respiratory excursions are accurately reproduced. The resistance to movement (inertia) of a counterweighted bell may be a consideration, especially in the measurement of FVC and flows. With systems in which the movement of the spirometer bell mechanically traces a spirogram, corrections must be made for changes in temperature and saturation of expired gas. Units in which the bell activates a potentiometer may be equipped with signal corrections from ATPS to BTPS. Individual manufacturers give specific details as to what corrections are necessary and how they are to be made for their particular instruments. Individual spirometer bells are supplied with volume displacement factors.

Two types of water-seal spirometers are in common use today. The Collins spirometer was the basic tool of pulmonary function testing for over a decade (Fig. 9-1). This water-seal spirometer was available in a variety of sizes. The older models feature a 9- or 13.5-liter bell, and the later modular units feature interchangeable 7- and 14-liter bells. The basic unit employs a bell counterweighted by a pulley and chain assembly that serves to move two recording pens, and a variable-speed kymograph. One pen records respiratory excursions during inspiration as well as expiration; the other records excursions during inspiration only, thus tracing accumulated volumes (VE, MVV, etc.). The kymograph has speeds of 32, 160, and 1920 mm/min, so that timed capacities can be conveniently recorded. The Collins type of water-seal spirometer can be fitted with a rotary potentiometer (on the pulley that supports the chain assembly) to provide analog output signals.

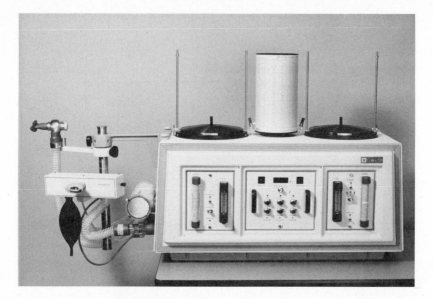

Fig. 9-2. Automated Stead-Wells water-seal spirometer. The Stead-Wells spirometer uses a lightweight plastic bell that is not counterweighted (shown here completely empty). The spirometer bell carries a pen that traces directly on a rotating kymograph. With appropriate circuitry and gas analyzers, foreign gas lung volumes and $D_{L_{CO}}$ are easily performed. (Courtesy Warren E. Collins, Inc., Braintree, Mass.)

The Stead-Wells type of water-seal spirometer (Fig. 9-2) operates on the basic principles just outlined, with the exception of employing a lightweight plastic bell not counterweighted or supported by pulleys. The Stead-Wells spirometer carries a recording pen mounted against a variable-speed kymograph, but, unlike the Collins spirometer, inspiratory excursions deflect the pen downward and expiratory excursions deflect it upward. The Collins spirometer traces the spirogram in an inverted manner because of the pulley-driven recording pens. The Stead-Wells spirometer offers less inertia and hence is somewhat more suitable for those tests measuring flow rates during the early part of an FEV maneuver, such as the $FEF_{200-1200}$. The Stead-Wells type of spirometer can also be directly attached to a linear potentiometer to provide analog signals proportional to volume and flow.

The problems encountered with water-seal spirometers usually arise from leaks in the bell or in the breathing circuit; gravity causes volume loss in the presence of such leaks. Inadequate water in the device may also lead to erroneous readings that are sometimes difficult to detect. The bulk of the water-seal spirometer makes it somewhat difficult to transport.

Dry rolling-seal spirometers

One of the more recent innovations in spirometry is the dry rolling-seal spirometer. A typical unit consists of a piston in a cylinder, which is supported by a rod resting on frictionless bearings (Fig. 9-3). The piston is coupled to the cyl-

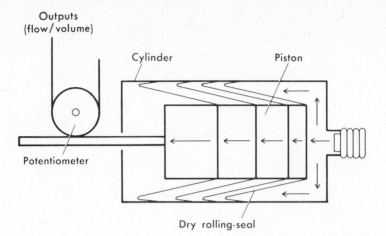

Fig. 9-3. Cutaway view of the main components of a dry rolling-seal spirometer. The figure gives an exaggerated view of the rolling-seal, which actually fits closely between the piston and the cylinder wall. The piston has a large surface area, so that its horizontal movement is minimized. This allows recording of normal breaths and maximal respiratory excursions with only a small amount of mechanical movement and hence little resistance. The piston rides on a rod that activates an electrical potentiometer, or the rod may drive a direct-recording pen. The rotational movement of the potentiometer is translated into analog signals for both flow and volume. (From Form 370, Ohio Medical Products, Madison, Wis.)

inder wall by a plastic seal that rolls on itself rather than sliding. The volume of the piston cylinder combination is usually 10 to 12 liters, but the piston has a large enough diameter that excursions of just a few inches produce large volume changes. The piston is normally lightweight aluminum, so that there is little inertia or mechanical resistance.

Dry-seal spirometers are suitable for the same tests as water-seal spirometers:

1. Lung volumes
2. Ventilation
3. Diffusing capacity
4. Pulmonary mechanics

Some dry rolling-seal spirometers employ mechanically driven graphing devices in which the piston moves a pen. Most, however, have a rotary potentiometer that is activated by the movement of the piston to provide an electrical output for volume and flow. Since the dry-seal spirometer is so readily adapted to producing analog outputs for both volume and flow, most of the currently available systems are interfaced with computers with digital display and graphics printers either built in or available in modular form (Fig. 9-4). Since the dry-seal spirometer travels in a horizontal plane, there is no need for counterbalancing. Most systems feature electronic corrections for temperature, thus eliminating a number of time-consuming calculations. One-way circuits and CO_2 removers are

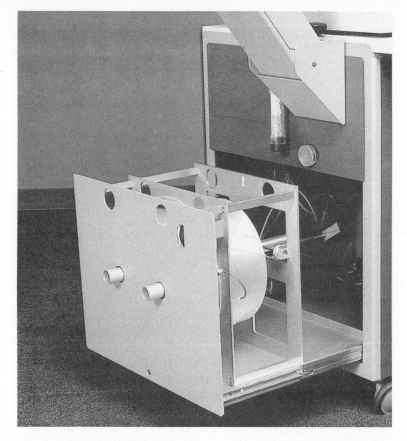

Fig. 9-4. Typical dry-seal spirometer consisting of a large aluminum piston mounted in a cylinder, with two ports to accommodate simple spirometry and rebreathing maneuvers (with a CO_2 absorber) (see Fig. 9-3). (Courtesy Gould Medical Instruments, Inc., Dayton, Ohio.)

available, so that dry-seal spirometers can be used for rebreathing tests in the same way as water-seal spirometers.

Dry rolling-seal spirometers, employing the basic design described, are available from several manufacturers. Most include analog BTPS corrections. Most units are compatible with computers that accept analog flow and volume input, as well as strip chart or X-Y recorders (see Recorders and Related Devices). The primary problem encountered with dry rolling-seal spirometers is sticking or other mechanical resistance in the piston-cylinder assembly. This can usually be avoided with adequate cleaning. Although somewhat more portable than the water-seal spirometer, the dry rolling-seal spirometer may be too cumbersome for transport to the bedside, particularly if a computer or X-Y recorder is included.

Bellows spirometers

A third type of volume displacement spirometer is the bellows or wedge bellows, which consists of a collapsible bellows that folds or unfolds in response to breathing excursions. The wedge bellows opens and closes somewhat like a fan with one side fixed (Fig. 9-5). Since one side of the bellows remains stationary, the other side moves with a pivotal motion around an axis through the fixed side, and this displacement of the bellows by a volume of gas is transmitted to a mechanical recording device. The recording chart is arranged to move at a fixed speed under the pen and thus traces a spirogram. The conventional bellows may be mounted either horizontally or vertically. Large horizontal bellows offer little mechanical resistance and are normally used in conjunction with a potentiometer to produce analog volume and flow signals. Several types of small vertically mounted bellows are currently available and are used widely for portable spirometry and bedside testing.

The wedge and conventional bellows (Fig. 9-6) are suitable for measurement of the VC and its subdivisions, FVC, and pulmonary mechanics, including inspiratory/expiratory flow rates and MVV. In conjunction with the appropriate gas analyzers and breathing circuitry, bellows systems may be used for lung volume determinations and DL_{CO}.

The most common problem with the bellows design is inaccuracy resulting from sticking of the folds of the bellow, due to dirt or moisture, or aging. Corrections for BTPS are made by either analog adjustment or software, or are included in the scale of the recording chart paper. As with water-seal and dry

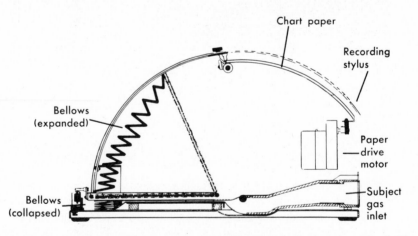

Fig. 9-5. Cross-sectional diagram of a wedge bellows type of spirometer. The fanlike movements of the wedge bellows produce mechanical movement, which is usually translated directly to a recording device. Some manufacturers suspend the bellows so that the primary movement is in a horizontal rather than vertical direction; large wedge bellows offer little mechanical resistance and are comparable to dry-seal or water-seal spirometers in accuracy and linearity. (Adapted from Vitalograph Medical Instrumentation: Product brochure, Lenexa, Kan.)

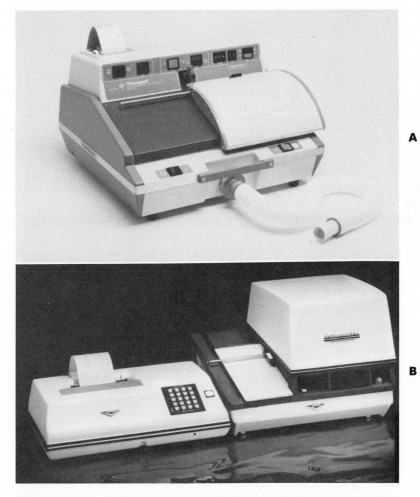

Fig. 9-6. Two types of bellows spirometers. **A,** Wedge bellows spirometer with direct-writing recorder, digital displays, and built-in printer for automated data reduction. **B,** Conventional bellows type of spirometer with the bellows mounted horizontally and the rod driving a pen across moving graph paper. A potentiometer allows analog output to a dedicated microprocessor with a built-in printer for automatic data reduction. (**A** courtesy Vitalograph Medical Instrumentation, Lenexa, Kan., **B** courtesy Jones Medical Instrument Co., Oakbrook, Ill.)

rolling-seal spirometers, bellows spirometers can be used for direct mechanical recording of volumes and flows or, by means of potentiometers, adapted to produce analog output for electronic recording or conversion to digital form (see Chapter 10). The combination of direct recording and computerized data handling are a distinct advantage of volume displacement spirometers, since they do not depend on the computer entirely.

PNEUMOTACHOMETERS

In contrast to volume displacement spirometers of the water-seal, dry rolling-seal, or bellows types is the pneumotachometer, or flow-sensing device. Pneumotachometers use various physical principles to produce an analog output that can be integrated for measurement of volumes and flows. Integration of the flow signal is a process in which flow (volume/time) is divided into extremely small intervals (time) and the volume from each interval summed. This can be performed quite easily by electronic means but depends on accurate flow signals and accurate timing. Although a wide variety of types of pneumotachometers are presently available, four basic designs are commonly used.

The first, and simplest, type of flow-sensing device is the rotameter or respirometer, which consists of a vane connected to a series of gears, such that gas flowing through the body of the instrument rotates the vane and registers a vol-

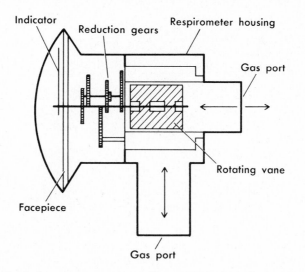

Fig. 9-7. Mechanical rotameter—cutaway diagram of the Wright respirometer. A large-bladed rotating vane mounted on jeweled bearings drives reduction gears connected to the main indicator arm. Two gas ports allow measurements of totalized volume, either inspiratory or expiratory, depending on the port to which the connection is made. Not pictured is a small indicator arm, which marks volumes larger than 1 liter on the facepiece; also omitted are instrument controls for engaging or disengaging the vane and for resetting the indicators to zero. (From British Oxygen Co., Ltd.: Operating instructions, Wright respirometer, print No. 630207, Issue **3**:6, Aug. 1971.)

ume (Fig. 9-7). The respirometer not only is suitable for measurement of lung volumes such as VC, but also is ideal for ventilation tests such as VT and V̇E. One such device, the Wright respirometer, can be used to measure volumes at flows between 3 and 300 L/min. At flows above 300 L/min the vane is subject to distortion and therefore should not be used to measure FVC when the subject is capable of flows greater than 300 L/min. At flows less than 3 L/min the inertia of the vane/gear system causes erroneous measurements. The special advantage of the respirometer is its compact size and practicality in the bedside setting. The respirometer registers tenths of liters up to 1 liter on one scale and liters up to 100 liters on another scale, which makes it ideal for measuring volumes over longer periods.

A newer adaptation of the rotameter includes a photo cell and light source that is interrupted by the movement of the vane. This interruption, or pulsing of the

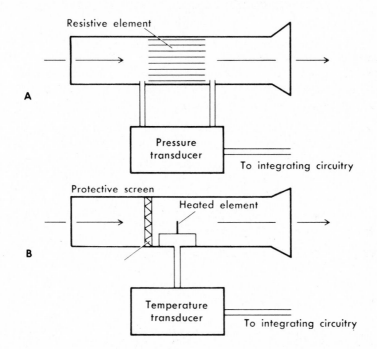

Fig. 9-8. Two conventional pneumotachometers. **A,** Pressure differential type of pneumotachometer in which a resistive element causes a pressure drop proportional to the flow of gas through the tube. Sensitive pressure transducers monitor the pressure before and after the resistive element and convert the differential into a signal that varies as the flow changes. The volume passing through the pneumotachometer can be calculated by integrating the flow over the time interval for which the flow occurred; this is done by an electronic integrating circuit. **B,** Heat transfer type of pneumotachometer in which a heated element of small mass responds to gas flow by heat loss. As the element cools, a greater current is needed to maintain a constant temperature; the current change is proportional to gas flow, and a continuous signal is supplied to an integrating circuit as for the pressure-drop pneumotachometer.

light beam, can be converted to an analog output that is converted to a flow signal. The flow signal can then be timed and integrated to produce volumes and FEVт measurements. The signal thus produced may not be linear at high or low flows, because of inertia or distortion of the rotating vane.

The remaining types of flow-sensing spirometers all use tubes through which laminar airflow is possible (see Appendix, Useful Equations). The second type of flow-sensing device is a tube with a resistive element that allows gas to flow through it but causes a pressure drop. The pressure differential is measured by means of a sensitive pressure transducer, which converts the difference in pressure into a signal that is proportional to the flow of gas (Fig. 9-8, *A*). The resistive element is usually a screen or similar device that allows gas to flow through without undue back pressure, while at the same time causing enough of a pressure drop to produce a signal. The signal from the pressure transducer is electronically integrated for a given interval to derive volume measurements.

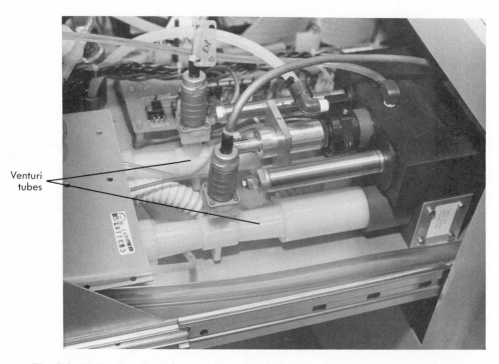

Venturi
tubes

Fig. 9-9. Thermal conductivity type of pneumotachometer. Venturi tubes contain paired stainless steel probe wires maintained at two different temperatures exceeding body temperature and connected by a Wheatstone bridge. The Venturi tube streamlines gas flow (into laminar flow), and the temperature of the wires is decreased in proportion to the mass of the gas and its flow. Two flow sensors are used; one measures expiratory flow, and the other serves as a reference. (Courtesy Gould Medical Instruments, Dayton, Ohio, and Missouri Baptist Hospital, St. Louis, Mo.)

The third commonly used type of pneumotachometer is that which is based on the cooling effect of gas flow. A heated element (usually a platinum wire or small bead of metal) is situated in a tube (Figs. 9-8, *B*, and 9-9). Gas flow past the element causes a temperature drop, so that more current is required to maintain the preset temperature of the element. The amount of current needed to maintain the temperature is proportional to the magnitude of the gas flow. The heated element is usually of very small mass, so that slight changes in gas flow can be detected. (Temperature change occurs more rapidly in objects of small mass.) The signal is applied to an integrator circuit, as with the pressure transducer pneumotachometer, to derive volume measurements.

A fourth type of flow-sensing instrument is designed according to the principle of vortex shedding. A flow tube is constructed with struts placed in the airstream so that gas flowing over the struts is broken up into waves called vortices. An ultrasonic crystal downstream of the strut transmits high-frequency sound waves through the turbulent gas flow to a receiving crystal on the opposite side (Fig. 9-10). The size of the strut and flow tube determine the size of the vortices and allow the device to be calibrated so that each vortex passing through the ultrasonic beam produces a pulse. The number of pulses is proportional to flow and, when combined with integrating circuitry, provides measurement of volumes. The ultrasonic pneumotachometer is relatively insensitive to gas composition, temperature, or humidity, although accumulation of moisture on the struts or ultrasonic transducers can cause erroneous readings.

Pneumotachometers with suitable analog outputs require integrating circuitry in order to produce volume and timed flow measurements. When used with suitable gas analyzers and breathing circuits, they may be used for the following measurements:

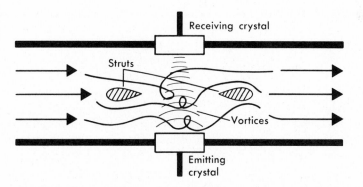

Fig. 9-10. Ultrasonic flow sensor. A beam of ultrasonic waves is emitted by one crystal and received by another crystal on the opposite side of the flow tube. Gas flowing in streamline passes over struts in the tube and forms vortices. This is called *vortex shedding* and changes the frequency of the transmitted ultrasound waves. Appropriate signals are processed electronically to derive flow and volume measurements. Flow (and volume) can be measured for gas moving in either direction.

1. Lung volumes, including TLC and RV
2. Ventilation, including V_T and $\dot{V}_E$
3. Distribution tests
4. Pulmonary mechanics, including MVV, FEV_T, $FEV_T\%$, and flow rates

Pulmonary function testing with the pneumotachometer offers some advantages over volume displacement spirometry setups. The most obvious of these is the ability to do precise testing with lightweight compact units. The fact that a signal is generated without the mechanical action of a spirometer or bellows allows for direct processing of information. Strip chart or X-Y recorders can be directly connected to the basic pneumotachometer/integrator setup to produce hard copy data along with a digital readout of test results. In addition, the electronics required for signal processing may be easily interfaced with a microprocessor or separate computer.

There are some disadvantages associated with flow-based testing units. Pneumotachography is based on the assumption that a certain flow will generate a proportional signal. However, at extremes of flow (low or high), the signal generated may become nonproportional, or nonlinear. This is true of almost every type of pneumotachometer. Some systems use two pneumotachometers, one for high flows, as in forced breathing, and one for low flows, as in V_T excursions. The signals from this type of system may be more linear across the range of the pneumotachometer because the range itself is reduced. Most units "linearize" the signal electronically or by software before any parameters are measured so that the values will be accurate to within acceptable limits. Other corrections, such as converting results to BTPS, can be done easily by electronic means. Most units that use resistive elements to cause a pressure differential include a means of heating the element to above body temperature to avoid deviations resulting from condensation of water in the element. Rotameter, pressure differential, and thermal conductivity types of pneumotachometers may all be affected by the composition of the gas being measured. Changes in gas density or viscosity most often require special corrections to the output of the transducer in order to obtain accurate volumes. For the most part, these corrections are performed by computer software. A flow-sensing spirometer may be calibrated with ambient air, but then used to analyze mixtures containing helium, oxygen, or other test gases, provided the software is designed to correct for differences in gas composition for each individual test.

The final results from any measurement done with a pneumotachometer can be only as accurate as the circuitry that converts the input signal to actual readout values or hard copy tracing. Those pulmonary function parameters that are measured on a time base (FEV_T, MVV, $FEF_{200-1200}$, etc.) require precise timing mechanisms as well as volume or flow measurements. The most common timing mechanism in pneumotachography is the initiation of a specific test interval by a minimum flow or pressure change. Recording flow or volume on a time base begins when the flow generated through the pneumotachometer has reached a threshold limit, usually around 0.1 to 0.2 L/sec. Instruments that initiate timing in response to a pressure change usually have a similar threshold that must be achieved to begin recording the input signal. Calibration and quality control techniques for spirometers and flow-sensing devices according to individual tests are included in Chapter 11.

PULMONARY GAS ANALYZERS

The determination of the composition of pulmonary gases is an integral part of tests for distribution of inspired gas, FRC, RV, diffusion, and exercise testing.

One of the most commonly used gas analyzers is that which determines the concentration of N_2 in respired gas. The single-breath and 7-minute N_2 distributions, as well as the open-circuit method of determining the RV (see Chapter 1), require N_2 analyzers. A common N_2 analyzer is the Giesler tube ionizer (Fig. 9-11). This instrument consists of a needle valve that samples the desired gas, an enclosed ionization chamber with two electrodes, and a photocell. A vacuum pump maintains a constant pressure in the ionization chamber by bleeding gas through the needle valve. When a current is supplied to the electrodes, the N_2 between them is ionized and emits light. This light, after being filtered, is collected by a phototube. The intensity of the light is directly related to the concentration of N_2 in the sample, provided that the current, distance between electrodes, and pressure remain constant. The phototube converts the light signal into an electrical signal, which is linearized and can then be used as input to an appropriate meter or computing circuit. The signal from the N_2 analyzer can be

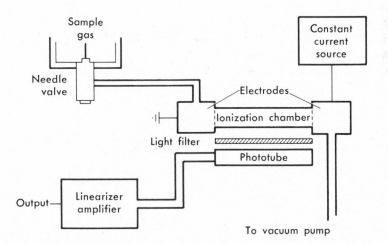

Fig. 9-11. Giesler tube gas analyzer. The Giesler tube gas analyzer is commonly used for nitrogen analysis. A vacuum pump draws a gas sample into an ionization chamber, where the ionized gas emits light (all except the desired gas if filtered), which is monitored by a phototube. The phototube transmits a signal proportional to the intensity of the light, and the signal allows rapid gas analysis. (From Hewlett-Packard: Application note AN 729, San Diego, Calif, 1973.)

combined with the volume signal from electronic units to provide instantaneous, or breath-by-breath, measurements of N_2 volumes as necessary for open-circuit determinations of the FRC. An older method of measuring the FRC by the open-circuit method depended on measuring the concentration of N_2 in a large volume of expired gas (washed out) in a Tissot spirometer. This method was susceptible to error because of the measurement of a small concentration of N_2 in a large volume. The accumulation of breath-by-breath measurements has obviated this difficulty to a certain extent, since the FRC calculation is not dependent on a single measurement.

The calculation of FRC and RV by the closed-circuit method requires an He analyzer or catharometer. The catharometer measures the concentration of He in the sample gas by means of a thermal conductivity sensing unit (Fig. 9-12). Two glass-coated thermistor beads serve as sensing elements and are connected by a Wheatstone bridge circuit. The sensors change temperature and hence electrical resistance as a function of the molecular weight of the gases surrounding them. One bead serves as a reference, so that a difference in the concentration of gases

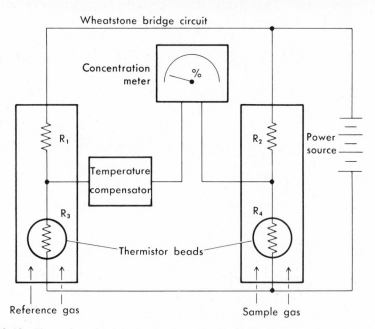

Fig. 9-12. Thermal conductivity analyzer (catharometer), such as is used for analysis of He. Two thermistor beads (temperature-sensitive electrical resistors) are connected in a Wheatstone bridge circuit. When the thermistors are subjected to the same gas, their electrical resistance decreases equally and the concentration meter registers zero (by calibration). When the sample gas is applied to the sample thermistor (R_4 in this example) and the reference thermistor is submitted to a reference gas, a potential occurs and deflects the concentration meter by a proportionate amount. (From Bourns, Inc.: Life systems operations instruction manual, Model LS114-5, Riverside, Calif.)

at the two sensors can be detected because of the differences in heat conducted away at either of the sensors. Since the closed-circuit technique mixes only a small volume of He in the larger volume of the lungs and breathing system (see Chapter 1), the catharometer usually is calibrated for measuring small fractional concentrations of He (0 to 10%). The small necessary range allows for good linearity and sensitivity.

Perhaps the most sophisticated means of measuring the concentrations of respiratory gases is the mass spectrometer. A sample of gas is drawn into a capillary tube by a vacuum pump, which simultaneously reduces the pressure to a preset level. An electron beam ionizes the sample gases, which are directed into a beam by an electrostatic lens. As the beam passes through a magnetic field, the ions of the various constituent gases separate according to their specific mass and electrical charge (Fig. 9-13). Ion collectors gather the various ions and amplify their charges into a usable signal for monitoring or analog computations. Analysis of the composition of a gas mixture on a breath-by-breath basis offers the possibility of performing several different tests requiring gas analysis with the same measuring device, as well as in vivo monitoring of respiratory gases. Although mass spectrometers allow gas analysis for such various tests as N_2 washout or CO diffusing capacity with a single analyzer, their relative cost is somewhat prohibitive. Mass spectrometers also require a certain degree of training and experience on the part of the technologist, so that they are probably better

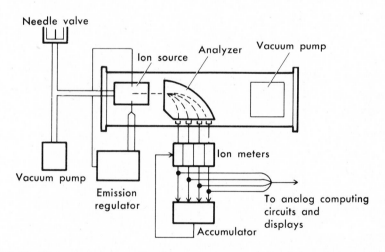

Fig. 9-13. Mass spectrometer. Respiratory gases are analyzed thus: a vacuum pump draws a small sample of gas into an ionizing chamber, where a current sufficient to ionize the desired gases is supplied; a magnetic analyzer separates the ion beam into constituent gases according to their charge/mass ratio; the separated beams of ions are collected by distinct detectors, and the relative concentration of each gas is determined in opposition to a reference gas. These parameters emerge as signals to computing and display circuits. (From Perkin-Elmer Medical Instruments: Advertising brochure for Model 1100, medical gas analyzer, Pomona, Calif.)

suited to monitoring multiple patients simultaneously, rather than being used for a single test. In areas such as exercise testing or anesthesia, where several gases need to be monitored at one time, the mass spectrometer may be the instrument of choice, despite its increased cost and upkeep.

Several respiratory gas analyzers are based on the principle of infrared absorption to measure gas concentrations. This technique is most often used in CO analyzers for the DL_{CO} tests and CO_2 analyzers for exercise testing and bedside monitoring in critical care. Two beams of infrared radiation pass through two parallel cells, one containing gas to be sampled and the other containing a comparison gas. The two beams converge on a single infrared detector (Fig. 9-14). Between the test cells and the infrared source an interrupter alternates beams to the cells. When the test gas and comparison gas are the same concentration, the radiation reaching the detector is constant; but when the sample gas is introduced, the amount of radiation reaching the detector varies in a rhythmic fashion. This causes a vibration in the detector that is translated into a signal proportional to the difference between the two beams. This type of system is readily adaptable to measurements involving small changes in gas concentrations such as those necessary in tests of diffusing capacity.

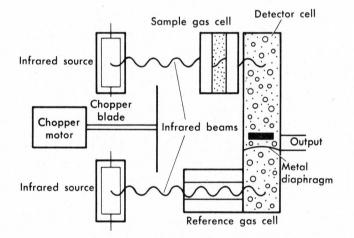

Fig. 9-14. Essential components of an infrared gas analyzer, such as is used for determination of CO_2 and CO concentrations. Infrared sources emit beams that pass through parallel cells, one containing a reference gas and the other the sample gas to be analyzed. A rotating blade "chops" the infrared beams in a rhythmic fashion, so that when both the reference and sample cells contain the same gas, there is no variation in the radiation reaching either half of the detector cell. When the sample gas is introduced, differing amounts of radiation reach the two halves of the detector cell, causing the diaphragm separating the compartments of the detector to oscillate. This oscillation is transformed into a signal proportional to the difference in gas concentrations. The infrared analyzer is ideal for determination of small concentration changes in gas samples. (From Beckman Instruments, Inc.: Medical gas analyzer LB-2: operating instructions, FM-149997-301, Schiller Park, Ill., 1972.)

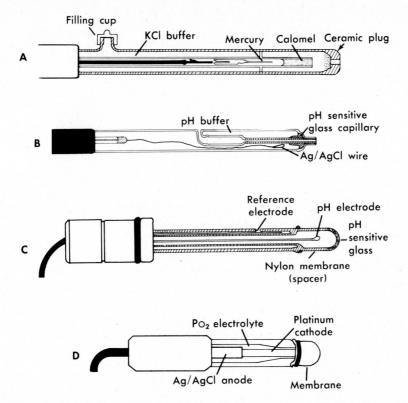

Fig. 9-15. pH, P_{CO_2}, and P_{O_2} electrodes. **A,** The reference pH electrode contains a sealed-in potassium chloride buffer and a porous ceramic plug that allow electrical contact to the exterior; the reference wire develops a constant potential. **B,** The pH-measuring electrode contains buffer and a silver–silver chloride wire. A thin capillary tube constructed of pH-sensitive glass allows a potential to develop, which varies with the pH of the solution in the capillary. The difference between the variable potential and the constant potential of the reference electrode indicates the pH of the sample. **C,** The P_{CO_2} (Severinghaus) electrode is an adaptation of the pH electrode. The pH electrode contains a sealed-in buffer, whereas the reference electrode is the other half-cell and is in communication with a P_{CO_2} electrolyte of aqueous bicarbonate. The entire glass electrode is encased in a Lucite jacket (not shown) containing the electrolyte and capped with a Teflon membrane that is permeable to CO_2. A nylon material covers the tip of the glass electrode to act as a spacer to keep the electrolyte in contact with the pH-sensitive glass. CO_2 diffuses through the Teflon membrane, dissolves in the electrolyte, and alters the pH. The pH change is displayed as partial pressure of CO_2. **D,** The P_{O_2} electrode contains a platinum cathode and a silver–silver chloride anode. The top is protected by a polyethylene or polypropylene membrance, which allows O_2 to diffuse. O_2 migrates to the cathode, which has a slightly negative charge. The O_2 is reduced by picking up free electrons that have come from the silver–silver chloride anode through the phosphate-potassium chloride buffer. Changes in the voltage result from changes in the amount of O_2 dissolved in the electrolyte, and this reflects the P_{O_2}. A voltmeter measures the amount of change and registers it as partial pressure of O_2.

BLOOD GAS ELECTRODES AND RELATED DEVICES

Measurements of arterial blood gases routinely include determination of P_{O_2}, P_{CO_2}, and pH, and calculation of $S_{a_{O_2}}$, HCO_3^-, total CO_2, base excess, and several other parameters dependent on one or more of the three primary electrodes.

The glass pH electrode contains a solution of constant pH on one side of the glass membrane. The solution from which pH is to be measured is brought into contact with the other side of the pH-sensitive glass (Fig. 9-15). The difference in pH on either side causes a potential difference, or voltage. To measure this potential, two half-cells are used: one for the constant solution and one for the unknown solution. The constant solution half-cell is usually a silver–silver chloride wire. The external half-cell in the unknown solution is usually a saturated calomel electrode and is called the reference electrode. These half-cells are connected to a millivolt display that is simply calibrated in pH units. The voltage difference between the two electrodes is proportional to the pH difference of the solutions. Since the pH of one solution is constant, the developed potential is a measure of the pH of the unknown solution.

The P_{CO_2} electrode (Severinghaus electrode) measures P_{CO_2} potentiometrically by an adaptation of a pH measurement. A combined pH glass and reference electrode is in contact with a solution behind a gas-permeable membrane. CO_2 diffuses across the membrane in both directions as partial pressure changes, causing equilibration between the electrolyte and the sample. CO_2 is hydrated in the electrolyte according to the equation:

$$CO_2 + H_2O \rightleftarrows H_2CO_3 \rightleftarrows H^+ + HCO_3^-$$

The change in H^+ concentration is proportional to the change in P_{CO_2}. The electrode senses the change in P_{CO_2} as a change in pH of the electrolyte and develops a voltage that is exponentially related to P_{CO_2}, so that a tenfold increase in P_{CO_2} is approximately equal to a decrease of 1 pH unit (Fig. 9-15).

The P_{O_2} electrode (Clark electrode) produces a current at a constant voltage that is proportional to the O_2 tension to which the electrode is exposed. This current is a result of the flow of electrons produced by the reduction of O_2 at the cathode according to the equation:

$$O_2 + 2H_2O + 4e^- \rightarrow 4OH^-$$

Fig. 9-16. A, Automated blood gas analyzer, including automatic flushing and calibration, tonometering of calibrating solutions, and on-line display of results and calibrations using a built-in computer and video display terminal; pH, P_{CO_2}, P_{O_2} and Hb are measured; HCO_3^-, total CO_2, standard bicarbonate, base excess, and saturation are calculated. **B,** Automated co-oximeter; a small sample (approximately 0.2 ml) of blood is aspirated, hemolyzed, mixed with diluent, and held in a cuvette while spectrophotometric measurements are made to determine $S_{a_{O_2}}$, vol% O_2, COHb, MetHb, and total Hb. Flushing and zeroing of the spectrophotometer are performed after each sample. (**A** courtesy Radiometer America, Westlake, Ohio; **B** courtesy Instrumentation Laboratories, Lexington, Mass.)

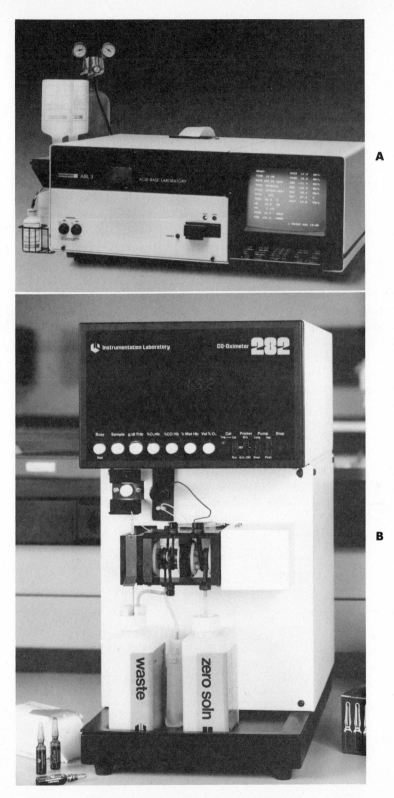

Fig. 9-16. For legend see opposite page.

Each O_2 molecule can take up 4 electrons, and the greater the number of O_2 molecules present (Po_2), the greater the current. The cathode of the electrode is covered by a membrane that is permeable to gases but not to other contaminants or ions (Fig. 9-15). Electrons are provided by a silver–silver chloride anode. A Po_2 electrolyte is enclosed in a reserve chamber around the anode and supplied to the tip by an annular capillary tube. Although the gas-measuring (Po_2 and Pco_2) electrodes and the pH electrode system can each be used separately, all three are usually implemented together in a blood gas analyzer (Fig. 9-16, *A*).

The transcutaneous O_2 electrode ($tcPo_2$) operates on a principle similar to that of the Clark electrode. The $tcPo_2$ electrode consists of a ring-shaped silver anode that is heated by a coil to cause hyperemia at the skin placement site. Inside the circular anode is a series of thin platinum cathodes (Fig. 9-17). All of the elements are enclosed in a plastic case, except for the face of the sensor, which is covered by a Teflon membrane. A KCl electrolyte is placed between the membrane and the sensor, and then another drop of electrolyte and a cellophane membrane are added to form a double membrane. The flow of current between the silver and platinum electrodes is proportional to the O_2 tension. A feedback mechanism keeps the temperature constant at the skin site to compensate for changes caused by capillary blood flow, thus stabilizing the measurement. $tcPo_2$ and Pa_{O_2} are not identical, but the gradient between them tends to be relatively constant, so that $tcPo_2$ can be a valuable measurement once the gradient has been established. Conditions that affect perfusion of the skin may alter the gradient between arterial and transcutaneous PO_2.

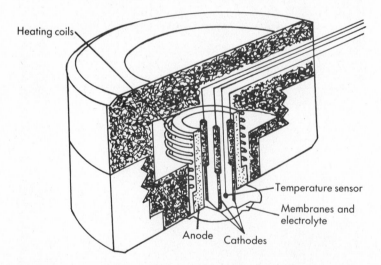

Fig. 9-17. Transcutaneous Po_2 electrode. A cross-sectional diagram of the components of the $tcPo_2$ electrode shows a circular anode around a series of cathodes and a temperature sensor. A heating coil causes local hyperemia so that surface Po_2 more closely resembles Pa_{O_2}. A double membrane separates the electrode proper from the skin (see text).

The spectrophotometric oximeter (Fig. 9-16, *B*) uses the principle of light absorption to analyze the saturation of Hb with O_2. In addition, the concentration of carboxyhemoglobin (COHb—the Hb bound with CO) can be determined. The oximeter analyzes the absorption of light at three different wavelengths; at each of these wavelengths two or more of the species of Hb have identical absorbances (Fig. 9-18). These common points are termed isobestic points. A wavelength that is isobestic for oxyhemoglobin, deoxyhemoglobin (reduced Hb), and COHb is 548 nm. At this particular wavelength the absorbance of a mixture of the three pigments is directly proportional to the total concentration of Hb. An isobestic point for oxyhemoglobin and deoxyhemoglobin is 568 nm. The absorbance of COHb at this point is considerably higher; thus a change in absorbance at 568 nm

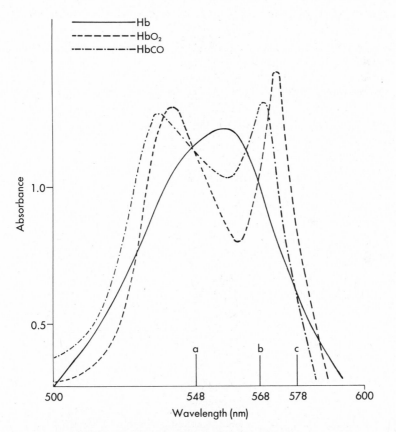

Fig. 9-18. Principle of spectrophotometric oximetry. Absorbance measurements are made at three distinct wavelengths (548, 568, 578 nm) as light passes through a blood sample. At 548 nm all three forms of Hb (Hb, HbO_2 and COHB) have identical absorbances. At 568 nm only Hb and HbO_2 coincide, whereas at 578 nm Hb and COHb coincide. The solution of three simultaneous equations provides the relative proportions of each species, as well as the total Hb (see text).

compared with 548 nm indicates a change in the concentration of COHb relative to the sum of the concentrations of the other two species. The isobestic point for deoxyhemoglobin and COHb is 578 nm, and oxyhemoglobin absorbance is considerably greater. The degree of difference indicates a change in the concentration of oxyhemoglobin relative to the other two pigments. By analyzing the values for absorbance and solving simultaneous equations, the total Hb concentration, oxyhemoglobin, and COHb saturation can be determined.

The spectrophotometric oximeter provides essential information regarding the O_2-Hb reaction, particularly in instances where increased concentrations of COHb are present. It should be noted that most automated blood gas analyzers calculate the saturation of Hb using the measured Pa_{O_2} and pH and predetermined values for temperature and partial pressure at which the Hb is 50% saturated (P_{50}). These estimates may result in a significant overestimation of the true saturation in the presence of COHb or abnormal hemoglobins, such as methemoglobin. The oximeter provides a more accurate estimate of the actual O_2 saturation of the blood but may give spuriously low Hb, HBO_2, and COHb readings if significant amounts of other pigments (such as methemoglobin) are present. Other substances that cause light scattering in the blood specimen may also cause false readings.

The fiberoptic ear oximeter (Fig. 9-19) is designed to analyze oxyhemoglobin saturation in vivo. The ear oximeter uses a flexible fiberoptic probe to transmit a narrow band of light through the antihelix or pinna of the ear. Measurements are made at multiple (as many as eight) separate wavelengths from 650 to 1050 nm. Light pulses at each of the desired wavelengths are transmitted through the earlobe approximately 20 times/sec. A second light path is used as a reference to

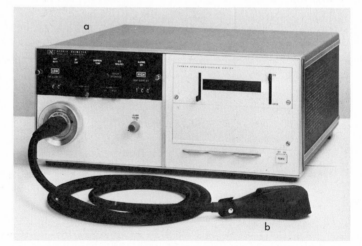

Fig. 9-19. Hewlett-Packard ear oximeter. *a,* Console containing the light source, filter detectors, analog and digital signal processors, and display; *b,* fiberoptic cable and ear probe (see text). (Courtesy Hewlett-Packard, Waltham, Mass.)

maintain the sensitivity of the instrument. An optical detector provides signals that are digitized and passed to a microprocessor. Simultaneous absorbance equations are then solved to determine the oxyhemoglobin concentration relative to the total Hb.

The ear oximeter allows discrete or continuous measurements of saturation. Calibration is accomplished automatically by measuring the light intensities at each of the light wavelengths without any light absorption and storing the measurements for reference. Certain pigments such as bilirubin or Cardio-green dye may affect the accuracy of the saturation measurement if they are present in sufficient concentrations. Normally saturation measured by ear oximetry correlates well with saturation determined spectrophotometrically over the ranges normally encountered clinically (70% to 100% saturation).

BODY PLETHYSMOGRAPHS

Two basic types of plethysmographs are in common clinical use: the traditional pressure plethysmograph and the newer "flow" box. The pressure box is based on the principle that pressure changes in the sealed box can be calibrated as volume changes, as long as the temperature is constant (see Chapter 11 for calibration techniques). Since the pressure plethysmograph is a closed system, volumes exchanged between the subject's lungs and the box do not directly cause pressure changes; pressure fluctuations result from the compression and decompression of gas within both the thorax and the box. By making V_{TG} and Raw measurements at rapid rates (panting), very small leaks are acceptable. "Slow" leaks are sometimes introduced to facilitate thermal equilibrium by connecting a long length of small-bore tubing to the atmospheric side of the box pressure transducer, or connecting it to a glass bottle within the box. Pressure plethysmographs are best suited to maneuvers that measure small volume changes (100 ml or less).

The flow box uses a flow transducer in the box wall to measure volume changes in the box. The subject breathes through a pneumotachometer that is connected to the room. Gas in the box is compressed or decompressed and the pressure change measured as gas flows out of the box through the flow opening. Flow through the wall is integrated, corrections applied, and the volume change recorded as the sum of the volume passing through the wall and the volume compressed. The flow type of plethysmograph requires computerization but does not need to be rigorously airtight. In addition, maximal breathing maneuvers, such as the VC, may be recorded with the subject in the flow box.

In each type of plethysmograph (Fig. 9-20, *B*) a pneumotachometer is necessary for measuring airflow at the mouth for the Raw maneuver. The flow signal is also used to determine the end-expiratory point for shutter closure in the V_{TG} measurement. The pneumotachometer must be linear across the range of flows typically measured (0-2 L/sec), for both spontaneous breathing and panting. Heated Fleisch or Silverman types of pneumotachometers (pressure differential) are usually implemented in the box. A mouth pressure transducer is normally coupled to an electronic shutter mechanism. The transducer records mouth pres-

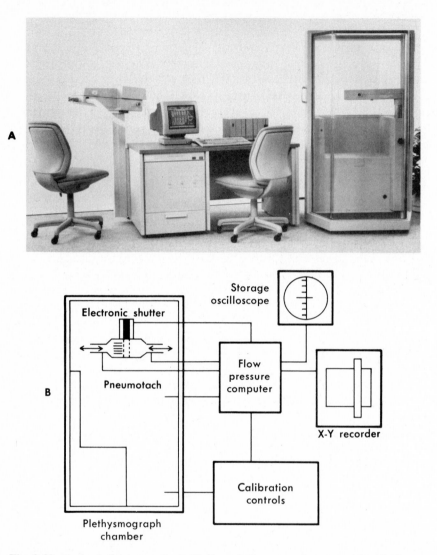

Fig. 9-20. Body plethysmograph. **A,** Modern plethysmograph setup, with a highly transparent box that can be used as a pressure or flow box, self-contained calibration equipment, and computerized data reduction and display. **B,** Diagram of plethysmograph components: pneumotachometer with automatic shutter mechanism; body box proper; interface/computer for reduction of pressure, flow, and volume signals; storage oscilloscope and X-Y recorder; and calibration instruments with controls (see text and Chapter 1). (**A** courtesy Medical Graphics Corporation, St. Paul, Minn.)

sures, usually in the range of 0 to 20 cm H_2O, when the airway is occluded. Some older systems require the technologist to close the shutter, by remote control, at end-expiration. This is accomplished by observing the tidal breathing maneuver on an oscilloscope and actuating the shutter at end-expiration. Most modern systems allow the shutter to be closed automatically at a preselected point in the breathing cycle.

Recording of the breathing maneuvers may be accomplished by one of several techniques. Most plethysmograph systems use a storage oscilloscope to record the breathing maneuvers. The tracings may then be photographed or transferred to a plotter or X-Y recorder. On computerized systems the breathing maneuvers may be stored as digital data and then displayed on the video screen. Calculation of tangents, or angles, from the standard oscilloscope is usually performed by rotating a graticule to align its axes with those of the loop and then reading the appropriate value. Most computerized systems allow the operator to select a "best fit" line drawn by the computer or to manipulate the tangent via the computer keyboard. Computerized plethysmographs offer the advantage of providing lung volume and airway resistance information immediately on completion of the maneuver. This aids the technologist in selecting appropriate maneuvers for averaging, as well as in repeating the test as required when spurious values are obtained.

Most plethysmographs include the necessary hardware to perform physical calibration (see Chapter 11). These typically include a pressure manometer for mouth pressure calibration, a flow generator for pneumotachometer calibration, and some sort of volume displacement device for box pressure (flow) calibration. Computerized systems allow automated calibration of transducers by means of software-generated correction factors, along with the actual physical calibration. A few manufacturers supply quality control devices such as the isothermal lung analog (see Chapter 11).

Subject comfort and ease in performing the required maneuvers are important features of the plethysmograph, since many subjects may become claustrophobic inside the box. Older boxes relied on solid materials (plywood, etc.) to provide the necessary rigidity to the enclosure; newer boxes made of durable plastics are largely transparent and less confining for the subject (Fig. 9-20, *A*). Also important is an adequate communication system to allow voice contact with the subject. Since panting against a closed shutter is somewhat difficult, some individuals require continuous coaching in order to elicit valid maneuvers.

RESPIRATORY INDUCTIVE PLETHYSMOGRAPHS

The most recent technique allowing measurement of pulmonary function is based on the principle of inductive plethysmography. The respiratory inductive plethysmograph (RIP) consists of two or more Teflon-insulated coils of wire sewn into elastic bands that are connected to oscillator circuits (Fig. 9-21). The elastic bands are then positioned around the chest and abdomen. Breathing excursions stretch the bands, causing a change in the inductance in the oscillator circuits. The distention of the coils within the elastic bands is proportional to the

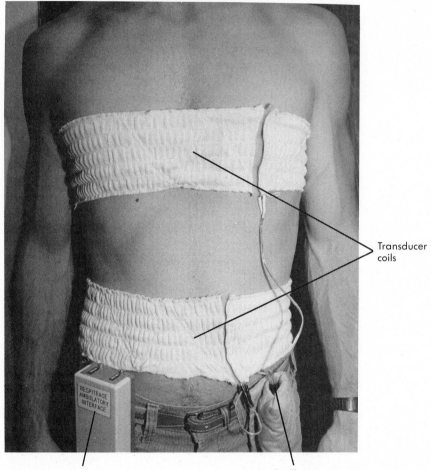

Transducer
coils

Interface   Oscillators

Fig. 9-21. Respiratory inductive plethysmograph (RIP). Two elastic bands with Teflon-coated coils sewn in are placed around the rib cage and abdomen; oscillators connected to the coils (hanging from the belt here) monitor changes in the cross-sectional areas of the two compartments as changes in inductance. By calibration, the changes in cross-sectional areas can be converted to volume changes in the two compartments to record V_T, rate, and timing of inspiration and expiration.

change in the cross-sectional areas of the rib cage and abdomen, respectively. Measurement of volumes (V_T, etc.) is accomplished by summing the signals from the two compartments. The validity of this technique is based on the assumption that lung volume change is described with two degrees of freedom— change in thoracic volume plus change in abdominal volume.

The respiratory inductive plethysmograph must be calibrated so that changes in rib cage and abdomen cross-sectional areas may be translated into volumes. This is usually accomplished by measuring the relative contribution of the inductances of the two coils as the actual volume change is recorded by means of a spirometer or pneumotachometer. If volumes are measured with two different breathing patterns, a "best fit" line can be generated, which is used to derive calibration factors for each of the transducers. This may be expressed:

$$\frac{RC}{SP} + \frac{AB}{SP} = 1$$

where

    RC = Rib cage contribution to the tidal volume
    AB = Abdominal contribution to the tidal volume
    SP = Volume as measured by spirometry

The calibration "factors" thus obtained are applied to the output of the two channels as gains, and the respiratory inductive plethysmograph may be used to measure V_T, respiratory rate, timing of inspiration, expiration, and total respiratory cycle time (T_I, T_E, and T_{tot}, respectively). Various indices relating the extent of paradoxical and asynchronous movement of the two compartments may also be quantified.

Because calibration is crucial to accurate measurement of volume change, a microprocessor or small dedicated computer is often used to derive calibration factors once the transducer bands have been placed. The computer may also be used to store and process data derived from the plethysmograph and to display graphic representations of the breathing pattern. Changes in body position may affect the calibration factors, so it is important to be able to calibrate quickly the inductive plethysmograph. Once calibration is complete, volume changes can be determined without physical connection to the subject's airway, as is the case with standard methods of assessing ventilation. Respiratory inductive plethysmography is ideally suited to the study of breathing patterns in a variety of disorders, as well as in those subjects in whom connection of a spirometer to the airway is impractical (infants, ventilated patients, etc.).

RECORDERS AND RELATED DEVICES

An integral part of pulmonary function testing is the recording of spirograms, the various distribution and ventilation tests, lung volumes, and $D_{L_{CO}}$ maneuvers. From its inception, pulmonary function testing has concerned itself with the spirogram. The kymograph, a rotating drum carrying chart paper, was the initial instrument for producing a hard copy record of respiratory movements (Fig. 9-1).

A kymograph is a mechanical recorder in the strictest sense, meaning that the physical movement of the bell or bellows is translated into an equivalent movement of the pen across the paper. Normally corrections for BTPS must be made. Calibrated chart paper eliminates some corrections, but the assumption is made that the subject is at 37° C and the spirometer is at 25° C, which may not always be accurate. Several of the most commonly used spirometers incorporate the kymograph recording system. A second common type of recorder includes those instruments that use mechanical recording on an X-Y type of graph. A constant-speed motor provides movement along the time axis (X), and the spirometer provides the volume (Y) input. This principle is used in many bellows types of spirometers and in some rolling-seal spirometers. For both kymographs and simple chart recorders, the accuracy of the timing motor driving the graph paper is essential for valid measurements of flow. The paper speed should be at least 2 cm/sec; higher speeds are preferable. The volume axis of the graph should have a scale of at least 10 mm/L. To accurately reproduce the "start-of-test," the paper should be moving at a constant speed before recording the volume deflection. Not all recorders fulfill this requirement. The recorder must be able to show at least 10 seconds of volume accumulation after recording begins, and it is preferable to use a little more paper than to prematurely terminate the maneuver.

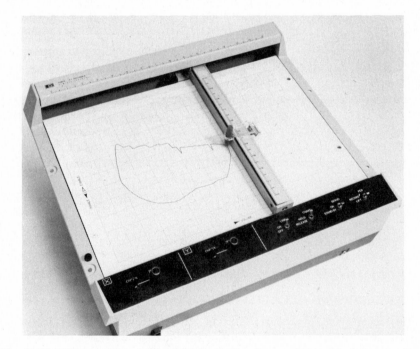

Fig. 9-22. X-Y type of recording device capable of accepting analog inputs for flow, volume, gas concentration, or other typical DC signals, and graphing either against a time base or by plotting one input against another. (Courtesy Hewlett-Packard, San Diego, Calif.)

The successor to the mechanical X-Y recorder is the electronic X-Y recorder. In this instance a two-axis recorder receives electrical input in the form of signals. The signals drive small motors that control the pen movement (Fig. 9-22). The advantage of this type of instrument is that several tests can be recorded by supplying an appropriate input signal, in addition to the volume-time spirogram. The signal generated by a simple pneumotachometer or analog device can be recorded in spirographic form. Gas analyzers coupled to such an instrument allow easy recording of tests such as the SB_{N_2} and multiple-breath N_2 washout. The electronic recorder is easy to calibrate; a known voltage can be applied and the recorder gains adjusted to produce an equivalent deflection (1 volt = 1 cm, etc.). Volume transducers that produce analog outputs can then be calibrated against the recorder so that a given volume change in the spirometer causes a proportional deflection on the recorder. Many recorders feature a third dimension for hard copy recording in the form of superimposed time measurements when the main input is not graphed on a time base. For instance, a flow-volume loop plots flow on the vertical axis and volume on the horizontal axis; an X-Y-T recorder can interpose time marks (tics) on the two-dimensional tracing, thus allowing timed volumes to be obtained as a third dimension. Most electronic recorders have variable sensitivity on both axes, which allows for greater flexibility than that provided by a mechanical tracing. Systems equipped with digital readouts or computer graphics as well as an electronic recorder allow for easy comparisons of measured values and the spirogram.

Many types of recorders, particularly strip chart and X-Y electronic types, can be used in conjunction with computer-stored data (see Chapter 10). Most automated pulmonary function systems provide for both computer-generated graphics and an alternate form of hard copy recording. If the computer is equipped with a digital-to-analog converter, then stored data can be used to drive a conventional recorder or plotter that accepts analog (voltage) input signals. A primary advantage of this type of data recording is that the data can be manipulated by the computer to provide corrections, linearization, etc., before being transformed into a hard copy tracing.

SELF-ASSESSMENT QUESTIONS

1. Which of the following are advantages of volume displacement types of spirometers over flow-sensing devices?
    I. They are easily portable.
    II. Direct mechanical recording of spirograms is possible.
    III. They are not affected by the composition of expired gas.
    IV. Unlike the case with flow-based spirometers, $DL_{CO}SB$ can be performed
    a. I, II, III, and IV
    b. I, III, and IV
    c. II and III
    d. III and IV
2. A subject has spirometry performed using a dry rolling-seal spirometer; the spirometry is then repeated using a bellows spirometer. His FVC measured with the bellows is 1.2 liters less than his FVC measured with the rolling seal. Which of the following might be a cause of this difference?

    a. This is normal variation in the FVC.

    b. The bellows may be cracked or sticking.

    c. Bellows-type spirometers typically measure volumes by 0.5 to 1.0 liter less.

    d. All of the above

3. Which of the following accurately describe flow-sensing types of spirometers?

    I. They are slightly more accurate than volume displacement devices.

    II. Volumes are derived by electronic integration of a flow signal.

    III. Lung volume determinations can be performed with appropriate gas analyzers.

    IV. Most types are influenced by gas composition.

    a. I, II, III, and IV

    b. I, III, and IV

    c. II, III, and IV

    d. II and III

4. Which of the following gas analyzers is (are) capable of measuring two or more gases simultaneously?

    a. Giesler tube analyzer

    b. Thermal conductivity type

    c. Mass spectrometer

    d. Wheatstone bridge catharometer

    e. b, c, and d

5. Which of the following gas analyzers is (are) commonly used for measurement of CO_2 and CO concentrations?

    a. Thermal conductivity type

    b. Infrared type

    c. Giesler tube

    d. Spectrophotometer

6. Which of the following measures the partial pressure of O_2 by means of a platinum electrode?

    a. Severinghaus electrode

    b. Clark electrode

    c. Calomel reference electrode

    d. Spectrophotometric oximeter

7. The transcutaneous O_2 electrode:

    a. Operates on a principle similar to the Clark electrode

    b. Uses a platinum cathode

    c. Measures the Pa_{O_2} directly

    d. All of the above

    e. a and b

8. The spectrophotometric oximeter determines the relative concentrations of saturated Hb, desaturated Hb, COHb, and MetHb by:

    a. Comparing absorbances at several wavelengths

    b. Dissociating the various Hb species with light

    c. Extracting O_2 molecules individually

    d. Exposing the Hb to infrared light

9. The Pco_2 electrode (Severinghaus) measures the partial pressure of CO_2 by:

    a. Chemically extracting CO_2 from HCO_3^-

    b. Measuring the change in H^+ as CO_2 is hydrated within the electrode

    c. Comparing the unknown CO_2 with the CO_2 in a sealed electrode

    d. Ionizing CO_2 molecules between two wires

10. Differences between the flow-type plethysmograph and the variable-pressure box include:
   I. The flow box need not be airtight.
   II. Volume changes are measured as pressure changes.
   III. Box volume is determined from flow.
   IV. Mouth pressure measurements are unnecessary.
     a. I, II, and IV
     b. I and III
     c. II and IV
     d. III only

11. The minimum paper speed acceptable for a direct recording of spirometry is:
     a. 2 mm/sec
     b. 10.0 mm/sec
     c. 2 cm/sec
     d. 10 cm/sec

12. The respiratory inductive plethysmograph monitors changes in lung volumes by measuring changes in the frequency of oscillations from transducers; these changes are proportional to:
     a. The cross-sectional area of the rib cage
     b. The transverse diameter of the thorax
     c. The cross-sectional area of the abdomen
     d. The transdiaphragmatic pressure
     e. a and c

SELECTED BIBLIOGRAPHY

Spirometers
Finucane, K.E., Egan, B.A., and Dawson, S.V.: Linearity and frequency response of pneumotachographs, J. Appl. Physiol. **32:**121, 1972.
Fitzgerald, M.X., Smith, A.A., and Gaensler, E.A.: Evaluation of "electronic" spirometers, N. Engl. J. Med. **289:**1283, 1973.
Food and Drug Administration: Proposed rule: medical devices; classification of diagnostic spirometers, Fed. Reg. **44:**63326, 1979.
Gardner, R.M., Hankinson, J.L., and West, B.J.: Evaluating commercially available spirometers, Am. Rev. Respir. Dis. **121:**73, 1980.
Permutt, S.: Office spirometry in clinical practice, Chest **74:**298, 1978.
Sullivan, W.J., Peters, G.M., and Enright, P.L.: Pneumotachographs: theory and clinical applications, Respir. Care **29:**736, 1984.
Wells, H.S., et al.: Accuracy of an improved spirometer for recording fast breathing, J. Appl. Physiol. **14:**451, 1959.

Gas analyzers
Fowler, K.T.: The respiratory mass spectrometer, Phys. Med. Biol. **14:**185, 1969.
Norton, A.C.: Accuracy in pulmonary measurements, Respir. Care **24:**131, 1979.

Blood gas electrodes and related devices
Brown, L.J.: A new instrument for the simultaneous measurement of total hemoglobin, % oxyhemoglobin, % carboxyhemoglobin, % methemoglobin, and O_2 content, IEEE Trans. Biomed. Engr. **27:**132, 1980.
Fahey, P.J., et al.: Clinical evaluation of a new ear oximeter, Am. Rev. Respir. Dis. **127**(suppl.):129, 1983.
Huch, A., and Huch, R.: Transcutaneous, noninvasive monitoring of Po_2, Hosp. Pract. **11:**43, 1976.
Linzmayer, I., Aghdasi, I., and Ishikowa, S.: Clinical applications of ear oximetry, Clin. Res. **23:**350A, 1975.

Rebuck, A.S., Chapman, K.R., and D'urzo, A.: The accuracy and response characteristics of a simplified ear oximeter, Chest **80:**860, 1983.

Rubin, P., Bradbury, S., and Prowse, K.: Comparative study of automatic blood-gas analyzers and their use in analyzing arterial and capillary samples, Br. Med. J. **1:**156, 1979.

Plethysmographs

DuBois, A.B., Bothello, S.Y., and Comroe, J.H.: A new method for measuring airway resistance in man using a body plethysmograph: values in normal subjects and in patients with respiratory disease, J. Clin. Invest. **35:**327, 1956.

DuBois, A.B., et al.: A rapid plethysmographic method for measuring thoracic gas volume: a comparison with nitrogen washout method for measuring functional residual capacity in normal subjects, J. Clin. Invest. **35:**322, 1956.

Leith, D.E., and Mead, J.: Principles of body plethysmography, National Heart, Lung, and Blood Institute—Division of Lung Diseases, 1974.

Respiratory inductive plethysmography

Chadhat, T.S., et al.: Validation of respiratory inductive plethysmography using different calibration procedures, Am. Rev. Respir. Dis. **125:**644, 1982.

Dolfin, T., et al.: Calibration of respiratory inductive plethysmography (Respitrace) in infants, Am. Rev. Respir. Dis. **126:**577, 1982.

Konno, K., and Mead, J.: Measurement of the separate volume changes of rib cage and abdomen during breathing, J. Appl. Physiol. **22:**407, 1972.

Sackner, M.A.: Monitoring of ventilation without physical connection to the airway: a review. In Scott, F.D., Raferty, C.V., and Goulding, L., editors: ISAM Proceedings of the Third International Symposium on Ambulatory Monitoring, London, 1982, Academic Press, Inc.

Recorders

Gardner, R.M., et al.: Spirometry—what paper speed? (abstract), Am. Rev. Respir. Dis. **125:**89, 1982.

CHAPTER TEN

Computers in the pulmonary function laboratory

Computers have become an integral part of almost every pulmonary function testing system because of the tasks typically involved in the reduction of pulmonary function data. These include the solution of many repetitive calculations, data storage and retrieval, printing of reports and graphs, manipulation of signals from various transducers, automated control of the instruments themselves, and various other applications, such as word processing. This chapter examines some of the general components and terminology used with small computer systems, automated data acquisition, important qualities in a pulmonary laboratory system, languages and programming, and some additional practical applications.

Several different levels of computerization are typically found in conjunction with pulmonary function testing systems. Numerous small, portable spirometers use a microprocessor to perform calculations and control various instrument functions such as digital display of data, graph paper control, etc. The next higher level is the microcomputer, either incorporated directly into the pulmonary function system or as a stand-alone instrument that is interfaced to the spirometer and gas analyzers. The microcomputer has replaced the minicomputer to a certain extent, except in laboratories where several instruments are managed by a single computer. Some laboratories use pulmonary function equipment that is interfaced as part of a multiuser system; such systems typically require a mainframe computer, particularly if a large number of users are supported.

The selection of a computerized pulmonary function system must be based on a careful evaluation of the number and complexity of the tests to be performed. Many applications, such as bedside testing, may require only minimal automation, particularly if the volume of tests performed is low. In general, choosing a pulmonary laboratory computer should follow these guidelines:

1. Define the *tasks* that the system will be expected to perform. What tests are required, how many subjects will be tested per month, what degree of sophistication in the reported data is necessary, and will the system be used for other purposes in addition to pulmonary function studies? It is important to identify these tasks in order of importance.

2. Once the tasks have been clearly defined, the *software* that best meets these objectives should be selected. Since pulmonary function software is often specific to a particular instrument, both software and instrument capabilities should be evaluated in reference to the required tasks.

3. *Hardware* that runs the selected software should be the final element in the selection process. In some instances there may be little choice as to the computer hardware, as noted above. If more than one hardware option is available, the system chosen should maximize functions offered by the software.

COMPUTER SYSTEMS

Most microcomputer and minicomputer systems can be divided into component parts similar to those depicted in Fig. 10-1. These components are typical of small computer systems in general, but some may have functions specific to pulmonary function testing.

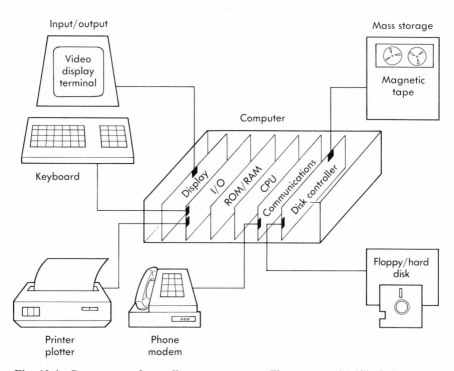

Fig. 10-1. Components of a small computer system. The computer itself includes a central processing unit (CPU) connected to various divisions of memory (ROM/RAM), input/output processors (I/O board), and controllers for the video display, disk drives, and communication devices. Typical input/output devices include the video display (sometimes referred to as the CRT), the keyboard (the standard input device), and printers or plotters. Communications usually include a modem for transmission of data over conventional phone lines. Mass storage devices include magnetic tape drives, and floppy and hard disk drives. Many small computer systems allow for addition of various components simply by plugging in different "cards." Not shown is an interface such as might be used with an analog-digital converter (see text and Fig. 10-2).

Computer or *microprocessor* refers to the "brain" of the system. Microprocessors are sometimes referred to as the central processing unit, or CPU. The microprocessor performs most, if not all, of the instructions provided by the software program. These instructions typically include calculations, storage and retrieval of data from memory, and control of peripheral devices such as printers and disk drives. Microprocessors are classified by the number of "bits" of information that can be handled at one time; a bit is a 0 or 1 in the binary number system. Commonly used in laboratory computer systems are 8-bit, 16-bit, and 32-bit CPUs. In general, 16-bit and 32-bit processors can address more memory and perform calculations more rapidly than smaller microprocessors.

Memory is usually classified as read-only memory (ROM) or random access memory (RAM). The computer's ROM usually contains often-used instructions, such as those for controlling the video display, etc. ROM cannot be changed by a user program but can be altered if the chip containing the instructions is replaced. PROMs (programmable ROM chips) or EPROMS (erasable programmable ROM chips) are often used in just this way in pulmonary function testing systems. By placing instructions to control a particular piece of equipment on a PROM, it becomes quite easy to change to different equipment—just install a new PROM. The RAM available in a computer refers to the amount of memory that is accessible to the user. For most application programs, a certain amount of RAM is necessary. The more complex the program, the greater the amount of RAM required. Many smaller computers maximize their use of available memory by breaking the application program into small segments and then loading only those segments that are required for a certain test; this technique conserves RAM but may slow down overall program execution. Both RAM and ROM are quantified in terms of the number of computer words or *bytes* that they can hold (1 byte = 8 bits). A kilobyte, or K, is the equivalent of 1024 bytes, and most small systems use from 32K up to 640K. In general, an 8-bit microprocessor can address only 64K of memory without special adaptations; a 16-bit CPU can address up to 640K. Although most application programs do not require this much memory in order to run, a large amount of data can be held in memory at one time and calculations speeded up with more available RAM. Mass storage devices (see below) are often classified in terms of megabytes of memory (Mbytes, millions of bytes), as well as in kilobytes).

Input/output (I/O) devices are those parts of the computer system through which data are either entered or displayed. These include the monitor (cathode ray tube, or CRT), the keyboard, mass storage devices such as disk or tape drives, printers, modems (for communications over telephone lines), and special interfaces between the computer and other analog output instruments (see below). While most devices perform either input or output, some function as both under software control (disk drives, modems, and interfaces). Because most of these peripheral devices are quite complex, they often employ highly specialized integrated circuits (chips), or even their own microprocessor, to carry out various tasks.

Mass storage devices include magnetic tape systems, as well as floppy and hard disks. Magnetic tape systems are usually employed on larger multiuser systems (mainframe computers) where a large amount of data must be maintained. Smaller tape drive units are sometimes used for data storage where a large volume of data is recorded but rapid or random retrieval is not required. Some tape units are employed as inexpensive backups to floppy or hard disk systems, as described next. On most dedicated pulmonary function laboratory systems, floppy disk drives (or a combination of floppy and hard disk drives) are used. Several different sizes of floppy disk drives are widely employed, the most common being the 5¼-inch, followed by the 8-inch. The volume of data that can be stored on a disk is described by the number of tracks available and the density with which the data is recorded. A typical 5¼-inch diskette normally accommodates 80 tracks (40 on each side of the disk) capable of holding about 360K of data. Recent advances in floppy disk technology have increased both the number of tracks and the density of the data, so that well over 1 Mbyte of data can be placed on a single diskette. The chief advantages of floppy disks for program and data storage is that they are relatively inexpensive, small, and portable. Their main disadvantage is that they can be damaged rather easily, and they eventually wear out. The hard disk, or fixed drive, uses a technology similar to that of the floppy disk, except that instead of a flexible plastic disk, a solid metal platter is employed. The hard disk drive allows a much greater amount of data to be stored in approximately the same space as a floppy disk drive. Hard disks are commonly described by the total storage space provided; 5- to 10-Mbyte disks are widely used in small laboratory systems, and 15- to 40-Mbyte disks are employed in some of the more sophisticated designs. The advantages of the hard disk over the floppy disk drive are the large amount of data that can be contained on a single device and the speed with which the data can be accessed. Some disadvantages of the hard disk include the necessity of backing up important information (usually on floppy disks or tape) and keeping track of hundreds or even thousands of files on a single drive. Also, since the hard disk is not easily portable, data cannot be exchanged between computers by simply moving a diskette.

A third type of pseudostorage device is the electronic disk, or RAM disk. The RAM disk is a disk drive defined in the memory of the computer; it has no physical parts but acts just like a regular disk drive, only much faster. RAM disks are ideal for programs that access the disk often, because they are so fast. However, since the RAM disk is not a permanent storage device, any data contained on it must be transferred to a floppy or hard disk before powering down the computer.

Software refers to all of the instructions contained in the memory (ROM and RAM) of the computer. These sets of instructions are referred to as programs. Most application programs are loaded into the computer from disk or tape, but many basic functions are contained on chips as ROM (operating system functions, etc.).

DATA ACQUISITION AND INSTRUMENT CONTROL

One of the greatest advantages of computerized pulmonary function systems is the ability to process analog signals from various transducers (spirometers, pneumotachometers, gas analyzers, etc.) to perform automated acquisition of data. Equally important is the computer's capacity for controlling certain instrument functions (valve switching, recording, etc.) to allow the technologist to easily manage complex maneuvers. These functions are implemented by means of an interface (Fig. 10-2) that permits the computer to communicate with the pulmonary function equipment.

One of the primary devices employed in interfacing pulmonary function equipment with computers is the analog-to-digital (A/D) converter. The A/D converter accepts an analog signal, usually a DC voltage in the range of 0 to 10 volts (or −5 to +5 volts), and transforms the signal into a digital value. A/D converters are classified by the number of bits (binary digits) into which they convert the signal; the greater the number of bits, the more sensitive the resulting digital number. An ''8-bit'' converter can transform a voltage into a number represented by 00000000 to 11111111 in binary numbers. In the decimal numbering system this corresponds to a range of 0 to 255 (2^8). A spirometer that produces an analog signal of 0 to 10 volts (equal to 1 volt/L), if connected to an 8-bit converter, will have the signal divided into 256 parts with a resolution of

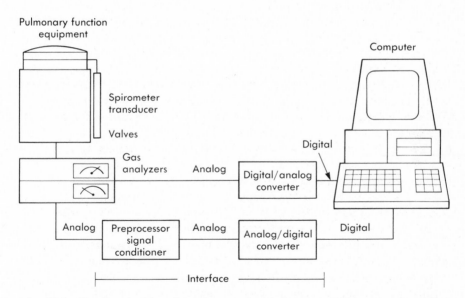

Fig. 10-2. Computer interface for pulmonary function testing. Components of a typical interface between a spirometer and gas analyzers and a small dedicated computer are represented. Analog signals from the pulmonary function equipment are first ''conditioned'' to allow the analog-to-digital converter to handle them. The A/D converter then transforms a voltage (usually DC) into digital data in the form of a binary or hexadecimal number. The digital data is then processed by the computer for display and/or storage. In order for the computer to control various instrument functions, a digital-to-analog converter transforms digital data into appropriate analog signals to open valves or start recorders (see text).

about 39 ml over the 10-liter volume range. For a more precise measurement (i.e., higher resolution), a 10-, 12-, or 16-bit converter must be used. For most laboratory systems, a 12-bit converter provides the necessary precision for instruments with outputs in the 0- to 10-volt range. In addition to converting voltages into numbers, the sampling rate at which conversions take place is important to the accuracy of the data gathered. Most A/D converter systems consist of from 8 to 16 distinct channels, each of which is capable of accepting a separate analog input. The highest sampling rates are attained when conversions are done on only one or two channels. For tests in which a great deal of accuracy is required and in which the signal changes very rapidly, such as a forced expiration, conversions may be performed on a single channel. High-speed converters can perform more than 20,000 conversions/sec; as more channels are included in the conversion scheme, the rate for each channel is reduced. The maximum accuracy is attained by matching the output of a particular transducer (spirometer, etc.) to a particular A/D converter with the appropriate sampling rate.

Some signals require special handling either before A/D conversion or by manipulation of the numeric data after conversion. These functions are often included in the interface between the test instrument and the computer and are referred to as preprocessing. Most transducers include amplifiers that allow setting of offsets and gains; these are primitive forms of signal preprocessing. A common example of signal preprocessing would include transforming a 10-volt signal into a 5-volt signal before A/D conversion or transforming a resistance into a voltage so that conversion would be possible. Other preprocessing functions of the interface might include such devices as a peak detector or counting and timing circuits. All of these functions reduce the work of the A/D converter and the controlling software. Many A/D converter systems have the capacity to process and store data on board until the computer is ready for it; this allows for rapid data acquisition while still permitting complex processing of the data as the computer requests it. In addition, the use of a ''smart'' interface permits the data to be transmitted in a standard format (ASCII codes)*; this allows any computer that can run the necessary software to be compatible with the interface. This is particularly important because the computer or software can be upgraded without replacing the testing equipment.

Another function of the interface between instruments and computer is the conversion of digital information into analog signals. This is accomplished by the digital-to-analog (D/A) converter. In its simplest form, the D/A converter acts as a computer relay switch. A nonzero value sent from the computer can be used to open an electrically operated valve or solenoid after the converter generates the required voltage (typically 5 volts DC). D/A conversion allows the computer to perform switching tasks such as activating kymographs or recorders, switching valves in automated circuits, and opening solenoids to add oxygen, helium, or other gases. Another common use for D/A signal conversion is to allow data

---

*American Standard Code for Interchange of Information.

stored in or generated by the computer to be plotted on a standard X-Y recorder (see Chapter 9). This method is particularly useful for plotting data that is generated too rapidly for direct recording or that requires some "conditioning." Flow-volume loop data and plethysmograph tangents can be stored in RAM in the computer and then plotted on an X-Y recorder at slow speed to produce accurate graphic representations. To translate digital data from breathing maneuvers into analog signals for plotting, the D/A converter must possess a resolution sufficient to accurately represent the data. Normally an 8-bit D/A converter is adequate to drive the servomotors of a conventional plotter. The use of highly accurate digital plotters (that accept digital data directly) has eliminated much of the need for high-resolution D/A conversion.

Many pulmonary function systems provide alternate means of controlling various functions that are normally under computer control. This type of manual control allows for use of the spirometer, gas analyzers, and valves, even if the computer becomes unavailable.

COMPUTERIZED PULMONARY FUNCTION TESTING SYSTEMS

The interdependence of pulmonary function testing equipment and computers makes the capabilities of the computer system especially important. Because the technology of small computers and peripherals is advancing so rapidly, users cannot always anticipate what the computer may be able to do in the future, but rather must ascertain that a particular system meets specific needs at the present. If both the computer hardware and software can be upgraded easily and the system performs all necessary functions properly, then the equipment will probably not become technologically obsolete.

Accuracy and dependability

The first and most important quality of any computerized pulmonary function system is its ability to perform the required measurements with acceptable accuracy. In addition to required accuracy of the transducers (spirometer, gas analyzers, etc.), the computer hardware and software must be designed in such a way that data acquisition maintains accuracy. The computer should not compromise the data that would be obtained if a manual system were being used. The best means of assessing the adequacy of the hardware/software is to test it against the same data calculated manually. The two basic questions to be answered are "Does the system do the job?" and "Is it free of bugs?" The combination of a software system with particular testing equipment should allow rapid testing with repetition of maneuvers as required for obtaining valid data. The software should accommodate the subject tested, as well as the technologist performing the test; this means that the software must handle "abnormal" occurrences, such as the subject interrupting the sequence of the test, without loosing data or locking up the system. Computerization of spirometry may be quite different from automation of lung volume determinations or $D_{L_{CO}}$, since these typically require computer control of circuits and valving. If the accuracy of any component test cannot be easily verified, then the system may be difficult to maintain in day-to-day use.

Because the software required to perform the task of data acquisition in spirometry, lung volumes, diffusing capacity, and plethysmography is complex, it is relatively rare that a program is "bug free." This requires that the program developer offer continuing upgrades and support, as well as ongoing software development. If the software is developed in-house, then a system for evaluation and modification should be included. In many instances a software "bug" may be a matter of preference of a particular laboratory. For example, the absence of a software hemoglobin correction to the DL_{CO} might be considered an omisssion by some laboratories, whereas other laboratories might not employ such a correction. The best software systems allow for maximum user modification. The simplest means of customizing software is to build modifiable parameters into the software and then allow the user to select the desired options and save them in a configuration type of file. Such program options allow the software to meet a wide variety of laboratory needs.

Computerized and manual testing

A second important quality of any automated system is its ability to perform nonautomated tests also. As noted above, manual performance of component tests is normally the best means of assessing the accuracy of the measurements, for both the input instruments and the software. Because of the complexity of even small computers and the number of peripherals (disk drives, printers, etc.) commonly used, the failure of a single component can often disable a computer-dependent system. This is particularly a concern in busy laboratories where a computer failure may mean cancellation of many procedures. A serious shortcoming of many computerized systems is that both graphic and tabular data are computer generated; that is, no secondary recording system is available. A computer malfunction under these circumstances means that no data can be produced. A similar consideration is that in some circumstances the technologist may need to alter the method or sequence that the automated system normally uses. A valuable asset is a computer system that allows user intervention for data verification or modification of the test maneuver.

Ease of use

The ease with which a computerized pulmonary function system can be used is one of the most desirable qualities of an automated system. In general, use of the computer should speed up testing as it enhances the quality of the data obtained. Unfortunately, poorly designed software may require the technologist to perform many more steps than would be required by the same procedure done manually; this typically occurs with lung volume or DL_{CO} tests where operator intervention is required for setting up special circuits or gas analyzers. Some systems employ a "turnkey" approach; that is, the software is designed so that the operator may perform tests with little or no knowledge of what the computer is doing. Such systems function best for simple maneuvers that do not require operator intervention; they also allow the technologist to concentrate on eliciting the best possible effort from the subject. In most instances, however, the turnkey approach does not completely eliminate the need for the technologist to perform some computer-related procedures, such as preparing new storage disks or backing up subject data. Another drawback of some turnkey types of systems is lack of flexibility in the choice of options that the operator may have. Perhaps the most widely used means of providing an easy-to-use software package is to employ menu-driven programs. Menu-driven programs are those that prompt the operator as to the sequence of steps that the computer will accept; the prompts are typically always displayed somewhere on the video display and can usually be selected by a single keyboard entry. A well-designed menu-driven program allows the technologist to perform even complex tasks rather simply and hence concentrate on obtaining adequate subject cooperation. In addition, since only single-key entries are required for most functions, the program can easily check for invalid input.

Documentation

Perhaps as important as any of the above-described attributes for computerized pulmonary function systems is the documentation provided by the manufacturer and/or programmer. The complexity of data acquisition programs such as those used in pulmonary function testing, as well as the complexity of the operating systems that run even small computers, necessitates thorough documentation. Good documentation of computer programs includes all the information necessary to get the system up and running, even for the novice computer (pulmonary function) user. This should include information describing the interconnection of all peripheral devices, as well as any initialization programs that must be run. If the system is provided in several different configurations (different computers, etc.), each should be clearly described. Every segment of the application program should be carefully outlined, including diagrams of what the screen displays and printouts will look like and what user input is required. Examples (either text or via sample data from the computer itself) are invaluable for training new users on complicated systems. Some commercially available software uses ''off-the-shelf'' operating systems(MS-DOS,* etc.), whereas other manufacturers support a proprietary operating system. In either case, the functions of the operating system should be fully documented, along with the pulmonary function application programs. An extremely useful adjunct is the ''on-line'' type of help function. This usually consists of a text file that the operator can access from within the pulmonary function testing program. On-line help functions greatly speed up orientation to a new system, as well as the use of functions that may not be performed on a routine basis. A glossary of computer terms is helpful, particularly if the application program redefines commonly used terms or keys on the computer keyboard. An explanation of error messages is important in tracking down software problems versus operator errors.

---

*MS-DOS is a trademark of Microsoft, Inc.

Data file handling

The file handling capability of the computerized laboratory system is the attribute that may require the most careful consideration. In selecting a system to manage subject data files, it is essential to consider the complexity of the raw data and reduced data to be saved, how many tests will be done per month or year, and what type of access to the data is required. Because of the large amount of raw data generated from multiple spirometric efforts, lung volume determinations, and DL_{CO} maneuvers, it is usually not realistic to store all raw data except in a research setting. For this reason, most systems reduce the data to a certain extent and then store it in a compacted form. It is possible to store a large amount of tabular and graphic data in this way. Because of the importance of hard copy tracings in a pulmonary function laboratory, a completely "paperless" filing system is usually not practical. A common limitation to the amount of subject data that can be saved is the media itself. The commonly used 5¼" floppy diskette can typically store the data from 20 to 100 subjects, depending on the types of tests performed and the graphic data saved. Hard disk systems of 5 to 10 megabytes can obviously store much more data; however, they also require a more sophisticated operating system to keep track of the files created and must be backed up periodically to prevent loss of a large amount of information should the drive fail. These considerations are magnified as the capacity of the hard disk system is increased. Individual laboratories must carefully decide on the most appropriate means of maintaining subject data files. Most situations require a combination of magnetic data storage for rapid retrieval on a short-term basis, along with traditional paper files for spirograms, flow-volume plots, or more extensive tabular raw data. Other important attributes of a computerized data filing system for pulmonary function studies include some means of (1) editing stored data easily, (2) copying (backing up) data quickly and reliably, and (3) transferring the data to other computers or for use with other programs. Most commercially available software packages allow for operator selection of the actual data to be saved, in addition to providing algorithms to assist in choosing valid data. If the software allows only one set of test data for each component test (spirometry, lung volumes, etc.) to be saved, then some type of file editor is useful for deleting incorrect data or manually entering data obtained by an independent means.

Printers and plotters

A primary consideration with any computerized system is the hard copy that is produced. One of the most noticeable advancements in computerized pulmonary function testing in the last several years is the capability of generating high-quality, high-resolution graphic representations of spirograms, F-V loops, and plethysmograph tangents, in addition to tabular data. Two commonly used peripherals are the dot matrix printer and the digital plotter. The dot matrix printer uses a series of pins (from 9 to 24) to generate both alphanumeric characters and graphics. Despite the fact that letters may not appear fully formed with all dot matrix printers, these printers are fast (80-200 characters per second) and less noisy than impact-type printers. Newer dot matrix printers, using more pins, produce near-letter-quality type, are relatively fast, and retain the ability to generate high-resolution graphic images. Some printers use multicolor ribbons so that color graphics can be generated. Other types of printers available include thermal transfer and ink jet. The thermal types are extremely quiet but require heat-sensitive paper that tends to discolor with time. Ink-jet printers apply a small jet of ink directly to the paper to form both characters and graphic images; they are very quiet and relatively fast. Digital plotters interface directly to many computers and, with appropriate software to drive them, can be used to produce high-quality, multicolor representations of almost any figure that can be generated on the video display. Plotters are generally slower than dot matrix printers, particularly when producing alphanumeric characters for labels on graphs. However, they are usually quiet, which may be an important consideration in a busy laboratory.

To speed up the generation of graphic images, and to allow the computer to be used while the printer is working, many systems use a hardware printer buffer or a software spooling program. The hardware buffer is a memory device, placed between the computer and the printer or plotter, that accepts data much faster than the printer alone. The data is then fed to the printer/plotter at a slower rate while the computer is freed to perform other tasks. Many printers have built-in memory that functions as a buffer. A software spooler is a program that resides in memory along with the pulmonary function testing programs and functions much like the hardware buffer. The spooler accepts data and then "spools" it to the output device at an appropriate rate. Spoolers are somewhat less efficient than hardware buffers, since the computer's microprocessor must control the spooler, whereas the hardware buffer has its own processor. Dumping graphic images, even with a buffer or spooler, is usually slow because of the large number of bytes required for high-resolution graphics. A valuable software enhancement available on many systems is a "screen-dump" program. Like a spooler, the screen-dump program resides in memory as part of the main program and allows a hard copy of the CRT to be made at any time.

Hardware and software compatability

One of the benefits of a computerized pulmonary function laboratory is that the computer can often be used for more than just performing automated testing. This perhaps explains the trend that many manufacturers are following of interfacing existing pulmonary function equipment with generic computers and peripherals (Fig. 10-3). Two important considerations, if the computer is to be used for additional tasks, are (1) whether the system will run "off-the-shelf" software, and (2) whether the pulmonary function software will work in conjunction with the other software. Whether the system can be used with "off-the-shelf" software can be easily determined, but the user must be familiar with specific programs in order to ascertain if the hardware will support the functions of the program (see Additional Applications). For example, a pulmonary function testing system that uses a plotter as its primary output device may not function

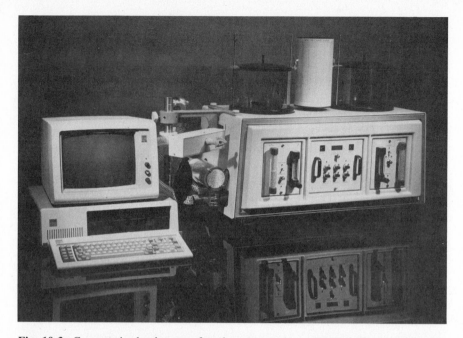

Fig. 10-3. Computerized pulmonary function system. An automated pulmonary function system, including a Stead-Wells spirometer, kymograph, and gas analyzers for performing lung volumes and DL_{CO}, is interfaced to a generic microcomputer. The microcomputer allows rapid processing of data with sophisticated displays of tabular and graphic information, as well as data storage on floppy or hard disks. The computer ''portion'' of the system can also be used for other tasks (see text). (Courtesy Warren E. Collins, Inc., Braintree, Mass.)

with a word processing program. Adapting pulmonary function software for use with other programs may be quite easy or may require rather high level programming, if it is possible at all. For example, if the pulmonary function software creates standard text files, then a simple text editor or word processor can be used to modify them or generate customized reports; similarly, if the pulmonary function software is well documented or the source code is available, then application programs in a higher-level language such as BASIC or PASCAL can be developed. Some manufacturers provide this type of customization as part of the original purchase, whereas others provide source codes and documentation so that customization can be provided by the user.

Communications

An application of pulmonary function testing that is becoming increasingly widespread is the ''outreach'' type of testing facility. Typically this consists of pulmonary function test equipment located at a remote site; this equipment communicates with a centralized laboratory computer via standard phone lines. The remote or satellite laboratory may be miles away or within the same building.

This type of telecommunications is usually implemented by means of a modem at both locations. The modem translates digital data from the computer into tones for phone line transmission, which can then be decoded back into digital data by the receiving computer. Many computers have an RS232C port (more or less an industry standard for communications) built in. The RS232C allows data to be transmitted serially (i.e., one bit at a time) and very rapidly either to a modem or to another device (computer, printer, etc.). The combination of RS232C port and modem allows a small computer at a remote site to transmit and receive data from a centrally located host. The host system supports specially designed software that allows communications with several remote terminals. In this way, tests are performed at the remote site and a copy of the data is transmitted to the host system, where it can be evaluated and interpreted. A related type of system is the multiuser computer, in which a large, centrally located computer communicates with smaller computers or simple terminals to share programs and data. This type of setup is referred to as a local area network. Such a multiuser system is ideal for large laboratories in which computerized pulmonary function testing, exercise testing, and blood gas analysis are all performed. A multiuser computer permits each station to be ''dedicated'' to a particular task while sharing programs that are needed in several areas and transferring data from one location to another. Multiuser systems are complex and somewhat difficult to implement but may save time and money in a high-volume laboratory if properly designed.

Maintaining the system

In a large, automated pulmonary function testing system that includes various input devices along with monitors, disk drives, printers, plotters, and modems, system maintenance becomes somewhat complex. In addition to the service to spirometers, gas analyzers, etc., the computer and peripherals likewise require preventive and sometime corrective maintenance. Perhaps the commonest source of problems is the software itself; even a program that is relatively free of bugs may load improperly or fail to read data correctly from a storage device or other peripheral. Most operating systems and languages provide ample error messages to assist in tracking down software errors. Good application programs report full error messages; some systems report only error codes, which must then be looked up in a manual. Careful evaluation or error codes or messages often provides an indication of the source of the error. Program failures quite often result when a peripheral device is not ready or is operating incorrectly. For example, if the program is expecting data from the A/D converter but the converter is not functioning, the program may try to process incorrect data or simply lock up. Well-designed software contains error traps to handle most types of input errors, but some problems cannot be anticipated. A trouble-shooting guide is invaluable in tracking down computer problems. Many systems contain diagnostic programs that allow memory checks, disk-drive checks, and related hardware evaluation. Such diagnostics allow the user to determine if the error is software or hardware based. Since most application programs are ''loaded'' from disk or tape, errors arising from the storage media are rather common. The simple solution to these errors is to maintain adequate backups of all programs and data, and to rotate disks or tapes on a regular interval. For hardware malfunctions (printer break-downs, disk-drive alignment problems, etc.), the usual course is to replace the suspected component. Many systems use components that are relatively easy, although not always inexpensive, to replace. Dirt, dust, smoke, and humidity quite often interfere with sensitive electronics but can be managed with a mini-mum of preventive care. Cabling and connectors between components are anoth-er source of hardware errors and should be evaluated whenever a peripheral begins functioning erratically or stops functioning suddenly.

Because of the number of computerized systems available, not every capabil-ity can be adequately described. Those discussed above include many of the important aspects related to automated data handling in the pulmonary function laboratory and may be considerations in the selection of a computerized testing system.

LANGUAGES AND PROGRAMMING

For the majority of pulmonary function technologists, the ability to use com-puterized pulmonary function testing does not require programming expertise. But to fully understand the process of data acquisition and processing, some background in programming concepts and computer languages is helpful. A sound understanding of how the computer controls various peripheral devices is useful for tracking down certain hardware malfunctions. Some programming skill may allow the development of utility routines to supplement a full-scale testing package. Understanding the operating system that controls most computer func-tions is probably the most valuable tool for the technologist, since it allows him or her not only to use the pulmonary function software, but also to enhance it by the use of various utility programs.

Computer languages

Each microprocessor recognizes a set of instructions, which are referred to as "machine language." These instructions are usually in binary form and represent the lowest-level language for controlling the computer. Since it is difficult to program using binary numbers, a special "assembly" language is used that applies mnemonics to each command. An assembly language program may be written using a text editor or word processor. This code is then processed by an assembler that converts the mnemonics into machine language instructions. The resulting program is usually stored in the form of hexadecimal bytes (*hexadeci-mal* refers to the number system with a base equal to 16 decimal). Assembly language (machine) programs are extremely fast and do not require a great deal of RAM. However, writing large programs in assembly language is a task that requires a great deal of programming expertise; the programmer not only must understand the machine language instructions, but also must be familiar with the specific hardware that the microprocessor will address. Most commercially avail-able general purpose programs (word processors, spreadsheets, etc.), as well as many pulmonary function packages, are written in assembly language. Modify-ing assembly language programs is done by "patching" the hexadecimal instructions either in memory or directly on the storage media. This technique is useful if the manufacturer or original programmer wishes to correct a program bug, particularly if only a few bytes must be changed. The correct code is supplied, and the user can then "patch" the existing program; most operating systems have a utility program designed just for such patching.

BASIC (Beginner's All-purpose Symbolic Instructional Code) has been used for about 20 years and has gained a lot of popularity with the scientific and technical community because of the ease with which it can be learned. High-level mathematic and text handling functions, as well as file management, are all possible in BASIC. Although it is relatively easy to write complex programs in BASIC, the language functions through an interpreter, which significantly slows execution. The BASIC interpreter translates each program line as the program is running into code, which the microprocessor can then execute. This causes BASIC to become too slow for many applications, particularly with regard to devices such as A/D converters. Two solutions to the slow execution problem with BASIC programs are widely applied. The first is to use a combination of machine language subroutines and BASIC code to speed up critical portions of the program. A machine language routine might be used to access the A/D converter and then pass the numeric values back to the BASIC program that called the subroutine. The second solution is to "compile" the BASIC program code into a form that is quite similar to native machine language. With careful programming, a speed-up of tenfold or more is often possible using compiled BASIC. One problem with this technique is that some BASIC commands cannot be compiled easily, particularly those that allow BASIC to function through the computer's operating system. Similarly, the compiled BASIC program cannot be modified easily without recompiling the source code. Nonetheless, many pulmonary function software packages use one or more of these techniques and support BASIC as the primary program language. For relatively short programs, especially when execution time is not critical, BASIC functions well because of its ease of use and rapid editing ability.

FORTRAN (FORmula TRANslation) has been the language implemented for most scientific and technical applications, particularly on minicomputers. FORTRAN is a compiled language. The source program is coded according to a structured format and then compiled before the program is actually run. In general, compiled programs can be executed much faster than interpreted programs (as in BASIC), since error checking is carried out during the compilation phase. FORTRAN supports calls to machine language subroutines, so that it can be used as high-level language and still mangage tasks such as reading data from A/D converters, etc. The recent widespread popularity of microcomputers (personal computers) with BASIC supplied as the user programming language has tended to reduce the popularity of FORTRAN somewhat. FORTRAN was designed primarily for numeric manipulations and does not allow for very easy handling of text characters. The large number of programs and subroutines already written and the fact that FORTRAN is available for most microprocessors make it practical for those laboratories developing their own software.

A third high-level language that is finding more implementations in pulmonary function laboratories is PASCAL. PASCAL is a compiled language that requires a highly structured source program. The source program is compiled into an intermediate form called p-code, which is then interpreted at the time the program is run. PASCAL supports a number of functions that allow complex programs to be written fairly easily, much like BASIC, but with the advantage of greater speed of execution. Because it is highly structured, PASCAL programs can be written in small parts, and then the parts are linked together as a series of procedures or used over and over as necessary. Other compiled, high-level languages such as C, FORTH, and MODULA-2 are becoming increasingly popular for complex programming applications but are not yet widely used.

Operating systems

Perhaps the "language" most often used in pulmonary function laboratories is DOS (Disk Operating System), or simply OS (for nondisk implementations). Many such operating systems are in use, but a few are quite common (CP/M, MS-DOS, etc.).* While some pulmonary function systems support their own operating systems, others use one or more of the "off-the-shelf" systems to provide compatibility with other commercially available software. The DOS is primarily responsible for supervising I/O functions of the computer as well as coordinating many functions from the application programs, no matter what language they use. The technologist may use the operating system for several important functions: copying files or programs, backing up data files, calling a directory of files on a particular device, sorting files, and so on. Most operating systems support automatic operations; this allows the user to perform multiple procedures by executing a single program. All of the commands normally entered from the keyboard are stored in a special file called a "batch" or "job control" file. Then, by calling the batch file, the same steps can be repeated as often as needed. Batch files are extremely helpful for initializing a small computer system; various different programs for controlling printers, screen displays, etc., can be loaded automatically so that the main program functions correctly. Batch files can also be used for tedious tasks such as backing up selected data files on a routine basis. Other utilities offered by most DOS systems include programs for formatting storage media (disks), editing files, protecting files with passwords, deleting files, and defining parameters for the operation of the video display and the printer.

While most pulmonary function laboratories use computers for performing tests, relatively few do extensive programming. Development of a complete pulmonary function testing package, complete with interfacing to all necessary laboratory instruments, is an involved task. Most laboratories developing their own software find it useful to engage professional programmers and consultants. The cost, in time and money, of producing a custom testing program is usually prohibitive, unless special computer resources are available (programmers and facilities). However, programming skills using languages such as BASIC, PASCAL,

---

*CP/M is a trademark of Digital Research, Inc.; MS-DOS is a trademark of Microsoft, Inc.

FORTRAN, or ASSEMBLY can allow in-house development of utilities and supplementary programs to enhance or extend commercially available software. A working knowledge of the operating system used by a particular computer can greatly enhance day-to-day functions of the laboratory. Finally, skill in using other application programs (spreadsheets, word processors, etc.) can increase the productivity of a system designed primarily for pulmonary function testing.

ADDITIONAL APPLICATIONS

In addition to pulmonary function software, several other types of application programs lend themselves to use in the pulmonary function laboratory. These include interpretation programs for pulmonary function tests, blood gas data and quality control programs, spreadsheets, database managers, word processing programs, and educational applications.

Pulmonary function interpreters

Many pulmonary function software packages include an interpretive program as an option. Most interpretive programs are based on one or more sets of algorithms for defining the presence of obstructive, restrictive, combined, or normal patterns on standard spirometry, lung volume, and DL_{CO} determinations. These interpretive programs analyze the results posted during standard pulmonary function studies using both the absolute values attained by the subject and the predicted normal values. Most algorithms are oriented along the same lines that a clinical interpreter might use. Depending on the sophistication of the program, computerized interpreters generally manage to point out the presence or absence of obstruction or restriction. Incorrect computerized interpretations may occur if test results are invalid due to inadequate effort or nonreproducible data. Computerized interpretation in no way substitutes for evaluation by a qualified interpreter but is helpful in situations where an immediate report of gross abnormalities is necessary, or for teaching purposes. If a computerized interpretation is included in the report to become part of the medical record, it should be clearly labeled as such. Computerized interpretations should never be used as the only interpretation; they should always be reviewed by a qualified reader.

Blood gas programs

Computerization in the blood gas laboratory includes several different categories of programs. Blood gas interpretation by computer is implemented by applying algorithms to evaluate acid-base status and oxygenation. Computerized blood gas interpretation can be useful in situations where an immediate interpretation for gross abnormalities is required. Since the computer routinely evaluates all the measured and calculated blood gas parameters, it can often suggest abnormalities that the casual interpreter might overlook. As with computerized pulmonary function interpretation, blood gas interpretations should always be held as preliminary and formally verified by a qualified interpreter. Other areas in which computerization is useful in the blood gas laboratory are quality control and data reporting. Because evaluation of multiple levels of controls requires statistical manipulation of large amounts of data (see Chapter 11), the computer is ideally suited to maintaining a quality assurance program. Most quality control programs require the calculation of means and standard deviations for each level of each component of control material (pH, Pco_2, Po_2). Since controls are usually run daily or more often, many times on multiple instruments, computerization of data files greatly reduces the record-keeping functions in a busy laboratory. A second advantage is that the computer can be used to interpret the results of quality control runs in real time, so that the technologist can immediately determine the status of each individual blood gas electrode (see Chapter 11). Quality assurance programs for various microcomputers are available from several professional organizations. Data reporting lends itself to computerization, since many patients receive multiple blood gas analyses. Most automated or semiautomated analyzers can be interfaced via the standard RS232C (see Communications above) or similar communication port so that blood gas data can be stored on disk or tape, with reports generated as required. Interfacing of the blood gas analyzer directly to a hospital information system allows blood gas data to be available wherever a terminal is located and tends to reduce transcription errors and lost results.

Databases

Database managing programs are available for almost every small computer. Most allow the user to design what information will be stored and how it will be arranged. Computer databases permit the user to save information in much the same manner as a conventional file might be used, but the computer can rapidly sort the information, search for records meeting specific criteria, and generate reports as required. The most common application in an area such as pulmonary function testing is maintaining lists of tests performed, patient demographics, diagnoses, and referral sources. Other uses include records of departmental inventory, expenditures, and similar operational information. Most databases can be customized so as to be used also for storing of test results from pulmonary function or blood gas studies. Reference lists and bibliographies can be maintained as a database. Many commercially available database management programs can be integrated so that information from spreadsheets or word processing programs can be easily exchanged.

Spreadsheets

Electronic spreadsheets were originally designed as a financial planning tool, replacing the ledger book. However, their ability to organize numeric data and perform repetitive calculations makes them ideal for many scientific and technical purposes. Most spreadsheets use matrix arithmetic; that is, numbers or formulas are placed in the cells of a two-dimensional matrix. A value or the result of an equation can then be accessed by referring to its location (row and column). By adding math and logic functions, rows or columns of numbers can be added, subtracted, averaged, or otherwise evaluated. The spreadsheet is quite useful for many statistical calculations, such as calculating means and standard deviations for blood gas quality control. Many spreadsheets have basic statistical functions built in. Similarly, reducing data from multiple-level procedures, such as exercise tests, can be performed quickly via the spreadsheet. Since formulas have only to be entered once and then replicated as often as needed, the spreadsheet handles repetitive calculations quite rapidly. Any data that is normally reduced using a calculator can be managed by the spreadsheet. Most spreadsheets can also be used for storing and editing numeric data, and for generating customized reports.

Word processing

Text handling or processing is one of the most widespread uses of small computer systems. In conjunction with an appropriate printer, a word processor can be used to generate almost any type of document that normally would require typing. In addition, the document is stored on magnetic media so that revisions or copies can be made as needed. In the laboratory environment word processors are ideal for maintaining documents such as procedure manuals, which typically require constant updating. In addition, word processors can be used to generate customized reports; in many instances data can be transferred directly from another program (spreadsheet, database, etc.) and incorporated into the report. Pulmonary function software that stores data in text files can usually be interfaced to a word processing program for custom report generation.

Educational programs

Computer-assisted instruction has several potential applications in the pulmonary function laboratory. Information that is normally taught by repetitive drill can usually be administered via computer. Many programs are available to allow multiple-choice and other types of questions to be administered via the computer; since the computer can easily score the results of a test taken, it becomes both an educational and an evaluation instrument for certain types of material. Computerized simulations are another teaching tool that can be adapted for laboratory personnel, particularly for interpreting the results of pulmonary function studies or blood gas analyses.

SELF-ASSESSMENT QUESTIONS

1. In selecting a computerized pulmonary function system, the first step is to:
   a. Identify the required hardware
   b. Select the necessary software
   c. Define the tasks the system must perform
   d. Determine the amount of memory required
2. Computer memory that is available to the user for programs and data storage is referred to as:
   a. RAM
   b. ROM
   c. PROM
   d. EPROM
   e. CPU

3. Which of the following accurately describe the hard disk type of mass storage system?
   I. More data can be stored than on a floppy disk.
   II. Data can be accessed more rapidly than with a floppy disk.
   III. The hard disk is easily portable.
   IV. The hard disk must be "backed up" to a floppy disk or tape.
   a. I, II, III, and IV
   b. I, II, and IV
   c. II, and III
   d. I and II

4. A typical interface between a computer and the pulmonary function testing equipment might contain:
   a. A D/A converter
   b. An A/D converter
   c. Electronics for signal "preprocessing"
   d. All of the above
   e. b and c only

5. The best means of determining the accuracy of software used to reduce pulmonary function data is:
   a. To perform frequent calibration checks
   b. To perform duplicate tests on a random basis
   c. To check results against the same data calculated manually
   d. Both a and b

6. Software that prompts the operator for required input is referred to as a:
   a. "Turnkey" system
   b. Menu-driven system
   c. Command interpreter
   d. Compiler

7. Which of the following correctly describes data file handling in the pulmonary function laboratory?
   I. Most raw data is reduced before storage.
   II. A paperless system is impractical because of the need for hard copy tracings.
   III. The number of patient tests stored is usually limited by the type of storage device used.
   IV. Some means of editing data files is usually required.
   a. I, II, III, and IV
   b. II, and III
   c. II and Iv
   d. III only

8. Which of the following devices may be used to speed up printing of reports and graphs?
   a. A hardware printer buffer
   b. A digital plotter
   c. A software spooler
   d. All of the above
   e. a and b

9. Which of the following computer languages may be "compiled" to speed up program execution?
   I. PASCAL

II. BASIC

III. FORTRAN

IV. ASSEMBLY

  a. I, II, III, and IV

  b. I, II, and III

  c. I and III

  d. III only

10. Computerized interpretation of blood gas analysis:

  I. May be used if a qualified interpreter is not available

  II. May be useful in detecting gross abnormalities

  III. May suggest subtle abnormalities that might have been overlooked

  IV. Uses a series of algorithms to evaluate acid-base and oxygenation status

  a. I, II, III, and IV

  b. I, III, and IV

  c. II, III, and IV

  d. II and III

SELECTED BIBLIOGRAPHY

Computerized pulmonary function testing

Black, K.H., Petusevsky, M.L., and Gaensler, E.A.: A general purpose microprocessor for spirometry, Chest **78**:605, 1980.

Dickman, M.L., et al.: On-line computerized spirometry in 738 normal adults, Am. Rev. Respir. Dis. **100**:780, 1969.

Gardner, R.M., et al.: Computerized decision-making in the pulmonary function laboratory, Respir. Care **27**(7):799, 1982.

Jones, N.L., et al.: Clinical exercise testing, ed. 2, Philadelphia, 1983, W.B. Saunders Co.

Computer data acquisition

Engleman, B., and Abraham, M.: Personal computer signal processing, Byte, p. 94, April 1984.

Mellichamp, D., editor: Real-time computing—with applications to data acquisition and control, New York, 1983, Van Nostrand Reinhold. Co., Inc.

Tompkins, W.J., and Webster, J.G., editors: Design of microcomputer-based medical instrumentation, New Jersey, 1981, Prentice-Hall, Inc.

Wyss, C.R.: Planning a computerized measurement system, Byte, p. 114, April 1985.

Computer applications

Byers, R.A.: Everyman's database primer, Culver City, Calif., 1984, Ashton-Tate.

Cohn, J.D., Engler, R.C., and DelGuercio, R.L.: The automated physiologic profile, Crit. Care Med. **3**:51, 1975.

Ellis, J.H., Perera, S.P., and Levin, D.C.: A computer program for the interpretation of pulmonary function studies, Chest **68**:209, 1975.

Gardner, R.M., et al.: Computerized blood gas interpretation and reporting system, Computer **8**(1):39, 1975.

Miller, H.: Introduction to spreadsheets, PC World **2**:66, 1984.

Silage, D.A., and Maxwell, C.: A spirometry/interpretation program for hand-held computers, Respir. Care **28**:62, 1983.

Languages and programming

Disk operating system—version 2.00, Boca Raton, Fla., 1983, IBM.

George, D.P.: Better and true BASICs, PC World **3**:161, 1985.

Leventhal, L.: Z80 assembly language programming, Berkley, Calif., 1979, Osborne & Associates.

Wolverton, V.: Running MS-DOS, Bellevue, Wash., 1984, Microsoft Press.

Zaks, R.: The CP/M handbook, Trenton, N.J., 1980, Sybex Inc.

CHAPTER ELEVEN

Quality assurance in the pulmonary function laboratory

ELEMENTS OF LABORATORY QUALITY CONTROL

Quality control is essential to the operation of the pulmonary function laboratory in order to produce valid and reproducible data. Four main components describe the necessary parts of a program to assure quality:

1. *Methodology*. The type of equipment used (spirometer, gas analyzer, recorder, etc.) determines to a certain extent the procedures that will be required for calibration and quality control, and how often such procedures must be performed. The particular methods used should be carefully matched to the testing regimens that the laboratory routinely employs, as well as to the number and complexity of the tests performed.

2. *Instrument maintenance*. As with the particular methodology employed, the type and complexity of the instrumentation will determine the extent of day-to-day maintenance that will be required. Familiarity with the operating characteristics of spirometers, gas analyzers, plethysmographs, and computers is best accomplished by manufacturer support and thorough documentation. Written procedures and accurate records are essential to an ongoing maintenance program and are required by most accrediting bodies.

3. *Control methods*. Test signals appropriate to each particular instrument (spirometers, analyzers, etc.) are necessary to determine both the accuracy and the precision of the data produced. In addition, since many laboratories use automated "systems," control signals are required to assure that both software and hardware are functioning within acceptable limits.

4. *Sampling technique*. A primary means of assuring the quality of data is to rigidly control the methods and procedures by which it is obtained. In the case of pulmonary function testing, *sampling technique* refers to the ability of the technician to manage the procedure and the subject's ability to cooperate in the test maneuvers. Technician and subject performance, as well as proper equipment functioning, must be evaluated on a test-by-test basis by applying appropriate criteria to determine the acceptability of the results.

This chapter deals primarily with the appropriate control signals for instrument maintenance and calibration, and with criteria for acceptability for various categories of pulmonary function tests (spirometry, lung volumes, DL_{CO}, etc.). The operating characteristics of various types of pulmonary function testing equipment are discussed in Chapter 9.

Two concepts that are central to quality assurance are the definitions of accuracy and precision. *Accuracy* may be defined as the extent to which measurement of a known quantity results in a value approximating that quantity. In most laboratory settings this is accomplished by taking repeated measurements and calculating the "mean" for the data. If the mean approximates the "known," then the instrument is considered accurate. *Precision* may be defined as the extent to which repeated measurements of the same quantity can be reproduced. If the same parameter is measured repeatedly and the resulting values are similar, the instrument may be considered precise. Accuracy and precision are not always present concurrently in the same instrument. A spirometer that consistently measures a 3-liter test volume as 2.5 liters is precise but not very accurate, whereas a spirometer that evaluates the same volume as 2.5, 3.0, and 3.5 liters on repeated maneuvers shows an accurate "mean" of 3.0 liters, but the individual measurements are not precise. Determination of the accuracy *and* precision of instruments such as spirometers is particularly important because many of the common pulmonary function parameters are "effort dependent"; that is, the largest value observed is often reported.

CALIBRATION AND QUALITY CONTROL OF SPIROMETERS

Calibration of spirometric devices is accomplished by one or more of several different methods:

1. Adjustment of the analog output signal from the primary transducer
2. Adjustment of the sensitivity of the recording device
3. Software correction (compensation)

Spirometers that produce an analog signal by means of a potentiometer (see Chapter 9) normally allow some form of "gain" adjustment so that the output can be matched to a known input. A related technique is the adjustment of the sensitivity of the recording device so that a known input produces a given deflection on the recording device. This method works well when the recorded tracing is to be measured manually. Perhaps the most common technique, because of the widespread use of automated data reduction, is to correct the signal produced by the spirometer by applying a compensation factor. This is usually accomplished by injecting a known volume into the spirometer and then calculating a correction factor based on the measured and expected values:

$$\text{Correction factor} = \frac{\text{Expected volume}}{\text{Measured volume}}$$

The correction factor derived by this method is then stored and applied to the subsequent volume measurements. This method assumes that the spirometer output is linear, so that the correction factor would be correct for any volume, large or small. Care should be taken that the measured volume is not "temperature corrected" (see below), since this would produce an erroneously high measured value.

Quality control of spirometric devices is closely tied to calibration; an important distinction is that calibration (adjustment) may or may not be needed, but quality control must be applied on a routine basis. Various control methods (signal generators) are available for spirometers: (1) simple large-volume syringes, (2) sine wave rotary pumps, (3) automatic syringes, (4) explosive decompression devices, and (5) normal subjects.

A *simple large-volume syringe* of 3 to 5 liters' volume may be used for generating a calibration signal, as well as for checking the volume deflection of volume displacement spirometers and the associated deflection of the recording device (Fig. 11-1, *a* and *b*). A large-volume syringe may also be used to check the volume accuracy of flow-sensing devices. A wide range of volumes should be used to assess the accuracy of the spirometer across its volume range (i.e., the spirometer should record 1 liter, 3 liters, and 5 liters with equal accuracy). Although a range of flows can be generated by varying the speed at which the syringe is emptied, it is impossible to reproduce those flows. However, applying a range of flows and measuring the resulting volume determinations may provide insight as to whether the device (and the software) remains accurate at low and high flows. It is important to note that simple volume checks and spirometer calibration are not identical; calibration implies that *adjustment* or *compensation* is performed, whereas application of a quality control signal is a means of checking the accuracy and/or precision of the device and software after calibration.

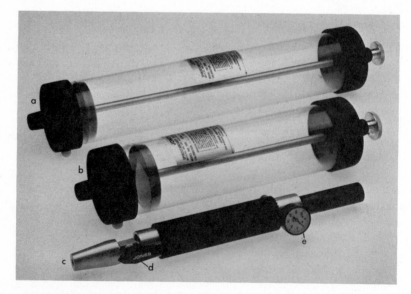

Fig. 11-1. Equipment for spirometer calibration. *a* and *b*, Large-volume syringes used for simple volume calibrations or for connection to FRC and DL_{CO} calibration setups (3 liters or more is recommended); *c*, FVC simulator that uses compressed gas (CO_2) released through a fixed orifice to produce an exponential flow curve; *d*, gas release valve; *e*, gas pressure indicator (see text). (Courtesy Jones Medical Instrument Co., Oakbrook, Ill.)

Simple volume checks should be applied as if a subject were being tested, with a few exceptions. For volume displacement spirometers, a leak check should be performed first. The device is filled with air to approximately half of its volume range and constant pressure applied by means of a weight or spring. No decrease in the volume tracing should be noted while the pressure is applied, and the volume should return to its original baseline when the pressure is removed. The large-volume syringe should be connected to the subject port with whatever circuitry is employed for the actual test. To prevent automatic correction to BTPS, the spirometer temperature correction should be set to 37° C. In some systems temperature correction cannot be overridden; the results of the check must then be converted to ambient values. Volumes may be injected as described above. For water-seal spirometers, the syringe should be filled and emptied several times to allow equilibration with the humidified air of the device. For some flow-sensing instruments, a length of tubing must be connected to the flow head (particularly those in which the flow head is close to the mouth) in order to avoid artifact caused by flow that is not laminar. The accuracy of the spirometer can be calculated:

$$\% \ \text{Error} = \frac{(\text{Expected volume} - \text{measured volume})}{\text{Expected volume}} \times 100$$

where

Expected volume = Actual volume of the syringe
Measured volume = Result recorded for the test

The maximum acceptable error (according to the American Thoracic Society recommendation—see Table 11-1) is 3% or 50 ml, whichever is larger. If the percent of error exceeds 3%, a careful examination of the spirometer, recording device, and testing technique should be carried out.

A second method of checking volume accuracy of spirometers is with a *sine wave rotary pump* (volumetric syringe or piston driven via a rotary drive motor). This type of device produces a biphasic volume signal that is useful for checking accuracy as the volume (and flow) simulates both inspiration and expiration. Although this type of device is of limited use for assessing the accuracy of a spirometer for most flow measurements, it is ideal for checking the frequency response, particularly at higher flow rates. This type of signal is necessary to evaluate a spirometer's ability to adequately record tests such as the MVV. The American Thoracic Society recommends that spirometers record a 2-liter sine wave within 5% accuracy from 0 to 250 L/min. Although tests such as this are impractical for most clinical laboratories, they should be available from manufacturers where necessary.

Automatic syringes are similar to the simple large-volume syringes that are used manually, but they have some type of computer-controlled motor drive, or electronic output. For the most part, computerized syringes are restricted to equipment manufacturers and to research applications centering on testing available clinical equipment. Other commercially available devices use sensors (mag-

Table 11-1. Minimum spirometry standards

Test	Range/accuracy (BTPS)(L)	Flow range (/sec)	Time (sec)	Resistance/ back pressure	Test signals
VC	7 L/±3% of reading or 50 mL, whichever is greater	0-12	60		Calibrated syringe
FVC	7 L/±3% of reading or 50 mL, whichever is greater	0-12	10.0		Two simulated FVC signals in range (1) FVC = 5 L, τ = 0.4 sec; (2) FVC = 3.5 L, τ = 2.4 sec
FEV_T*	7 L/±3% of reading or 50 ml, whichever is greater	0-12	τ	Less than 1.5 cm H_2O/L/sec at 12 L/sec flow	Same as FVC
$FEF_{25\%-75\%}$	7 L/±5% of reading or 0.1 L/sec, whichever is greater	0-12	10.0	Same as FEV_T	Same as FVC
Flow ($\dot{V}$)	12 L/sec ±5% of reading or 0.2 L/sec, whichever is greater	0-12	10.0	Same as FEV_T	Manufacturer proof
MVV	Sine wave 250 L/min at 2 L to ±5% of reading	0-12 ±5%	12-15 ±3%	Less than ±10 cm H_2O at 2 L V_T, 2 Hz	Sine wave pump 0-8 Hz ±10% at 12 L/sec

Data from Workshop on Standardization of Spirometry, sponsored by the American Thoracic Society, Snowbird, Utah, 1977.
*Determination of the "start-of-test" must be made by backward extrapolation of the initial part of the volume-time curve to a point of intersection with the volume baseline.

netic, etc.) coupled to simple microprocessors to calculate various flows ($FEF_{25\%-75\%}$, etc.).

Explosive decompression devices simulate the exponential flow pattern of a forced expiratory maneuver. Such devices use a known volume of gas compressed to a fixed pressure and then released through an orifice. One commercially available device (Fig. 11-1, *c*) uses CO_2 as the compressed gas. The primary advantage of this type of device is that it allows measurement of volumes and flows to be reproduced, thus allowing quality assurance checks on most spirometric parameters, for both hardware and software. In addition, the fact that the test signal can be reproduced as often as necessary allows not only accuracy, but precision as well, to be assessed. Explosive decompression devices may be of limited use with automated systems that require a particular pattern of respiration in order to trigger recording (such as inspiration-expiration-inspiration). Another potential limitation is the use of CO_2 as the compressed gas. Flow-sensing spirometers that use a physical principle that is affected by the gas composition may yield unacceptable values (see Chapter 9). These include pressure differential, thermal conductivity, and rotameter-type devices.

A semiquantitative means of assessing the accuracy and precision of spirometric devices is the repeated measurement of *normal, known subjects*. This is best accomplished by performing all routine spirometric measurements on subjects who will be available for future comparison, such as laboratory personnel. Although individual signals for FVC, FEV_1, and $FEF_{25\%-75\%}$ show a good deal of variability when test subjects are used, all aspects of the testing protocol are evaluated, including hardware, software, and testing procedure. This allows for a gross, but readily available, check of the overall function of the spirometer; it does not, however, replace the checking of accuracy by means of a known-volume syringe. To provide meaningful comparisons, the mean and standard deviation of 5 to 10 spirometric measurements for each reported parameter should be recorded.

In addition to checking the volume and flow accuracy of spirometers, there are several other important aspects of quality control that require routine evaluation:

1. *Flow resistance.* Normally the "back pressure" from a spirometer should be less than 1.5 cm H_2O at 12 L/sec flow. Resistance to flow is measured by placing an accurate manometer or transducer at the subject connection and applying a known flow. This is easily accomplished with flow-sensing devices but somewhat difficult with volume displacement devices and is normally performed only when there is some reason to suspect that the spirometer is causing undue resistance.

2. *Frequency response.* Frequency response is the ability of the spirometer to produce accurate volume (and flow) determinations across a wide range of frequencies. This applies most notably to the MVV, since the frequency varies with the individual subject. Frequency response is usually evaluated by means of a sine wave pump and is performed only if the spirometer is suspect.

3. *Flow*. Since flow-sensing spirometers directly measure flow and indirectly measure volume (by integration), it is sometimes useful to assess the accuracy of such devices. Inaccurate measurement of flow almost always results in inaccurate volume determinations. A flow rater may be used in conjunction with a compressed gas source to apply gas to the device at a known flow. Many flow-sensing spirometers use a volume signal to perform software calibration (correction as described above). However, it may be useful to check the flow output of the device at several different known flows if the volume accuracy of the device seems to vary with flow.

4. *Recorders*. Recording devices are perhaps as important as the volume/flow transducers themselves in providing accurate spirometric tracings. The American Thoracic Society has recommended a volume sensitivity of 10 ml/mm and a paper speed of 20 mm/sec as minimum values for hard copy recorders. Hard copy recordings of volume/time or flow/volume tracings should be recorded as a standard procedure with all spirometry. Accurate paper speed and volume sensitivity are particularly important when the results to be reported are obtained by manual calculation. Paper speed can be checked easily with a stopwatch. With the paper moving, a volume signal is applied at regular intervals so that deflections are placed on the tracing. The intervals between the deflections are then measured and compared with the speed of the recorder. Electronic or strip chart recorders can usually have their speed adjusted; kymographs and similar mechanical recording devices may require more sophisticated repair.

Common problems

Some of the common problems detected by routine quality control of spirometers include:
1. Cracks or leaks
2. Low water level (water seal)
3. Sticking or worn bellows
4. Inaccurate or erratic potentiometers
5. Obstructed or dirty flow tubes (flow sensors)
6. Mechanical resistance (volume displacement)
7. Leaks in tubes and connectors
8. Faulty recorder timing
9. Inappropriate signal correction (BTPS)
10. Improper software calibration (corrections)
11. Defective software or computer interface

CALIBRATION AND QUALITY CONTROL OF GAS ANALYZERS

Accurate analysis of both inspired and expired gases is required for measurements of lung volume (foreign gas techniques), $D_{L_{CO}}$, and gas exchange during exercise testing. In most instances the accuracy of the final results of these tests depends on the accuracy of the spirometer and gas analyzers used. Although various types of gas analyzers are commonly used in pulmonary function testing, some general principles apply to both their calibration and quality control. As noted above, *calibration* refers to the process of adjusting the output of the instrument to meet certain specifications, whereas *quality control* refers to a method of routine checking of the accuracy and precision of the device.

Calibration techniques for gas analyzers:

1. *Physiologic range*. Since many analyzers are not linear over a wide range, it is important to calibrate the device to match the physiologic range over which measurements are to be performed. Oxygen analyzers are commonly used to measure fractional concentrations of 0.21 to 1.00, which represent a wide physiologic range. However, if the analyzer is to be used for exercise testing of subjects breathing room air, the analyzer should be calibrated over the range of 0.12 to 0.21, since this represents the typical physiologic range of expired O_2. Reducing the physiologic range of the analyzers generally improves accuracy and precision. Many types of analyzers provide range adjustments just for this purpose, as well as for user-selectable amplification. Test gases used for calibration should represent the extremes of the physiologic range.

2. *Sampling flow rate*. As a general rule, gas analyzers must be calibrated under the same conditions as will be encountered during the actual testing procedure. In those types of analyzers that sample gas by pumping it from the breathing circuit (O_2, CO_2, CO, N_2), the sampling flow rate *must* be adjusted before calibration and then left unchanged during sampling, unless gas flow is stopped before the measurement is actually performed. A common problem is to calibrate the analyzer and then change the configuration of the sampling circuit (i.e., add tubing, three-way stopcocks, etc.). Any absorber circuits (CO_2, H_2O, dust filters, etc.) should be in place during calibration as well.

3. *Two-point calibration*. The most common technique for analyzer calibration involves exposing the device to two known gases, one of which does not contain the test gas; the other contains a known concentration of test gas, usually at the upper end of the physiologic range. This technique is employed for calibration when the test involves measuring the concentration of a gas that is not normally present in the expirate. The He dilution FRC and $DL_{CO}SB$ are examples of such maneuvers; both the He and CO analyzers are "zeroed" by drawing room air into the sensor cells, assuming, of course, that no helium or carbon monoxide is present in the atmosphere. Then a test gas containing a known concentration of the gas to be analyzed is admitted to the sensor. The analyzer gain is adjusted to match the known concentration. The test gas approximates the concentration to be analyzed during the test. The analyzer may then be rezeroed or the entire process repeated to verify the calibration. Depending on the stability of the analyzer, calibration may have to be repeated before each test application. A similar technique may be employed using two gases of known concentration if the expirate normally contains varying concentrations of the gas.

For example, room air and 12% oxygen might be used to perform a two-point calibration for an O_2 analyzer for exercise testing. The precision of the calibration gas should reflect the necessary accuracy of the measurements involved. For the most exacting analyses, calibration gases should be verified by an independent method.

4. *Three-point calibration*. An assumption made by the simple two-point technique is that the output of the analyzer is linear between the points used for calibration. To verify linearity or to determine the pattern of nonlinearity, three or more calibration points must be determined (Fig. 11-2). The multiple-point calibration is performed in a manner similar to that of the two-point calibration, except that the concentrations of known gases across the range to be analyzed are checked and then plotted. If the analyzer is indeed linear, the points plotted fall in a straight line; if nonlinearity is present, a calibration curve may be constructed to correct analyzed samples. In most instances an equation describing the nonlinear curve can be generated and then used either manually or by software to correct meter readings.

Quality control of gas analyzers can be performed by submitting the analyzer to various concentrations of known test gases or using a lung analog or test subject. Several test gases with concentrations in the range of the analyzer can be

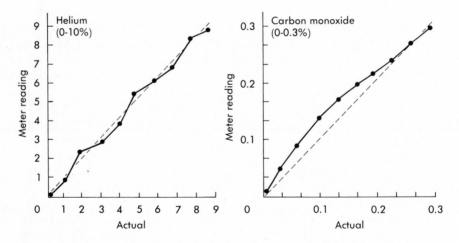

Fig. 11-2. Calibration/linearity check of gas analyzers—typical plots of varying gas concentrations in relation to the meter readings of the analyzers for two gases (He and CO). In each case different dilutions of a known gas are prepared (see text) and submitted to the analyzer. The meter reading is then compared with the actual (calculated) value. In the example the He analyzer shows good linearity in the comparison of measured versus expected concentrations. The CO analyzer shows a nonlinear pattern (as might be expected for an infrared analyzer). If enough points are determined, a "calibration" curve can be generated for correction of the meter readings; by mathematically fitting the curve, an equation can be generated for subsequent correction of meter readings.

maintained but may be a rather complex quality control method for most clinical laboratories. A simpler technique is to prepare serial dilutions of a known gas using a large-volume syringe, such as the type used for simple volume calibration. For example, 100 ml of He and 900 ml of air may be mixed in a 1-liter syringe and then injected into the analyzer sampling device. Subsequently, 100 ml of He might be diluted in 1000 ml, then in 1100 ml, and so on, with the expected concentrations calculated:

$$\text{Expected \% test gas} = \frac{\text{Volume of test gas}}{\text{Total volume of gas}} \times 100$$

As each dilution is analyzed, the meter reading is recorded and plotted against the expected percentage (Fig. 11-2). This method is simple and available to most laboratories; care must be taken when preparing samples in this way so that air does not enter the syringe and further dilute the test gas.

A second method of verifying analyzer performance involves simulating either lung volume or $D_{L_{CO}}$ maneuvers. This may be accomplished using a fixed- or variable-volume lung analog, which is simply a closed container with a known volume (Fig. 11-3). The lung volume simulator is connected at the subject connection with the system prepared as for lung volume or $D_{L_{CO}}$ determination. A large-volume syringe may then be used to "ventilate" the simulator just as a

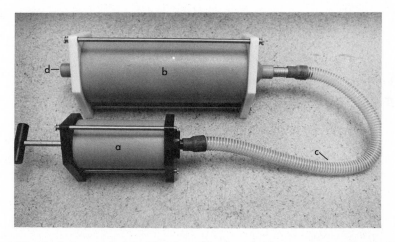

Fig. 11-3. Typical setup for checking the calibration of either an open- or closed-circuit FRC system, or a $D_{L_{CO}}SB$ system. *a,* Large-volume syringe; *b,* variable-volume closed container (the volume is varied by setting the internal piston); *c,* connective tubing so that the syringe can be used to "ventilate" the closed container; *d,* system connection for attachment to the subject port. The system volume is determined by adding the volume set on *b* plus the volume of *c* (determined by filling with water and measuring), plus any dead space contained in the connections. The large-volume syringe is then used to simulate breathing for the specific test being checked (see text).

subject would. At the end of the test the result is compared with the known volume of the analog system. This method tests not only the gas analyzer, but the volume transducer, breathing circuit, and software as well. Temperature corrections should be overridden or not performed. Simulation of the $D_{L_{CO}}SB$ maneuver in this way should produce values very near zero, since both He and CO are diluted in the simulator, but their relative concentrations remain identical. If the two analyzers are not linear in relation to one another, the resulting gas concentrations will vary. If the volume of the simulator can be varied, a linearity check at several different dilutions can be performed.

Testing known subjects is a third means of quality checking gas analyzers, but it may not detect small changes in performance, since the entire lung volume, $D_{L_{CO}}$, or exercise system is used. Despite the natural variability occurring with testing of known subjects, gross malfunctions of systems involving gas analyzers can be detected.

Some of the common problems occurring with gas analyzers that may be detected by routine quality control checks include:

1. Leaks in sampling tubes or connectors
2. Blockage of sampling tubes
3. Exhausted water vapor or CO_2 absorbers
4. Contamination of photocells or electrodes
5. Improper mechanical zeroing (taut band display)
6. Inadequate warm-up time
7. Poor vacuum pump performance (mass spectrometer or N_2 analyzers)
8. Chopper motor malfunction (infrared analyzers)
9. Electrolyte exhaustion (O_2 analyzers)
10. Aging of detector cells (infrared analyzers)
11. Poor optical balance (infrared analyzers)

CALIBRATION AND QUALITY CONTROL OF PLETHYSMOGRAPHS

The calibration techniques described here apply primarily to a "pressure" type of plethysmograph. Users of "flow" plethysmographs should perform the calibration procedure for the box transducer according to the manufacturer's instructions.

1. *Mouth pressure transducer*—is physically calibrated by directly connecting it to a water (or mercury) manometer that encompasses the range of pressures normally measured ($\pm$ 25 cm H_2O). Air is injected into one port of the manometer to cause a deflection of 5 cm (for example), thus creating a difference of 10 cm between the two columns of the manometer. The gain of the mouth pressure amplifier is then adjusted so that the display device (oscilloscope, recorder, or both) deflects by a given amount equivalent to 10 cm H_2O (1 inch, for example). This deflection then becomes the calibration factor for the mouth pressure transducer (in this example, 10 cm H_2O/inch).

2. *Box pressure transducer*—is physically calibrated by closing the box and applying a volume signal comparable to that which occurs during subject testing. In a 500-liter plethysmograph a volume signal of 25 to 50 ml is typical. A sine wave pump connected to a small syringe is ideal, since the same volume can be added and removed from the box at varying frequencies. With the pump operating, the gain of the box pressure transducer is adjusted so that the changing volume of the syringe causes a given deflection on the display device. For example, a 30 ml syringe might be adjusted to cause a 1-inch deflection on the oscilloscope; the box pressure calibration factor then is 30 ml/inch. This procedure can be repeated at varying frequencies from 0.5 to 5.0 cycles/sec (Hz) in order to verify adequate frequency response (the deflection should not change with different frequencies). Flow-type plethysmographs may be calibrated similarly, except the box flow transducer is adjusted rather than a pressure transducer. The box is normally calibrated empty, and then a volume correction for the subject is applied to the final calculation (see Appendix).

3. *Flow transducer*—the pneumotachometer is physically calibrated by applying a known flow of gas via a rotameter or similar type of flow device. The gain of the pressure transducer connected to the pneumotachometer is adjusted in a manner similar to that of the others, so that the flow causes a given deflection on the display. For example, a flow of 1 L/sec may be set to cause a 1-inch deflection, and thus the calibration factor for flow becomes 1 L/sec/inch. By using an adjustable flow rater, the linearity of the pneumotachometer can be verified by checking the deflections at various flows. A weighted spriometer may also be used to generate a known flow.

Some automated plethysmograph systems provide for electronic or software adjustment of the transducers. The known physical signals are similarly applied, but gain adjustments are done electronically or by generating a "correction" factor. Another check provided by some systems is a calibrated voltage signal applied to the display device; this should not be confused with the actual physical calibration described above but may be used to check the oscilloscope or recorder after physical calibration.

Quality control of the body plethysmograph is usually accomplished by use of an isothermal lung analog, a known subject, or comparison with foreign gas dilution or radiologic lung volumes.

An isothermal volume analog can be constructed from a 4- to 5-liter glass bottle that has been filled with metal wool (usually copper) to act as a heat sink (Fig. 11-4). The mouth of the bottle is fitted with two connectors, one to be attached to the subject connection of the mouth shutter, the other to a rubber bulb with a volume of 50 to 100 ml. The actual volume of the device can be determined by subtracting the volume of the metal wool (weight × density) from the volume of the bottle or by filling the device with water from a volumetric source. The dead space of the connector and rubber bulb should also be added to the total volume. The check is performed by a subject seated in the sealed box with the isothermal volume device connected and the mouth shutter closed. While breath-holding, the subject squeezes the bulb; a P_{mouth}/P_{box} tangent is recorded and the volume calculated as usual, except that the P_{H_2O} is not subtracted. The measured volume should equal the volume of the isothermal lung analog (bottle plus connector and bulb minus metal wool) ±5%. The entire procedure may be repeated at various frequencies from 0.5 to 5.0 cycles/sec to ascertain adequate frequency response from the box (the tangents or angles should not change).

A second means of checking the accuracy of the plethysmograph is to measure parameters from a known subject (a series of 10 measurements provides an adequate mean value with which subsequent results may be compared). Despite day-to-day variability in subjects, this method allows checking of both the VTG

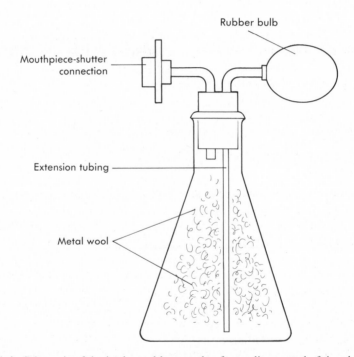

Mouthpiece-shutter connection

Rubber bulb

Extension tubing

Metal wool

Fig. 11-4. Schematic of the isothermal lung analog for quality control of the plethysmograph. A large (approximately 4-liter) jar is fitted with a stopper with two openings. One opening connects to the mouthpiece shutter apparatus of the plethysmograph, and the other is connected to a rubber hand bulb with an extension deep into the bottle. Metal wool (copper) is used to fill the container and acts as a heat sink, so that pressure changes in the bottle cause only minimal changes in gas temperature. By having a subject in the plethysmograph squeeze the bulb (while breath-holding), the VTG maneuver is simulated. A P_{mouth}/P_{box} tangent may be recorded and the volume of the container calculated. The calculated volume should be within 5% of the volume of the device. The true volume is determined by filling the container with water and subtracting the volume of the metal wool. The volumes of the connectors and rubber bulb should be considered as well.

and airway resistance, and quality controlling the box, the transducers, the recording device, and software. Unfortunately, discrepancies between the mean of previous measurements and an individual quality control trial do not indicate from which section of the equipment the problem has arisen. However, with some practice, the source of the problem can usually be uncovered.

A third method of checking the accuracy of the plethysmograph is to compare the VTG with lung volumes from a normal subject determined by foreign gas or radiologic technique. Good correlations (greater than 0.90) have been demonstrated between foreign gas, radiologic, and plethysmographically determined lung volumes in normal subjects. Large differences (greater than 10%) in volumes measured by the plethysmograph and by one of the other methods are nonspecific but may serve as a gross indicator of equipment malfunction. Because this method and the known subject technique described above are based on measurements of individuals, it is important that the subject performs the breathing maneuvers correctly (see Criteria for Acceptability of Lung Volumes and Plethysmography).

Some of the common problems that are identified by routine quality control of plethysmographs include:

1. Leaks in door seals or connectors (pressure boxes)
2. Improperly calibrated transducers
3. Excessive thermal drift
4. Poor frequency response
5. Excessive vibration (poorly mounted transducers)

CALIBRATION AND QUALITY CONTROL OF BLOOD GAS ANALYZERS

Blood gas analyzer systems may be divided into two categories on the basis of the type of calibration employed: manual or automatic. Although the principles involved in both automatic and manual calibrations are similar, some important differences do exist, particularly in the role of the technologist maintaining the instrument.

Manual calibration of the blood gas electrodes involves exposing the gas-measuring electrodes (P_{O_2}, P_{CO_2}) to two or more gases with known partial pressures of oxygen and carbon dioxide and bringing two or more known buffers into contact with the pH-measuring electrode. Calibration gases spanning the physiologic range of the P_{O_2} and P_{CO_2} electrodes are used in much the same fashion as for gas analyzers described above. Typical combinations might include a "high" calibration gas with an F_{O_2} of 0.20 (20%) and an F_{CO_2} of 0.05 (5%); a "low" calibration gas would have an F_{CO_2} of 0.10 (10%) and an F_{O_2} close to zero. The descriptions "high" and "low," applied to the calibration gases, do not always describe the gas tensions of both oxygen and CO_2. After the gases are bubbled through water at 37° C to saturate them with water vapor, they are allowed to flow into the measuring cuvette. The partial pressures of the calibration gases are dependent on the ambient barometric pressure; each calibration gas tension is calculated:

$$P_{gas} = F_{gas} \times (P_B - 47)$$

where

P_{gas} = Partial pressure of calibration gas
F_{gas} = Fractional concentration of the same gas
P_B = Ambient barometric pressure
47   = Partial pressure of water vapor at 37° C

Each calibration gas is allowed to remain in the measuring chamber until equilibrium is reached. Once the partial pressure reading has stabilized, the appropriate control is adjusted to match the electrode to the calculated pressure. As with expired gas analyzers, the "low" gas is used to zero the electrode; the "high" gas is used to adjust the gain on the electrode. Zeroing the electrode does not necessarily mean using a gas with a partial pressure of zero, but rather setting the low range of the electrode. As noted previously, two-point calibrations are commonly used to calibrate gas analysis devices; more than two calibration gases, however, must be used to prove the linearity of the electrode system. On most blood gas systems a combination of calibration gases is used, so that the PO_2 is calibrated over a range of 0 to 150 mm Hg and the Pco_2 from approximately 40 to 80 mm Hg. Because some systems use gases to calibrate the gas tension electrodes but measure gas tensions in a liquid (blood), some difference may exist between analysis of the same partial pressure in gas or liquid. This is particularly true with the polarographic oxygen electrode used in most blood gas analyzers and is related to the consumption of O_2 at the electrode tip. Since O_2 molecules diffuse much faster in a gaseous medium than in blood, if the analyzer is calibrated with gas, a correction factor must be applied to provide accurate measurement in a liquid. This is usually accomplished by calibrating the electrode using a liquid that has been tonometered (see below) with the calibration gas and then measuring the calibration gas itself and deriving a ratio factor based on the difference between the two. Some systems use tonometered solutions for routine calibration of the gas electrodes, thus avoiding the necessity of determining the gas/liquid ratio.

Manual calibration of the pH electrode system is performed by exposing the measuring electrode to two (or more) known buffers. The "low" buffer typically has a pH of 6.840 (similar to the sealed-in buffer used in the measuring electrode), with a "high" buffer in the range of 7.38 (close to normal adult blood pH). The zero and gain of the pH voltmeter is adjusted to match these known points.

Automatic calibration of blood gas analyzers differs slightly from manual calibration, not in the gases or reagents involved, but in the role of the technologist in assuring that the procedure achieves the desired outcome. In general, the gas tension electrodes are balanced and sloped using two (or more) gases of known fractional concentrations. Adjustment of the output of each electrode's amplifier is performed by a microprocessor that not only reads the calibration values, but also compares the measured values to expected values. Automatic calibration of the pH system is performed similarly, with the microprocessor adjusting the electrode output to match two or more known buffers. Most automated systems include checks of various other parameters that are fundamental to blood gas analysis, such as barometric pressure and the temperature at the measuring cuvette. Some automated systems tonometer their own calibrating solutions for calibration of both the gas and pH electrodes. Because automatic calibration occurs at predetermined intervals, and because adjustments are performed based on the response of the electrodes, it is important that all the necessary conditions for an acceptable calibration be met before the procedure occurs. During the automatic calibration, inadequate buffer or calibration gas may cause the microprocessor to adjust the output of the electrode(s) excessively. A similar problem arises when blood or protein clots at the tip of the electrode, altering its sensitivity, and then an automatic calibration occurs. The microprocessor again adjusts the electrode output to attempt to bring it into range. Although this process works well for minor changes in electrode function, it may not adequately calibrate the electrode if there is an excessive buildup of debris at the measuring surface. The technologist must maintain the buffers, gases, and electrodes so that automatic calibration can occur successfully. Inappropriate adjustments that occur are usually detected easily by routinely checking the results of the auto-calibration.

Two general methods of quality control for blood gas analysis are in widespread use: (1) tonometry and (2) commercially prepared controls. In general, the interpretation of blood gas quality control is the same with either of these methods, with a few minor differences.

A *tonometer* is a device that allows precision gas mixtures to be equilibrated with either whole blood or a suitable buffer. One commonly used tonometer creates a thin film of blood or buffer by spinning the sample in a chamber that is flooded with the precision gas. Another type bubbles the gas through the sample to create a large surface for gas exchange. The tonometer is maintained at 37° C, and the gas is humidified; after an equilibration period determined by the gas flow rate and the size of the sample being prepared, the sample may be transferred to the blood gas analyzer. The expected gas tensions are calculated from the fractional concentrations of the precision gas, just as described above for manual calibrations. If whole blood is used as the control material, then Po_2 and Pco_2, but not pH, can be checked. Blood is ideal for controlling the gas electrodes, since its viscosity and gas exchange properties are the same as patient samples, but unless the buffering capacity of the blood to be tonometered is known, the pH cannot be accurately calculated. Tonometry of a bicarbonate-based buffer using a known fractional concentration of CO_2 allows both gas and pH electrodes to be controlled, although the gas exchange characteristics of the buffer differ from those of whole blood. Tonometry can be performed inexpensively using pooled waste blood and small amounts of precision gas, with control of pH accomplished by tonometry of a buffer. Normally three levels of control materials are used to provide checks over the physiologic range of the electrodes, so three precision gas mixtures are required. Accuracy of tonometry is highly dependent on a standardized technique. Sampling syringes must be lubricated and then flushed with the precision gas. Careful attention to the preparation and sampling from the tonometer is required to obtain reliable results and, as might be expected, is somewhat dependent on individual technique.

Commercially prepared controls fall into two general categories: blood based and aqueous/fluorocarbon based. The blood-based matrix consists of buffered fixed human red cells. The aqueous-based control is a bicarbonate-containing buffer; the fluorocarbon-based control is a perfluorinated compound that has enhanced oxygen-dissolving characteristics. These control materials are packaged in sealed ampules of 2 to 3 ml volume and require minimal preparation for use. The blood-based material requires refrigerated storage, incubation at 37° C for several minutes, and agitation before use. The aqueous/fluorocarbon–based controls have typical shelf lives of 1 year and simply require agitation for 10 to 15 seconds. Multiple levels of these controls are used to provide control over the range of values clinically seen. Although commercially available controls are considerably more expensive than tonometered samples, they are convenient to use and less susceptible to handling errors. One difficulty associated with aqueous controls (and to a lesser extent with fluorocarbon solutions) is poor reproducibility of the Po_2, especially at low partial pressures. This results in such a wide range of "normal" values that the control may be of limited clinical usefulness. Some of these difficulties may be overcome by careful statistical handling of the Po_2 quality control data as described below.

With all of the quality control methodologies described, a sound method of interpretation of the results of "control runs" is necessary to translate the derived data into information that will allow the technologist to maintain or repair a poorly operating instrument. The most common method for detecting "out-of-control" blood gas electrodes is to use the sample mean ±2 standard deviations (SD) statistical concept, with a sample population of at least 20 to 30 data sets. One standard deviation on either side of the mean in a normal distribution will include about 67% of the points, whereas 2 SD will include 95%, and 3 SD 99.7%. For any particular quality control sample that falls within ±2 SD of the mean, the run can be considered "in control." If the control sample falls between 2 and 3 SD from the mean, there is only a 5% chance that the run is in control; nevertheless, because of random error in sampling, 1 of 20 control runs can be expected to be in the 2 to 3 SD range and still be acceptable. To distinguish true out-of-control situations from random errors, more complex sets of rules have been developed. The most widely used rules are those proposed by Westgard (see Selected Bibliography). These rules are a subset of many statistical models that are used together to provide the greatest probability for detecting real errors and rejecting false errors. This approach to quality control is termed the multiple-rule method and usually requires that two or more control levels be evaluated on the same measurement device (electrode). The multiple-rule method is applied as follows:

1. When one control observation exceeds the mean ± 2 SD, a "warning" condition exists.
2. When one control observation exceeds the mean ± 3 SD, an out-of-control condition exists.

3. When two consecutive control observations exceed the mean $+ 2$ SD or the mean $- 2$ SD, an out-of-control condition exists.
4. When the range of differences between consecutive control runs exceeds 4 SD, an out-of-control condition exists.
5. When four consecutive control observations exceed the mean $+ 1$ SD or the mean $- 1$ SD, an out-of-control condition exists.
6. When ten consecutive control observations fall on the same side of the mean ($\pm$), an out-of-control condition exists.

One problem with using a strict statistical approach is that when outliers (more than 2 or 3 SD) are rejected, the SD tends to become smaller, so that eventually good data may be rejected. This situation can be managed by including data into the database that is clinically acceptable. With the multiple-rule approach, it is necessary not only to evaluate the mean and standard deviation of the current control run, but also to keep a control history. This is usually accomplished by means of a control chart (Fig. 11-5). To adequately control an instrument such as a blood gas analyzer, three levels of control materials are normally used. Having three levels of control for each of the three electrodes (pH, PCO_2, and PO_2) dictates that nine mean and standard deviation values must be calculated for each instrument, and tracking consecutive runs can become quite cumbersome. To automate this procedure, computerized quality control data reduction programs are commonly employed. Such programs are available from professional organizations as well as commercial vendors. The chief advantages of such programs is that data storage is simplified, all necessary statistics can be maintained, and sets of rules such as those outlined can be applied easily to each control run to detect errors. This type of record keeping for quality control and instrument maintenance is required by many accrediting agencies and by some states.

Several other techniques related to quality control of blood gas analyzers are commonly employed. Interlaboratory proficiency testing consists of the analysis of unknown control specimens from a single source so that an individual laboratory can be compared with other laboratories using both the same and different methodologies. Results of proficiency tests are reported as means and standard deviations for each type of instrument participating in the program. Proficiency testing does not provide day-to-day quality control but acts as a means to verify that the values reported by an individual laboratory are within a commonly accepted range. Multiple levels of unknowns are usually provided to check the typical ranges of values seen in clinical practice. Proficiency testing programs are available from professional organizations (College of American Pathologists, American Thoracic Society), as well as commercial vendors, and are required by most accrediting agencies.

Comparison of either controls or random samples on multiple instruments provides another means of quality control. Since many blood gas laboratories have two or more instruments, comparisons between instruments provide a type of proficiency testing that yields immediate information. Along the same lines, monitoring either controls or samples by independent methods may provide a means of checking the accuracy of a particular instrument. For example, measurement of pH by means of an automated blood gas analyzer and a manual pH

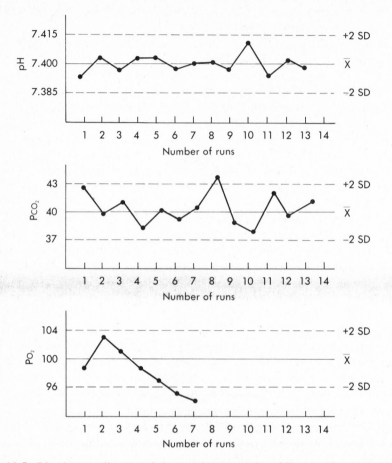

Fig. 11-5. Blood gas quality control charts—three examples of Shewhart/Levey-Jennings charts (pH, P_{CO_2}, and P_{O_2}) on which the mean for a specific control material is plotted as a solid line and the $\pm$ 2 SD lines are dotted. The left axis on each graph is labeled with the actual mean and 2 SD values. Consecutive control "runs" are plotted along the horizontal axis. On the pH control chart all of the values vary about the mean in a regular fashion—the electrode appears "in control" for the 13 measurements plotted. The P_{CO_2} chart shows a slightly different pattern: individual control values vary more than the pH, and run 8 shows a value outside of the 2 SD range. In this case the value is probably a "random" error, since 1/20 of normal values still fall outside the $\pm$ 2 SD limits. The P_{O_2} chart shows a "trend" of decreasing control values until runs 6 and 7 both produce values less than -2 SD; this pattern indicates that the electrode is malfunctioning and needs to be serviced. By applying strict rules to the interpretation of consecutive control runs (with or without charts) most "out-of-control" situations can be detected (see text).

electrode could be used to determine the accuracy of the automated calibration system.

Some of the common problems encountered in the blood gas laboratory that are detected by adequate quality control are:

1. *Electrode malfunction.* The most common causes of out-of-control situations relate to problems arising from the gas and pH electrodes. Protein and blood product buildup on the membranes covering the electrodes is quite common and can usually be remedied by careful cleaning. Leaks in the membranes themselves and depletion of electrolyte solution also commonly lead to electrode drift.

2. *Temperature control.* Failure of the water or air bath to maintain the measuring cuvette at $37°$ C or thermometer inaccuracy may lead to unacceptable electrode performance. Temperature control systems should be checked routinely against a certified thermometer (National Bureau of Standards).

3. *Improper calibration.* Improper manual calibration, either one- or two-point, is often related to operator error. Analysis of quality control data may determine if the technologist is performing calibration or sampling incorrectly. Problems arising from automatic calibration almost always relate to the instrument—performing a calibration with inadequate buffer or a poorly functioning electrode.

4. *Reagent contamination or loss.* Contamination of calibration buffers and gases leads to inaccurate calibration and sample analysis. Quality control values that are consistently high or low may indicate a problem with reagents. Analysis of the buffers or reagents by an independent method may be required to detect deficiencies.

5. *Mechanical problems.* A common source of error is the mechanism responsible for pumping or aspirating the sample into the measuring cuvette. Leaks in pump tubing or poorly functioning pumps allow calibrating solutions, controls, and patient samples to be contaminated. If air bubbles are introduced during analysis, gas tensions may be in error whereas pH determinations may be acceptable, but large changes in P_{CO_2} can cause alterations in the pH. Inadequate rinsing of the measuring chamber may also occur with pump problems. This usually results in blood clotting in the transport tubing or measuring chamber.

6. *Improper sampling technique.* Failure to collect arterial specimens anaerobically, to properly store the sample in ice water, and bubbles in the specimen may result in questionable results. Excess heparin typically results in a decrease in pH. Improperly iced blood gas specimens exhibit changes in pH, P_{CO_2}, and P_{O_2}; red and white blood cells consume O_2 and produce CO_2 with a reduction in the pH. Air bubbles in the specimen shift the gas tensions in the sample toward room air; low P_{O_2} values move toward 150 mm Hg, whereas P_{O_2} values above 150 are reduced. Another common problem related to sampling is obtaining a venous specimen inadvertently. Adequately functioning electrodes, as demonstrated by good

quality control, can detect poor sampling techniques, in distinction to actual clinical abnormalities.

CRITERIA FOR ACCEPTABILITY OF PULMONARY FUNCTION STUDIES

Quality assurance in the pulmonary function laboratory focuses not only on the instrumentation used, equipment calibration, and application of control signals, but also on careful attention to the *sampling method* employed. In terms of pulmonary function testing, *sampling technique* is best defined as the procedures used to obtain patient data. This includes the effort and cooperation of the subject, the instruction and encouragement provided by the technologist, and the proper performance of the equipment. Application of objective criteria to help decide on the validity of the data is one means of providing high-quality results.

The criteria described below are divided by test category. Standards for spirometry have been set forth by the American Thoracic Society, but guidelines for other tests are much less standardized. In each of the test categories a common method is employed; in applying the criteria, the following steps should be generally followed:

1. Examine the hard copy tracing whenever available. The best hard copy for this purpose is a direct recording such as a kymograph tracing for spirometry; computer-generated graphics, either on paper or video display, may be used as well. Compare the observed tracing with the characteristics of an acceptable curve.
2. Look at the numerical data. Are the results reproducible? Are the best two or three values within 5% of one another?
3. Are key points in the particular test procedure present (e.g., minimum change in gas concentration or timing of the maneuver)? The key points to look for vary with the exact methodology employed for each category of test.
4. Are the results of different categories of tests consistent (i.e., do spirometry, lung volumes, DL_{CO}, and blood gas analysis all point to a similar interpretation)?

These general guidelines are the basis for applying the criteria to individual sets of patient data.

CRITERIA FOR ACCEPTABILITY OF SPIROMETRY

The following criteria may be used to judge the acceptability of tests derived from the forced expiratory volume maneuver:

1. The volume-time tracing should show maximal effort, with a smooth curve; the tracing should show at least 6 seconds of forced effort. A volume plateau with a volume change of less than 25 ml in a 0.5-second interval should be achieved. Some subjects with severe obstruction may continue exhalation well past 10 seconds, so 6 seconds is simply a minimum. Similarly, in severe obstruction, very low flows may be observed at the end of expiration.

2. The start-of-test should be abrupt and unhesitating; on any maneuver that displays a "slow" start, the back-extrapolated volume should be calculated and the FEV_1, etc., adjusted (Fig. 11-6). If the volume of back extrapolation is greater than 10% of the measured FVC, then the maneuver is not acceptable and should not be included for reporting purposes.
3. A minimum of three acceptable tests should be obtained; the FVC values of the two "best" acceptable tests should be within 5%, or 100 ml, whichever is larger. This may be calculated:

$$\frac{\text{Second-best FVC}}{\text{Best FVC}} \times 100$$

If the two "best" acceptable tests are not within 5% (or 100 ml), then the maneuver should be repeated until the criteria are met. The "best" test is usually obtained within the first five attempts.
4. The MEFV curve, if obtained, should show reproducible flows at similar lung volumes. The PEFR (peak flow) should be consistent and is a good indicator of subject effort. Superimposing MEFV curves or displaying

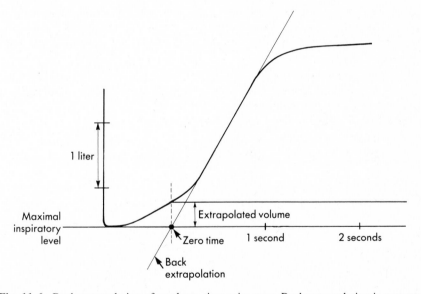

Fig. 11-6. Back extrapolation of a volume-time spirogram. Back extrapolation is a means of correcting measurements made from a spirogram that does not show a sharp deflection from the baseline maximum inspiratory level. A straight line drawn through the steepest part of a volume-time tracing is extended to cross the baseline. The point of intersection is the back-extrapolated time zero, and timed intervals (such as FEV_1) are measured from this starting point rather than from the initial deflection from the baseline. The perpendicular distance *(slashed line)* from the zero time point to the volume-time tracing defines the back-extrapolated volume. To accurately determine the zero time point, the extrapolated volume should be less than 10% of the FVC or 100 ml, whichever is greater. Tracings with larger extrapolated volumes may be considered invalid.

them side-by-side offers a simple means of checking reproducibility. Complete loops should be close; that is, inspiratory and expiratory VC values should be similar.

The "best" test (i.e., the values to be reported) should come from an acceptable maneuver with the largest sum of FVC and FEV_1; the FEV_1 (and other FEVx values) may be taken from another acceptable maneuver if they are larger. The rationale for this is that if the maneuver was performed correctly, a larger FEV_1 should not be discarded just because the FVC was lower. Spirometric parameters that are determined by the FVC (such as the $FEF_{25\%-75\%}$) should come from a single maneuver with the largest FVC and FEV_1 sum (Table 11-2). One serious problem with using these criteria for spirometry reporting is that if a single tracing is stored for inclusion in the final report, it may not contain all of the data appearing on the report. It is advisable to maintain hard copy recordings (or raw data) of all acceptable maneuvers. Other methods of selecting the "best" test include using the PEFR as an indicator of maximal effort or combining raw data from several MEFV loops to create an "envelope" loop. Using the peak flow may result in error if the FVC and FEV_1 are not also evaluated, since the PEFR is largely effort dependent and occurs at the beginning of the forced expiration. Combining loops to generate an envelope will provide the maximum flow achieved at any lung volume, but again not all reported data may be depicted.

Spirometry may be performed with the subject in either the sitting or standing position for adult subjects; in children less than 12 years of age, results of spirometry may be significantly larger when the subject is in the standing position. The use of noseclips is recommended for spirometric measurements that entail rebreathing, even if just for a few breaths. Some spirometers record only expiratory flow and require the subject to place the mouthpiece into the mouth after inspiring to TLC; if such is the case, noseclips are usually unnecessary. Care should be taken, however, that the subject places the mouthpiece into his or her mouth rapidly before beginning the forced expiration to avoid unmeasurable loss of volume. It is usually impossible to calculate the volume of back extrapolation

Table 11–2. Comparison of spirometry efforts

Test	Trial 1	Trial 2	Trial 3	"Best" test
FVC	5.20	5.30	5.35*	5.35
FEV_1	4.41*	4.35	4.36*	4.41
FEV_1/FVC (%)	85	82	82	82
$FEF_{25\%-75\%}$	3.87	3.92	3.94	3.94
$\dot{V}_{max\ 50}$	3.99	3.95	3.41	3.41
$\dot{V}_{max\ 25}$	1.97	1.95	1.89	1.89
PEFR	8.39	9.44	9.89	9.89

*These values are the key to selecting the "best" test results. The FEV_1 is taken from Trial 1, even though the largest sum of FVC and FEV_1 occurs in Trial 3. All FVC-dependent flows (average and instantaneous flows) come from Trial 3. It should be noted that the $FEV_{1\%}$ (FEV_1/FVC) is calculated from the FEV_1 of Trial 1 and the FVC of Trial 3. The MEFV curve, if reported, would be the curve from Trial 3 as well.

manually from a tracing that displays only expiratory flow. In either type of recording system (rebreathing or expiratory flow only) the mechanical recording device should have its pen (or paper) moving at recording speed when the forced expiration begins. Systems that initiate pen or paper movement at the same time as expiration are typically unable to adequately record the start-of-test.

CRITERIA FOR ACCEPTABILITY OF THE MVV

The maximum voluntary ventilation maneuver may be considered acceptable if the following criteria are met:

1. The tracing (volume versus time) should show a continuous, rhythmic effort for at least 12 seconds. The end-expiratory level should remain fairly constant unless significant air trapping occurs. Most subjects show changes in the end-expiratory level on the first few breaths of the MVV as they adjust to a mechanically efficient lung volume; this usually shows up on the tracing as a decrease in spirometer volume. The first three to five breaths may be discarded if the maneuver was continued long enough for a 12-second interval to be measured. Performing the test for 12 to 15 seconds is usually adequate.

2. The measured MVV should exceed the largest FEV_1 multiplied by 35. Since there is a good correlation between the two parameters, the effort put forth by the subject can be judged against an acceptable FEV_1 maneuver. Similarly, if the MVV exceeds the $FEV_1 \times 35$ by a large amount, the validity of the FEV_1 itself may be questioned.

3. At least two acceptable maneuvers should be obtained; the results should not differ by more than 10%. If a difference greater than 10% is observed, the test should be repeated until the two best maneuvers are reproducible. Other, less strenuous, tests may be interposed in order to minimize fatigue that may accompany repeated MVV trials.

The ''best'' test should be the largest MVV observed from an acceptable maneuver. If the subject is unable to perform the MVV for 12 seconds because of coughing, fatigue, or shortness of breath, that fact should be noted on the final report.

CRITERIA FOR ACCEPTABILITY OF THE SVC

The slow vital capacity maneuver may be considered acceptable if the following criteria are met:

1. The end-expiratory volume during the three breaths immediately preceding the VC maneuver should not vary by more than 100 ml. Increasing or decreasing end-expiratory levels usually indicate that the subject is not breathing consistently near FRC or that a leak is present. It should be noted that even if the end-expiratory level is constant, the tidal volume usually increases when the subject is asked to breathe through the spirometer circuit with a noseclip in place. This increase in V_T will influence the inspiratory capacity (IC) and expiratory reserve volume (ERV), depending on the pattern of breathing.

2. The subject should expire smoothly to residual volume (RV) and then inspire without interruption to total lung capacity (TLC). A plateau (volume) should occur at both maximal expiration and maximal inspiration. The SVC may be measured either from maximal inspiration (inspiratory VC) or from maximal expiration (expiratory VC).

3. At least two acceptable SVC maneuvers should be obtained. The volumes on these trials should be within 5% of one another, or the maneuver repeated until the two best results are reproducible.

4. The SVC should be within 5% of the previously measured best FVC. An SVC much less than 95% of the FVC may be due to poor effort on the part of the subject. An SVC much larger than the FVC may be due to dynamic compression of the airways during the FVC maneuver, insufficient effort, or poor understanding of the test. It should be noted that an SVC that is significantly larger than the FVC may mean that the $FEV_{1\%}$ was overestimated.

It is important to obtain an acceptable SVC, particularly if the subdivisions (IC and ERV) are to be used to calculate RV and TLC. These same criteria should be applied to the SVC if it is done alone or as part of the lung volume determination (by foreign gas or plethysmography). SVC maneuvers done during the He dilution FRC measurement may show slightly lower ERV values, since the subject exhales through the CO_2 absorber. The IC and ERV may be recorded from the FVC maneuver if tidal breathing is also recorded; the end-expiratory level should be well defined as described above.

CRITERIA FOR ACCEPTABILITY OF LUNG VOLUMES AND PLETHYSMOGRAPHY
He dilution FRC

The helium dilution functional residual capacity determination may be considered acceptable if the following criteria are met:

1. The "system" baseline should be flat, and the He concentration should be stable up to the point of subject switch-in; this indicates that no system leaks are present.

2. The rebreathing pattern should be regular; in either the stabilized volume or oxygen bolus method the tidal breathing pattern should be regular, with successive breaths showing a gradually falling end-tidal level (as O_2 is consumed). A pattern of increasing tidal volume and rate usually indicates inadequate CO_2 absorption; this is uncomfortable and dangerous for the subject and may affect the He analyzer readings.

3. The test should be continued until the He concentration changes by less than 0.02% over a 30-second interval. If the He analyzer is incapable of readings as small as 0.02%, then 0.05% in 30 seconds may be used. If the He concentration is reported only every 30 seconds (as in some automated systems), the test should be continued for at least 3 minutes, even if the equilibration criteria above are met before then. This avoids the "false" equilibrium that may occur with irregular breathing patterns or frequent addition of oxygen.

4. The oxygen consumption (either measured or estimated) should be appropriate for a quietly breathing subject (200 to 400 ml/min). Some systems estimate O_2 consumption during the rebreathing by noting the volume added divided by the time of the test. In the stabilized volume method the O_2 consumption can be estimated by noting how often (and how much) oxygen is added. During the oxygen bolus method the rate of fall of the spirometer volume is proportional to the O_2 consumption rate. High O_2 consumption usually indicates a leak; very low or no O_2 consumption means that the subject is receiving oxygen outside the system, also usually an indication of a leak.

5. The He wash-in curve (if plotted) should be smooth and regular. The exact pattern will depend on the evenness of ventilation, but the curve should show gradually decreasing He concentrations. The curve should be flat at equilibrium.

The time to reach equilibrium should be reported; if the subject fails to achieve equilibrium, that also should be reported. Extremely large or small FRC values (especially in normal subjects) should be examined carefully in regard to the above criteria. Comparison of the He washout lung volumes to those obtained by an independent method is helpful. In normal subjects or those with mild to moderate restrictive diseases, lung volumes determined by plethysmograph, chest x-ray method, or single-breath dilution (as done with $D_{L_{CO}}$) should be similar. In obstructed subjects He lung volumes should be less than plethysmograph volumes and greater than single-breath volumes.

N_2 washout FRC

The nitrogen washout lung volume determination may be considered acceptable if the following criteria are met:

1. The washout should show a regular pattern without noticeable increases or abrupt jumps in end-tidal N_2. Individual breaths may vary, particularly in subjects with irregular breathing patterns or uneven ventilation, but the general trend should show gradually falling N_2 concentrations. Leaks in tubing, the sampling head, or at the mouthpiece usually allow room air, containing N_2, to enter the system. If a Tissot collection system is used, the volume of the spirometer should be constant when the valves are closed to the subject, indicating no leak in the spirometer.

2. Washout times should be appropriate for the type of subject being tested; normal subjects should wash out in approximately 3 minutes or less. Washout should be complete (i.e., down to approximately 1% N_2) in subjects without obstruction. Incomplete washout in unobstructed subjects usually indicates a small leak or a contaminated oxygen source.

The washout time should be reported; failure to wash out within 7 minutes (or more) should also be noted. Extremely large or small FRC values should be questioned in regard to the above criteria. Lung volume determinations by an independent method should compare as described above for He dilution FRC.

Body plethysmography (VTG)

The thoracic gas volume determined using the body plethysmograph may be considered acceptable if the following criteria are met:

1. The oscilloscope or recorded tracing should indicate that the subject panted correctly; the P_{mouth}/P_{box} loop should be closed or nearly so. The loop should be contained in the pressure range for which the transducers were calibrated; that is, if full-scale deflection is $\pm$ 10 cm H_2O on the mouth pressure axis, then the mouth pressure deflection should not exceed $\pm$ 10 cm H_2O. If the oscilloscope or recorder is calibrated appropriately, pressure signals that exceed the calibration limits will go "off-screen" and be easily detected. Open loops may indicate compression of gas in the oropharynx, especially with the cheek muscles, or leaks at the mouth.

2. A minimum of three acceptable panting maneuvers should be obtained. The tangents should agree within 5% of the average of the tangents measured. This may not always be practical, especially if only three acceptable tangents are obtained and all three vary significantly. In such cases the average may be used without rejecting individual maneuvers, but the variability of the tangents should be considered when interpreting the final results.

Similar criteria may be applied to measurements of tangents for calculation of airway resistance (Raw), except that the tangents for open-shutter and closed-shutter maneuvers are not averaged. Since the $\dot{V}/P_{box}$ tangent and P_{mouth}/P_{box} tangent are interdependent, the airway resistance is derived for each maneuver separately, and then the results of several maneuvers are averaged. In most instances the closed-shutter tangents (volume) measured during the resistance maneuvers will be less than those measured to derive VTG, since the typical subject pants *above* FRC. If the subject cannot perform at least three acceptable maneuvers, it should be noted on the report. The VTG should be determined from the average of three or more acceptable maneuvers. As described for the foreign gas techniques above, it is often instructive to compare lung volume determinations by two or more independent methods. In subjects with obstructive disease, plethysmographically determined lung volumes usually exceed those measured by the foreign gas techniques but compare favorably with radiologic volumes.

CRITERIA FOR ACCEPTABILITY OF DLCOSB

The modified Krogh technique—single-breath maneuver may be considered acceptable if the following criteria are met:

1. The volume-time tracing (see Fig. 5-2) should show a smooth, rapid inspiration from RV to TLC. The breath-hold baseline should be flat, and the exhalation of dead space gas should be rapid and smooth. The tracing should indicate the switch-in to alveolar sampling.

2. The volume inspired (VC) should exceed 90% of the largest previously measured VC: either FVC or SVC. If the subject inspires less than 90% of the known VC, then it may be assumed that the subject either did not exhale to RV or did not breath-hold at TLC, or both. For purposes of

standardization, the breath-hold should be as close to the true TLC as possible. If the inspired volume exceeds the best previously determined VC, then that VC should be questioned and may need to be repeated.
3. The breath-holding time should be between 9 and 11 seconds. Various methods of timing are employed with the single-breath D_{LCO} (see Chapter 5). Again, for purposes of standardization, the breath-holding time should be kept close to 10 seconds. Rapid inspiration and expiration tend to reduce differences produced by the method of timing employed. In subjects with obstruction, prolonged expiration adds to the time for diffusion to occur and may result in an overestimation of diffusing capacity. Reducing the washout volume may shorten the measured breath-hold time but may also lead to inaccuracies; sampling earlier will add more dead space gas to the "alveolar" sample, particularly in those subjects who may have increased dead space.
4. Duplicate determinations should be within 5% of one another. The reported value should be the average of two or more acceptable maneuvers.

The number of acceptable maneuvers that are averaged should be included in the report. If the subject is unable to perform acceptable maneuvers, that fact should be reported as well, particularly if a D_{LCO} value is reported anyway. If a washout volume other than the "standard" 1000 ml is used, it should be noted. The lung volume calculated from the D_{LCO} maneuver (V_A) may be compared with previously measured lung volumes. In normal and even moderately restricted subjects the V_A correlates reasonably well with the TLC if the single-breath maneuver is performed acceptably. In obstructed subjects the single-breath lung volume is typically smaller than lung volumes by multiple-breath foreign gas techniques, radiologic estimation, or plethysmography. It is often helpful to report the alveolar volume estimated by the $D_{LCO}SB$ for purposes of comparison. Similarly, the D_{LCO} itself may be reported using the standard single-breath technique and also recalculating the diffusion capacity using an independently determined lung volume in a similar equation.

SELF-ASSESSMENT QUESTIONS

1. A spirometer is tested by injecting a 3-liter volume from a large syringe several times; the results look like this:

Trial	Volume
1	3.5
2	3.6
3	3.6

Which of the following descriptions are true?
I. The spirometer is accurate.
II. The spirometer is precise.
III. The spirometer is accurate within 3%.
IV. The spirometer is not precise.
a. I, II, and III
b. I and II
c. I and IV
d. II only

2. Calibration relates to quality control in that:
   a. The two are identical
   b. Calibration includes "adjustment" of the output to match a known input
   c. Both use some sort of known test signal
   d. b and c
3. A 3-liter syringe is used to perform quality control on a spirometer; the results of several maneuvers are:

Trial	Volume
1	2.95
2	2.90
3	2.93
	2.93 AVERAGE

   What is the percent of error of this spirometer?
   a. 2.3%
   b. 5.0%
   c. 9.8%
   d. Cannot be determined
4. Which of the following is adequate for checking the accuracy of the FEV_1 measurement?
   a. A 3-liter syringe
   b. A sine wave rotary pump
   c. An explosive decompression device
   d. All of the above
5. A CO_2 analyzer is set up to monitor a subject's exhaled gas; what gas(es) should be used to calibrate the analyzer for this purpose?
   a. 5% CO_2
   b. 10% CO_2
   c. Room air and 5% CO_2
   d. a and b
6. To demonstrate the linearity of a gas analyzer, _____ gas(es) is (are) required?
   a. One
   b. Two
   c. Three or more
   d. Room air plus one
7. Physical calibration of the body plethysmograph requires:
   a. Calibration of the mouth pressure transducer
   b. Calibration of the pneumotachometer for flow
   c. Calibration of the box pressure (or flow)
   d. All of the above
   e. a and c
8. To manually calibrate a blood gas analyzer, a "high" calibration gas with 20% oxygen and 5% CO_2 is used; if the local barometric pressure is 753, the respective calibration pressures are:
   a. 151 and 38 mm Hg
   b. 151 and 40 mm Hg
   c. 141 and 38 mm Hg
   d. 141 and 35 mm Hg

9. Which of the following are true regarding the use of tonometry for quality control of blood gas analyzers?
    I. Tonometered blood may be used to check Po_2 and Pco_2 electrodes.
    II. Tonometered blood may be used to check pH electrodes.
    III. Three precision gases are required for three levels of controls.
    IV. Tonometry is independent of technician sampling technique.
      a. I, II, III, and IV
      b. I, III, and IV
      c. I and III
      d. II and IV

10. Quality control runs for a Pco_2 electrode have produced a mean of 38 mm Hg with a standard deviation of 1 mm Hg; according to the multiple-rule method, if the next two control runs produce values of 43 and 44 mm Hg, the electrode:
      a. Is "out of control"
      b. Is "in control"
      c. Displays only "random" error
      d. Is "in control" but showing an "out-of-control" trend

11. An individual forced expiratory volume maneuver may be rejected if:
    I. The volume of back extrapolation is greater than 10% of the FVC
    II. The end of the test does not plateau (volume continues to change by more than 25 ml in 0.5 second)
    III. The maneuver lasts less than 6 seconds
    IV. The volume-time tracing does not show smooth, continuous effort
      a. I, II, III, and IV
      b. I, III, and IV
      c. II, III, and IV
      d. II and III

12. According to the recommendations of the American Thoracic Society, the "best" test (i.e., the test from which flows will be reported) is the test with the:
      a. Largest of three acceptable FVC values
      b. Largest PEFR (peak flow)
      c. Largest sum of FEV_1 and FVC
      d. Largest FEV_1

13. A subject with normal spirometry values performs an He dilution FRC maneuver; after 7 minutes, equilibrium is still not attained and the test is terminated. The FRC is reported as 9.1 liters (BTPS). Which of the following would be appropriate to determine if the result is erroneous?
    I. Examine the hard copy tracing to see if any leaks were present.
    II. Check to see how much O_2 was added during the maneuver.
    III. Calculate the TLC (and derive the FRC) from the chest x-ray film.
    IV. Compare the V_{TG} from the plethysmograph.
      a. I, II, III, and IV
      b. II, III, and IV
      c. I, III, and IV
      d. II and III

14. Which of the following would be indications for rejecting a $DL_{CO}SB$ maneuver?
    I. The breath-hold time is 9.6 seconds.
    II. The volume inspired is 77% of the FVC.

III. The volume-time tracing shows a rapid inspiration.

IV. The volume-time tracing shows a rapid exhalation.

a. I, II, III, and IV

b. I, III, and IV

c. II only

d. III and IV

15. A subject performs spirometry, SVC, and MVV maneuvers; these results are reported:

	Measured
FVC	4.1 L
FEV_1	2.7 L
$FEF_{25\%-75\%}$	0.9 L/sec
MVV	59.5 L/min
SVC	3.9 L
ERV	1.9 L
IC	2.0 L

Which statement best describes the accuracy of these results?

a. The values are consistent and reproducible.

b. The SVC is invalid.

c. The MVV is invalid.

d. The FVC is invalid.

e. b and c

SELECTED BIBLIOGRAPHY

General references

Clausen, J.L., editor: Pulmonary function testing guidelines and controversies, New York, 1982, Academic Press, Inc.

Morris, A.H., et al.: Clinical pulmonary function testing, ed. 2, Salt Lake City, 1984, Intermountain Thoracic Society.

Calibration and quality control

Clausen, J.L., et. al.: Interlaboratory comparisons of blood gas measurements, Am. Rev. Respir. Dis. **123** (suppl.):104, 1981.

Gardner, R.M., Hankinson, J.L., and West, B.J.: Evaluating commercially available spirometers, Am. Rev. Respir. Dis. **121**:73, 1980.

Gardner, R.M., et al.: Spirometry: what paper speed? Chest **84**:161, 1983.

Glindmeyer, H.W., et al.: A portable adjustable forced vital capacity simulator for routine spirometer calibration, Am. Rev. Respir. Dis. **121**:599, 1980.

Hankinson, J.L., and Gardner, R.M.: Standard waveforms for spirometer testing, Am. Rev. Respir. Dis. **126**:362, 1982.

Leary, E.T., Graham, G., and Kenny, M.A.: Commercially available blood-gas quality controls compared with tonometered blood, Clin. Chem. **26**:1309, 1980.

Leith, D.E., and Mead, J.: Principles of body plethysmography, Bethesda, Md., 1974, National Heart, Lung, and Blood Institute—Division of Lung Diseases.

Shigeoka, J.W.: Calibration and quality control of spirometer systems, Respir. Care **28**:747, 1983.

Shigeoka, J.W., Gardner, R.M., and Barkham, H.W.: A portable volume/flow calibrating syringe, Chest **82**:598, 1982.

Westgard, J.O., et. al.: Performance characteristics of rules for internal quality control: probabilities for false rejection and error detection, Clin. Chem. **23**:1857, 1977.

Criteria for acceptability of pulmonary function studies

Ferris, B.G., editor: Epidemiology standardization project: recommended standardized procedures for pulmonary function testing, Am. Rev. Respir. Dis. **118**(suppl. 2):55, 1978.

Nathan, S.P., Lebowitz, M.D., and Knudson, R.J.: Spirometric testing: number of tests required and selection of data, Chest **76**:384, 1979.

Office spirometry in clinical practice: ACCP Committee on clinic and office pulmonary function testing, Chest **74**:298, 1978.

Sorensen, J.B., et al.: Selection of the best spirometric values for interpretation, Am. Rev. Respir. Dis. **122**:802, 1980.

Standardization of spirometry, Am. Rev. Respir. Dis. **119**:831, 1979.

Townsend, M.C., Duchene, A.G., and Fallat, R.J.: The effects of underrecorded forced expirations on spirometric lung function indexes, Am. Rev. Respir. Dis. **126**:734, 1982.

CHAPTER TWELVE

Case studies

The following cases are presented to illustrate the use of pulmonary function testing to aid in the diagnosis and treatment of various types of pulmonary disorders. Attention should be directed to the subject history accompanying each set of test values in order to better understand the numerical results. Readers are encouraged to evaluate the History and Test Results sections and then to write down an interpretation and compare their assessment with the one given in the Interpretation section. The Discussion section explains the comments given in the Interpretation. The first five cases deal with the types of pulmonary function tests typically performed in most hospital laboratories; Case 6 is an inhalation challenge test; Cases 7, 8, and 9 include exercise test data, interpretations, and discussions.

CASE 1
History

M.B. is a 27-year-old high school teacher whose chief complaint is dyspnea on exertion. The subject states that his breathlessness has worsened over the past several months. He has smoked one pack of cigarettes a day for approximately 10 years (10 pack/years). He denies a cough or sputum production. No member of his family has ever had emphysema, asthma, chronic bronchitis, carcinoma, or tuberculosis. There is no history of exposure to extraordinary environmental pollutants.

Pulmonary function testing
A. Personal data

    Sex: Male
    Age: 27 yr
    Height: 65 in
    Weight: 297 lb
    BSA: 2.28 m^2

B. Spirometry

	Before drug	Predicted	%	After drug	%
FVC (L)	2.90	4.70	62	3.01	64
FEV_1 (L)	2.47	3.86	64	2.40	62
$FEV_{1\%}$ (%)	85	82	—	80	—
$FEF_{25\%-75\%}$ (L/sec)	4.62	4.35	106	4.55	105
$\dot{V}_{max\ 50}$ (L/sec)	4.94	5.82	85	4.89	84
$\dot{V}_{max\ 25}$ (L/sec)	2.49	3.22	77	2.57	80
MVV (L/min)	178	137	130	177	130
Raw (cm H_2O/L/sec)	1.24	0.6-2.4	—	1.33	—

C. Lung volumes (by plethysmograph)

	Before drug	Predicted	%
VC (L)	2.90	4.70	62
IC (L)	1.96	2.91	67
ERV (L)	0.94	1.80	59
FRC (L)	1.87	3.29	57
RV (L)	0.93	1.49	57
TLC (L)	3.83	6.20	62
RV/TLC (%)	25	24	—

D. Diffusing capacity

	Before drug	Predicted	%
DL_{CO}SB (ml CO/min/mm Hg)	18.8	31.4	60

E. Blood gases (FI_{O_2} 0.21)

pH	7.44
Pa_{CO_2}	35
Pa_{O_2}	67
Sa_{O_2}	91%
HCO_3^-	23.6

Interpretation

Spirometry shows a moderately decreased FVC and FEV_1; flows are within normal limits, as are the MVV and Raw.

Lung volumes are moderately decreased, with the RV/TLC ratio preserved.

The DL_{CO} is moderately reduced. The pH and Pa_{CO_2} are within normal limits, but the Pa_{O_2} is mildly decreased, representing a widened A-a difference.

Impression. Moderate restrictive lung disease without evidence of obstruction, with mild hypoxemia.

Discussion

This case offers a good example of what might be considered a "pure restrictive defect." Characteristic of a restrictive process is the fact that all lung volumes, including FVC and FEV_1, are proportionately decreased, with little or no decrease in any of the flow measurements ($FEF_{25\%-75\%}$, $\dot{V}_{max\ 50}$, etc.). Also typical is the well-preserved ratio between FEV_1 and FVC, indicating that the volume expired in the first second was in correct proportion to the total volume exhaled, despite the decreases in the absolute volumes of each. The MVV demonstrates the subject's ability to move a normal maximum volume. This can be accomplished even in the face of moderately severe restriction by an increase in the rate rather than the V_T.

The DL_{CO} confirms the effect of the decreased lung volume's impaired gas transfer. It should be noted that the reduction in DL_{CO} is approximately proportional to the decrease in TLC. Another way of expressing this relationship is to divide the DL_{CO} by the TLC (sometimes called the DL/VL). The ratio in this case is 4.91 ml CO transferred per liter of lung volume. Similarly, if the predicted DL_{CO} is divided by the predicted TLC, a ratio of 5.06 ml CO transferred per liter of lung volume is derived. The DL/VL is sometimes useful for defining the extent of obstructive or restrictive components in reduced DL_{CO}. In restriction the ratio is preserved, but in obstruction it falls.

The widened A-a gradient (approximately 40 mm Hg) is again consistent with reduced lung volumes and is significant, particularly in view of the subject's complaint of exertional dyspnea and his age.

The explanation for the restrictive pattern may well lie in the subject's weight of 297 lb. For his height, he is at approximately 200% of his ideal weight. Obesity is one of the most common causes of restrictive patterns. Further evaluation of this subject might include testing his response to hypoxia and hypercapnia, since chronically obese individuals often display patterns of decreased ventilatory drive, resulting in CO_2 retention. The subject does not appear to be retaining CO_2 at this point, and treatment of the obesity might avoid future complications.

CASE 2
History

P.R. is a 21-year-old man in good health. He plays college football and has a chief complaint of shortness of breath following "wind sprints" and similar vigorous exercises. He denies any other symptoms, including cough or sputum production. He has never smoked. His grandfather had "lung problems," but there is no other history of pulmonary disease involving the family. He does state that several brothers and sisters have "hay fever." There is no history of exposure to extraordinary environmental pollutants.

Pulmonary function testing
A. Personal data
   Sex: Male
   Age: 21 yr
   Height: 73 in
   Weight: 180 lb
B. Spirometry

	Before drug	Predicted	%	After drug	%
FVC (L)	6.85	6.04	111	6.73	111
FEV$_1$ (L)	4.65	4.78	97	5.45	114
FEV$_{1\%}$ (%)	70	79	—	81	—
FEF$_{25\%-75\%}$ (L/sec)	3.90	5.00	78	4.88	97
$\dot{V}_{max\ 50}$ (L/sec)	5.01	6.52	77	6.10	94
$\dot{V}_{max\ 25}$ (L/sec)	2.79	3.75	74	3.25	87
MVV (L/min)	218	166	131	215	130
Raw (cm H$_2$O/L/sec)	2.10	0.6-2.4	—	1.60	—

C. Lung volumes (open-circuit method)

	Before drug	Predicted	%
VC (L)	6.58	6.04	109
IC (L)	4.63	3.65	127
ERV (L)	1.95	2.39	82
FRC (L)	3.60	4.33	83
RV (L)	1.65	1.94	85
TLC (L)	8.23	7.98	103
RV/TLC (%)	20	24	—

D. Diffusing capacity

	Before drug	Predicted	%
D$_{LCO}$SB (ml CO/min/mm Hg)	28.2	34.5	82

E. Blood gases (FI_{O_2} 0.21)

pH	7.41
Pa_{CO_2}	39
Pa_{O_2}	94
Sa_{O_2}	97%
HCO_3^-	24.4

Interpretation

Spirometry is within normal limits except for a slight decrease in the $FEV_{1\%}$. There is a significant increase in the FEV_1, $\dot{V}_{max\ 50}$, $\dot{V}_{max\ 25}$, $FEV_{1\%}$, and $FEF_{25\%-75\%}$ following administration of the bronchodilator. The MVV and Raw are normal. All lung volumes are within normal limits, as are the blood gas levels and DL_{CO}.

Impression. Mild obstructive defect with significant response to bronchodilator; otherwise normal lung function.

Discussion

The subject is a good example of an individual with essentially normal (or slightly above normal) values for almost every parameter. The exception is the $FEV_{1\%}$, which is consistent with a mild obstructive process. It is important to note that simply evaluating the FVC and FEV_1 in relation to their predicted values might give the impression that this subject is normal. But the $FEV_{1\%}$ indicates that the subject, whose lung volumes are slightly larger than normal, expired a disproportionately small volume in the first second. The borderline values for $FEF_{25\%-75\%}$, $\dot{V}_{max\ 50}$, and $\dot{V}_{max\ 25}$ also point to an obstructive process. In addition, there is a significant (17%) increase in FEV_1 following administration of a beta-adrenergic bronchodilator. This is particularly noteworthy in view of the subject's main symptom of shortness of breath following exericse. The subject would appear to exhibit reversible airway obstruction triggered by exercise.

Further evaluation of P.R. included an exercise test to try to demonstrate exercise-induced asthma (EIA). After 6 minutes of treadmill jogging, the subject's FEV_1 began to fall; it reached a low value of 4.10 ($FEV_{1\%}$ of 62%) 5 minutes after termination of the test. Scattered wheezes were heard on auscultation. The obstruction was readily reversed by inhaled bronchodilator.

Measurement of the CV by the SBN_2 method revealed a CV/VC ratio of 16% (predicted 8.1%), further pointing to the presence of small airway abnormality. Methacholine challenge testing was deferred, since the obstructive defect was adequately demonstrated by the exercise test.

CASE 3
History

F.H. is a 47-year-old loading dock foreman whose chief complaint is shortness of breath on moderate exertion. He claims that his dyspnea has become worse recently, but that it has been present for over 5 years. F.H. has smoked 1½ packs of cigarettes a day since age 15 (48 pack/years). He admits to a cough on arising and states that he produces a "small amount of grayish sputum," usually in the morning. F.H.'s father had tuberculosis, and one brother had multiple cases of pneumonia as a child and now has bronchiectasis. He denies any extraordinary exposure to environmental dusts or fumes.

Pulmonary function testing

A. Personal data

　　Sex:　　　Male
　　Age:　　　47 yr
　　Height:　　70 in
　　Weight:　　185 lb

B. Spirometry

	Before drug	Predicted	%	After drug	%
FVC (L)	4.01	4.97	81	4.49	90
FEV_1 (L)	2.05	3.67	56	2.20	60
$FEV_{1\%}$ (%)	51	74	—	49	—
$FEF_{25\%-75\%}$ (L/sec)	1.20	3.69	33	1.30	35
$\dot{V}_{max\ 50}$ (L/sec)	1.35	5.54	24	1.67	30
$\dot{V}_{max\ 25}$ (L/sec)	0.55	2.58	21	1.02	40
MVV (L/min)	71	136	52	85	63
Raw (cm H_2O/L/sec)	3.10	0.6-2.4	—	2.90	—

C. Lung volumes (by plethysmograph)

	Before drug	Predicted	%
VC (L)	4.01	4.97	81
IC (L)	2.71	3.18	85
ERV (L)	1.30	1.76	74
FRC (L)	4.60	3.94	117
RV (L)	3.30	2.18	151
TLC (L)	7.31	7.12	103
RV/TLC (%)	45	31	—

D. Diffusing capacity

	Before drug	Predicted	%
$DL_{CO}SB$ (ml CO/ min/mm Hg)	6.7	29.1	23

E. Blood gases (FI_{O_2} 0.21)

　　pH　　　　　7.37
　　Pa_{CO_2}　　　51
　　Pa_{O_2}　　　　54
　　Sa_{O_2}　　　　86%
　　HCO_3^-　　　32
　　Hb　　　18.3 vol%

Interpretation

The subject has a moderately decreased FEV_1 with only a slightly decreased FVC. The $FEF_{25\%-75\%}$ is markedly decreased, as are the $\dot{V}_{max\ 50}$ and $\dot{V}_{max\ 25}$. The MVV is moderately reduced, and the Raw is slightly above the expected value. There is little or no response to the bronchodilator.

Lung volumes show a marked increase in RV, with mild increases in the FRC and TLC. The RV/TLC is mildly elevated.

The DL_{CO} is severely reduced. The arterial blood gases reveal a compensated respiratory acidosis with moderate hypoxemia and elevated Hb.

Discussion

F.H. typifies a smoker who has developed a moderate degree of airway obstruction. His spirometry values reveal the extent of the obstruction: FEV_1, 56% of the predicted value; $FEF_{25\%-75\%}$, 33% of the predicted value; and MVV, 52% of the predicted value. The FVC is relatively well preserved and even increased somewhat following the bronchodilator. It should be noted that the $FEF_{25\%-75\%}$, despite being 33% of the predicted value, must be interpreted cautiously because of the variability in normal subjects for this measure. (The 95% confidence limits for this subject would include values between 1.45 L/sec and 5.93 L/sec—a large range. See the Appendix for predicted values and the SEE). There is not a significant response to the bronchodilator. The $FEV_{1\%}$ actually decreases as a result of a larger increase in the FVC than in the FEV_1. This occurs rather commonly in irreversible obstructive disease. The MVV is reduced, as might be expected. To ascertain that a valid MVV maneuver was obtained, the FEV_1 may be multiplied by a factor of 40; if the MVV approximates the resulting value (as it does here), it represents good effort on the part of the subject. The Raw is slightly increased, consistent with moderate airway obstruction and a productive cough.

The lung volumes reveal air trapping, as indicated by the increased RV and RV/TLC ratio. The increase in RV has been largely at the expense of the VC; hence the remaining lung volumes (TLC, FRC, etc.) are not far from the expected values.

The DL_{CO} is markedly reduced, presumably as a result of mismatching of ventilation and perfusion, caused by airway obstruction. If diffusing capacity is expressed per liter of lung volume, a ratio of 1.09 ml CO/min/mm Hg/L of lung volume is obtained. This DL/VL may be contrasted to the value presented in Case 1, where the ratio was close to the expected (restrictive defect); in the present case the ratio is low; hence the decreased DL_{CO} must be attributed to something other than loss of lung volume. In addition, the low DL_{CO} (23% of the predicted value) may indicate that oxygenation may be further impaired during exercise, although it is not possible to predict the extent of desaturation that might occur. Although the DL_{CO} is sometimes used to distinguish "pure" emphysema (decreased DL_{CO}) from "pure" bronchitis (normal DL_{CO}), in many instances the diseases overlap in such a way as to seriously limit the usefulness of this type of distinction.

The blood gas results reveal moderate hypoxemia consistent with ventilation-perfusion mismatching. There is a slightly elevated Hb, presumably secondary to the hypoxemia. In addition, there is a mild degree of CO_2 retention with renal compensation.

The lung function of this subject exemplifies the pattern seen in chronic obstructive airway disease of the mixed emphysematous and chronic bronchitic type. Although air trapping (increased RV) is consistent with emphysematous changes, it may be present in bronchitis and asthma, particularly during acute exacerbations.

Further evaluation of F.H. included a chest x-ray film and a ventilation-perfusion scan. The chest film showed increased hilar markings and right ventricular enlargement. The $\dot{V}/\dot{Q}$ scan showed areas of low $\dot{V}/\dot{Q}$ in both lower lobes, perhaps explaining the hypoxemia. He was recommended for exercise evaluation to determine whether further desaturation occurred with an increased work load and to determine his potential for pulmonary rehabilitation.

CASE 4
History

R.B. is a 37-year-old pipe fitter whose chief complaint is shortness of breath at rest and on exertion. His dyspnea has worsened in the past 6 months, so much so that he is no longer able to work. Additional symptoms include a dry cough, and he admits to some sputum production when he has a "chest cold." He has smoked one pack of cigarettes a day since age 18 (19 pack/years). He quit smoking about 3 weeks prior to the tests. His father died of emphysema and his mother of lung cancer. An only brother is in good health. His occupational exposure includes working for the past 13 years in the assembly room of a boiler plant, where boilers are put together. He admits to seldom using the respirators provided despite the "dusty" environment.

Pulmonary function tests

A. Personal data

Sex: Male
Age: 37 yr
Height: 69 in
Weight: 143 lb

B. Spirometry

	Before drug	Predicted	%	After drug	%
FVC (L)	3.04	5.05	60	3.10	61
FEV_1 (L)	2.03	3.90	52	2.26	58
$FEV_{1\%}$ (%)	67	77	—	73	—
$FEF_{25\%-75\%}$ (L/sec)	1.30	4.09	32	1.60	39
$\dot{V}_{max\ 50}$ (L/sec)	2.12	5.78	37	2.42	42
$\dot{V}_{max\ 25}$ (L/sec)	0.78	2.95	26	1.20	41
MVV (L/min)	83	141	59	91	65
Raw (cm H_2O/L/sec)	2.51	0.6-2.4	—	2.47	—

C. Lung volumes (by plethysmograph)

	Before drug	Predicted	%
VC (L)	3.04	5.05	60
IC (L)	1.62	3.18	51
ERV (L)	1.42	1.87	76
FRC (L)	2.75	3.81	72
RV (L)	1.33	1.94	69
TLC (L)	4.37	6.99	63
RV/TLC (%)	30	28	—

D. Diffusing capacity

	Before drug	Predicted	%
$DL_{CO}SB$ (ml CO/ min/mm Hg)	8.1	30.6	25

E. Blood gases (FI_{O_2} 0.21)

pH   7.43
Pa_{CO_2} 36
Pa_{O_2} 52
Sa_{O_2} 87%
HCO_3^- 23

Interpretation

Spirometry shows a moderately reduced FVC and FEV_1. The $FEF_{25\%-75\%}$, $\dot{V}_{max\ 50}$, and $\dot{V}_{max\ 25}$ are all severely reduced. The MVV is moderately low, and the Raw is at the upper limit of normal. Response to the bronchodilator is minimal except for the $\dot{V}_{max\ 25}$, which improved somewhat more than the other flows.

The lung volumes are consistent with moderate restrictive disease; the RV/TLC ratio is normal.

The DL_{CO} is severely reduced, and the blood gas results indicate moderate hypoxemia with a normal acid-base status.

Impression. Combined obstructive and restrictive pattern without significant bronchodilator response.

Discussion

R.B. typifies the subject with combined obstructive and restrictive disease. His spirometry indicates that a rather serious obstructive component is present ($FEF_{25\%-75\%}$, $\dot{V}_{max\ 50}$, etc.). However, the $FEV_{1\%}$ is close to the normal limit, in this case because the FVC is also reduced. Airway narrowing as a result of restriction is sometimes responsible for decreased flows, particularly if the restriction is severe, but R.B.'s symptoms of cough and sputum point to a genuine obstructive process. In addition, he has a smoking and family history that place him at risk. Because the FVC can be reduced in both obstructive and restrictive processes, spirometry alone does not adequately define the exact nature of this subject's disease.

The lung volume measurements confirm the presence of a restrictive component. Notably, all lung volumes are reduced in similar proportions. In this case the reduced VC parallels decreases in FRC, RV, and TLC. The reduced diffusing capacity is presumably a result of the combined process, as is the moderate hypoxemia with room air. The subject's history and symptoms point to the possibility of either restrictive or obstructive disease, or both. The obstructive component may be related to the subject's smoking history, but the restrictive component is more interesting. On investigation, it was learned that the subject's occupation involved exposure to asbestos, which can cause fibrosis. Chest x-ray films revealed linear calcifications of the diaphragmatic pleura and pleural thickening, as well as fibrotic changes, all consistent with asbestos exposure.

Asbestos bodies were identified from the subject's sputum. Open lung biopsy was deferred, since the causes of both the obstructive and restrictive components were considered adequately identified.

CASE 5
History

P.W. is a 27-year-old auto mechanic whose chief complaint is "breathing problems." He describes "attacks" of breathlessness that occur suddenly and then subside. He has no other symptoms and no personal history of lung disease. No immediate family member has had any lung disease. He has smoked a pack of cigarettes a day for the last 10 years (10 packs/years). He has no unusual environmental exposure, but he claims that gasoline fumes sometimes bring on the episodes of shortness of breath.

Pulmonary function tests

A. Personal data

    Sex: Male
    Age: 27 yr
    Height: 68 in
    Weight: 150 lb

B. Spirometry

	Before drug	Predicted	%
FVC (L)	3.80	5.15	74
FEV_1 (L)	3.70	4.13	90
$FEV_{1\%}$ (%)	97	80	—
$FEF_{25\%-75\%}$ (L/sec)	4.62	4.49	103
$\dot{V}_{max\ 50}$ (L/sec)	4.81	6.01	80
$\dot{V}_{max\ 25}$ (L/sec)	3.12	3.33	94
MVV (L/min)	162	146	111

C. Lung volumes (closed-circuit technique)

	Before drug	Predicted	%
VC (L)	4.97	5.15	97
IC (L)	3.30	3.17	104
ERV (L)	1.67	1.98	84
FRC (L)	3.72	3.68	101
RV (L)	2.05	1.70	121
TLC (L)	7.02	6.85	102
RV/TLC (%)	29	25	—

D. Diffusing capacity

	Before drug	Predicted	%
$DL_{CO}SB$ (ml CO/ min/mm Hg)	18.8	32.2	58

E. Blood gases (FIO_2 0.21)

pH	7.44
Pa_{CO_2}	36
Pa_{O_2}	92
Sa_{O_2}	87.1%
COHb	8.3

Interpretation

Spirometry show a mildly reduced FVC, with all other flows and the MVV being normal. Lung volumes are normal, with a slight increase in the RV. The DL_{CO} is moderately reduced. Blood gases are within normal limits except for a markedly elevated carboxyhemoglobin level and concomitant reduction in Sa_{O_2}.

Impression. The spirometry is inconsistent. The FVC and SVC differ markedly, and the DL_{CO} is not consistent with the blood gas data. Inadequate subject effort or technical errors are present.

Discussion

These test values are a good example of poor reproducibility, particularly on some of the maneuvers that tend to be influenced most by subject effort.

The spirometric values are seemingly consistent with a mild restrictive process. However, the FVC is much smaller than the SVC; since the subject cannot "overshoot" on the VC maneuver, the FVC can be presumed to be inaccurate. The FVC might be less than the SVC in severe obstruction, but all of the subject's other flows and MVV appear normal. It is similarly important to note that flows whose measurement depend on the FVC ($FEF_{25\%-75\%}$, $\dot{V}_{max}$, etc.) might also be erroneous if the FVC is incorrect. The FEV_1 and MVV do not depend on the FVC, and they appear to be normal.

The lung volumes appear normal. Since the closed-circuit technique for determination of FRC requires only tidal breathing, it is unlikely to be influenced by poor effort unless the subject introduces a leak. If the SVC is used to calculate the $FEV_{1\%}$, the ratio becomes 74%, in comparison with the 97% estimated from the FEV maneuver itself.

The DL_{CO} is much lower than one might expect in relation to the "normal" blood gases. An adequate $DL_{CO}SB$ manuever depends largely on the subject rapidly inspiring a VC breath from RV. Again, a poor VC effort could result in an underestimate of the true diffusing capacity. The effect of the elevated COHb would be to reduce the driving pressure of CO across the lung and to further reduce the measured DL_{CO}.

Because of the inconsistencies in the reported data, further evaluation of the available raw test data was performed. On closer examination, it was noted that during the spirometry the subject terminated each maneuver after approximately 2 seconds, hence the discrepancy between FVC and SVC. In addition, each of the three recorded spirograms had widely varying FVC values, confirming poor subject cooperation. The DL_{CO} maneuver also showed inconsistent VC efforts, with the largest VC equaling only 66% of the SVC. Careful attention to these inaccuracies at the time of the test might have prevented such inconsistencies from reaching the final report. The subject was requested to return for a second test. (Criteria for determining acceptability of various tests may be found in Chapter 11.)

CASE 6
History

M.M. is a 39-year-old secretary who has recently begun experiencing episodes of "choking and coughing." She was referred by an industrial health specialist who suspected some sort of reactive airway involvement. She relates that cigarette smoke and strong odors seem to bring on the episodes. She has never smoked and has no history of lung disease. She had some childhood allergies that disappeared at puberty. There is no history of any lung involvement in her immediate family. She is not currently on any medications.

Pulmonary function tests

A. Personal data

Sex:	Female
Age:	39 yr
Height:	66 in
Weight:	130 lb

B. Spirometry

	Before drug	Predicted	%
FVC (L)	3.71	3.80	98
FEV_1 (L)	2.80	2.97	94
$FEV_{1\%}$ (%)	75	78	—
$FEF_{25\%-75\%}$ (L/sec)	2.99	3.34	90
$\dot{V}_{max\ 50}$ (L/sec)	3.93	4.62	85
$\dot{V}_{max\ 25}$ (L/sec)	1.01	2.36	43
MVV (L/min)	106.40	109.70	97
Raw (cm H_2O/L/sec)	2.51	0.6-2.4	—

C. Lung volumes (by plethysmograph)

	Before drug	Predicted	%
VC (L)	3.70	3.80	97
IC (L)	2.03	2.60	78
ERV (L)	1.67	1.20	139
FRC (L)	3.11	3.00	104
RV (L)	1.44	1.80	80
TLC (L)	5.14	5.60	92
RV/TLC (%)	28	32	—

D. Diffusing capacity

	Before drug	Predicted	%
DL_{CO}SB (ml CO/ min/mm Hg)	18.9	21.9	86

E. Blood gases (FI_{O_2} 0.21)

pH	7.43
Pa_{CO_2}	37
Pa_{O_2}	98
Sa_{O_2}	97.3%
HCO_3^-	23.3

Methacholine challenge

Mecholyl (mg/ml)	FEV$_1$	% Control	Cumulative breaths	Cumulative units/5 breaths
Baseline	2.97	—	—	—
Control	2.92	100	—	—
0.075	2.93	100	5	0.375
0.150	2.90	99	10	1.125
0.310	2.75	94	15	2.680
0.620	2.41	83	20	5.780
1.250	1.99	68	25	12.000

One mecholyl unit is arbitrarily defined as 1 mg/ml of methacholine in diluent.

Interpretation

Spirometry is within normal limits, except for the $\dot{V}_{max\,25}$, which is reduced, consistent with small airway abnormality. The Raw is elevated also, consistent with airflow obstruction. Lung volumes are within normal limits, although the ERV is larger than expected. The DL_{CO} and blood gases are normal.

The methocholine challenge test is positive, with a PD_{20} of 1.25 mg/ml, representing a total dose of 12 methacholine units. The test was terminated because the subject's FEV$_1$ fell below 80% of the control value. Wheezing was present on auscultation for the last two methacholine doses and the subject experienced symptoms similar to her chief complaint when the test became positive.

Impression. Positive methocholine challenge consistent with reactive airway disease, probably in the small airways.

Discussion

This subject is a good candidate for an inhalation challenge type of test. Her baseline pulmonary function studies are normal, with possible small airway involvement. Because of her complaint of episodic coughing and choking, some form of hyperreactive airway abnormality is likely. Many subjects who develop an asthmatic response to inhaled irritants complain of cough as the primary symptom, and wheezing may or may not be present (usually heard on auscultation).

If obvious airway obstruction were present on the baseline spirometry, the challenge test would have been contraindicated. A simple before and after bronchodilator trial might have sufficed to demonstrate reversible obstruction. The FEV$_1$ is commonly used as the index of obstruction for inhalation challenge tests, but other parameters may also be evaluated, since the FEV maneuver is repeated at each level of dosage. The $FEF_{25\%-75\%}$, $\dot{V}_{max\,50}$, $\dot{V}_{max\,25}$, Raw, and SGaw may all be used to define the extent of airway reactivity. In some instances the peak flow (PEFR) may fall as the challenge is performed, particularly if the large airways are involved.

Some caution must be applied in interpreting the results of the methacholine challenge test. The subject should be largely symptom free at the time of the test and should not be using beta-adrenergic or methylxanthine bronchodilators, which might influence the results. These conditions were met in this subject, and because the FEV_1 fell precipitously at a moderate methacholine dosage, the test can be interpreted as positive with some certainty. To better manage this patient, a portable peak flow meter was dispensed. The subject was instructed in its use, and her peak flow correlated well with that from baseline spirometry. She was requested to use the device when the symptoms appeared, followed by a metered-dose inhaler. Subsequent reports indicated that her peak flow fell in excess of the level demonstrated on the challenge, but the symptoms were promptly relieved with use of the inhaler.

CASE 7
History

T.S. is a 65-year-old man with a history of COPD who was referred for exercise evaluation for pulmonary rehabilitation. He admits experiencing shortness of breath and dyspnea on exertion and claims that these have grown worse over the last year. He has a smoking history of 72 pack/years and has recently quit smoking. A chest x-ray film is normal except for some flattening of the diaphragms. Family history and occupational exposure were not significant.

Pulmonary function tests

A. Personal data

    Sex: Male
    Age: 65 yr
    Height: 69 in
    Weight: 125 lb

B. Spirometry

	Before drug	Predicted	%
FVC (L)	2.42	4.35	56
FEV_1 (L)	1.20	3.01	40
$FEV_{1\%}$ (%)	59	69	—
$FEF_{25\%-75\%}$ (L/sec)	0.77	2.83	27
$\dot{V}_{max\ 50}$ (L/sec)	1.37	4.94	28
$\dot{V}_{max\ 25}$ (L/sec)	0.59	1.80	33
MVV (L/min)	45	118	38
Raw (cm H_2O/L/sec)	2.80	0.6-2.4	—

C. Lung volumes (by plethysmograph)

	Before drug	Predicted	%
VC (L)	2.42	4.35	56
IC (L)	1.74	2.96	59
ERV (L)	0.68	1.39	49
FRC (L)	5.11	3.81	134
RV (L)	4.43	2.42	183
TLC (L)	6.85	6.77	101
RV/TLC (%)	65	36	—

D. Diffusing capacity

	Before drug	Predicted	%
$DL_{co}SB$ (ml CO/min/mm Hg)	11.8	25.7	46

Interpretation (pulmonary function study)

The spirometry is consistent with severe obstructive lung disease. Lung volumes show marked air trapping with residual volume replacement of the VC. The diffusing capacity is severely reduced. Bronchodilator studies were not done, because the subject had taken his medications immediately before the test.

Interpretation (exercise evaluation)

The exercise test (see Table 12-1) was terminated because the subject exceeded 85% of his age-related predicted maximum HR, and he was experiencing shortness of breath. His maximum $\dot{V}E$ exceeded his MVV slightly. VT increased with exercise, as did VD, and the VD/VT fell slightly. His gas exchange shows a $\dot{V}O_2$ of 1.2 L/min, which is approximately

Table 12–1. Exercise test—Case 7

Exercise level	1	2	3	4	5	6
Work load						
MPH	0	1.5	2	2	2.5	3
% Grade	0	0	4	8	8	8
Duration	10	3	3	3	3	3
METS	1	3.144	3.365	4.030	4.459	5.082
Ventilation						
f	30	24	26	30	36	39
$\dot{V}E$ (BTPS)	13.52	24.83	27.57	33.30	48.08	51.98
$\dot{V}A$ (BTPS)	5.99	14.37	17.34	21.57	31.64	34.31
VT (BTPS)	0.451	1.035	1.055	1.110	1.335	1.340
VD (BTPS)	0.251	0.436	0.391	0.392	0.457	0.456
VD/VT	0.556	0.421	0.371	0.352	0.342	0.340
Gas exchange						
$\dot{V}O_2$	0.237	0.745	0.797	0.954	1.056	1.204
$\dot{V}CO_2$	0.206	0.655	0.733	0.896	1.044	1.298
R	0.868	0.880	0.920	0.940	0.989	1.078
$\dot{V}E/\dot{V}O_2$	57	33.35	34.60	34.90	45.53	43.18
$\dot{V}O_2$/HR	2.786	7.838	8.390	9.090	8.516	8.916
Blood gases						
pH	7.47	7.43	7.42	7.39	7.39	7.38
Pa_{CO_2}	33	35	34	36	33	35
Pa_{O_2}	74	72	72	70	73	68
Sa_{O_2}	95.5	95	95	94	94	93
$P(A-a)O_2$	36	31	38	38	41	46
Hemodynamics						
HR	85	95	95	105	124	135
Systolic BP	124	162	178	194	200	210
Diastolic BP	90	86	90	100	104	108

57% of the expected value. $\dot{V}_{CO_2}$ rose, so that an R slightly greater than 1 occurred at the highest work load. The ventilatory equivalent ($\dot{V}E/\dot{V}O_2$) is elevated, and the O_2 pulse ($\dot{V}O_2$/HR) is slightly reduced.

Blood gas studies reveal a mild hypoxemia that worsened slightly with exercise. Saturation remained adequate. No hypercapnia or acidosis occurred.

No arrhythmias or ischemic changes were observed. Maximum HR achieved was 88% of his predicted maximum. There was mild systolic hypertension.

Impression. (1) Marked aerobic impairment; (2) ventilatory limitation with hypoxemia; (3) inappropriate cardiovascular response for the work load achieved.

Discussion

T.S. walked a total of 15 minutes on the treadmill, reaching a rate of 3 MPH at 8% grade. This equaled an energy production of 5.08 METS as a maximum.

His ventilatory pattern is characteristic of a subject with moderate airway obstruction. His respiratory rate is elevated at the beginning of the procedure, falls slightly, and then increases, particularly at the last two levels of work. The $\dot{V}E$ increases dramatically from level 1 (rest) to level 2, then increases slowly until the last two levels. The $\dot{V}A$ also increases in approximately the same fashion. The VT increases to about 1 liter and stays near that level throughout the test. This is a fairly normal response. Healthy subjects generally accomplish increases in ventilation by increasing their VT until they are using about 60% of the VC. Further increases are obtained by increasing the rate of breathing. In this case the subject immediately increased his VT to 50% to 60% of his VC, then increased his $\dot{V}E$ by raising his rate, particularly at the end of the test. Since his MVV was measured as 45 L/min (and the $FEV_1 \times 35$ was 42 L/min), the subject exceeded the maximum level of total ventilation that might have been expected. The VD rose during the exercise and fluctuated somewhat. The VD/VT ratio decreased slightly, as might be expected (even with moderate obstruction), since the VT increased more rapidly than the VD.

His gas exchange shows a steady increase in both $\dot{V}O_2$ and $\dot{V}CO_2$, with an R exceeding 1 at the final level. The subject may have reached his anaerobic threshold at this point. The marked increase in $\dot{V}E$ during the last two levels is presumably a result of the increased $\dot{V}CO_2$ from anaerobic metabolism. The ventilatory equivalent ($\dot{V}E/\dot{V}O_2$) is inappropriately high at rest (level 1), as might be expected for someone with moderate airway obstruction. The $\dot{V}E/\dot{V}O_2$ falls to lower levels during the first few stages of exercise but rises again at the higher work loads. At all levels the subject is performing an abnormally high level of ventilation for the amount of work being performed, consistent again with airway obstruction. The O_2 pulse ($\dot{V}O_2$/HR) rose with exercise, but not as high as might be expected (10 to 15 ml/beat). This points to an inappropriate cardiovascular response. Since the O_2 pulse is a function of the SV and the C(a-v)O_2, it is uncertain which factor was responsible for the low ratio of $\dot{V}O_2$/HR in this case. Cardiac pathology usually results in a decreased SV, whereas deconditioning results in a low C(a-v)O_2, caused by poor extraction of O_2 at the muscle level. Since the subject's HR and BP rose to near maximal levels without arrhythmias or S-T segment changes on the ECG, there may be some element of deconditioning involved.

In spite of a ventilatory limitation to exercise, the arterial blood gas levels did not change dramatically. The pH was slightly alkalotic at rest (hyperventilation); it fell with exercise but remained within a normal range. The Pa_{CO_2} stayed fairly constant, whereas the Pa_{O_2}, slightly low at rest, fell minimally. The subject used his remaining cardiopulmonary reserves to maintain normal blood gas levels.

In summary, the subject demonstrated a marked reduction in his exercise capacity ($\dot{V}O_{2max}$ = 57% of predicted), caused primarily by a ventilatory limitation, but with possible evidence of deconditioning. His rehabilitation program was subsequently directed toward conditioning exercises within the limits of the subject's pulmonary system.

CASE 8
History

J.Y. is 69-year-old woman with a history of chronic bronchitis who was referred for exercise evaluation. She has complained of shortness of breath on exertion. Her smoking history is 56 pack/years, but she quit over 1 year prior to this test. Her chest x-ray film is consistent with chronic bronchitis, showing increased vascular markings and an enlarged heart. She has no significant family history or occupational exposure. She admits to a morning cough that produces thick white sputum.

Pulmonary function tests

A. Personal data

   Sex: Female
   Age: 69 yr
   Height: 64 in
   Weight: 128 lb

B. Spirometry

	Before drug	Predicted	%
FVC (L)	1.30	2.85	46
FEV$_1$ (L)	0.73	2.04	36
FEV$_{1\%}$ (%)	56	72	—
FEF$_{25\%-75\%}$ (L/sec)	0.43	2.32	18
$\dot{V}_{max\ 50}$ (L/sec)	0.55	3.80	14
$\dot{V}_{max\ 25}$ (L/sec)	0.25	1.27	20
MVV (L/min)	31	85	36
Raw (cm H$_2$O/L/sec)	2.77	0.6-2.4	—

C. Lung volumes (by plethysmograph)

	Before drug	Predicted	%
VC (L)	1.30	2.85	46
IC (L)	1.08	1.99	54
ERV (L)	0.23	0.86	26
FRC (L)	3.78	2.77	137
RV (L)	3.55	1.91	186
TLC (L)	4.85	4.76	102
RV/TLC (%)	73	40	—

D. Diffusing capacity

	Before drug	Predicted	%
D$_{LCO}$SB (ml CO/ min/mm Hg)	8.3	17.4	48

Interpretation (pulmonary function study)

Spirometry is consistent with severe obstructive airway disease. Lung volumes indicate air trapping with a normal TLC. The diffusing capacity is severely reduced. Blood gas analysis and bronchodilator studies were deferred because this study immediately preceded the exercise test.

Interpretation (exercise evaluation)

A multistage exercise test was performed with a treadmill and an arterial catheter in place. Level 1 was a 10-minute baseline at rest (see Table 12-2).

The reason for termination of the test was a systolic BP of 250. The subject's respiratory rate increased from 12 to 33/min, with an increase in ventilation from 8 to 22 L/min. The V_T was relatively fixed at about 700 ml. $\dot{V}_A$ increased in proportion to $\dot{V}_E$.

Her $\dot{V}_{O_2}$ rose to only 0.548 L/min, which was 34% of the predicted maximum (1.634). Her ventilatory equivalent ($\dot{V}_E/\dot{V}_{O_2}$) for O_2 remained elevated. Her O_2 pulse ($\dot{V}_{O_2}$/HR) was low but elevated normally with exercise, though not to maximal levels.

Table 12-2. Exercise test—Case 8

Exercise level	1	2	3
Work load			
MPH	0	1.5	2
% Grade	0	0	0
Duration	10	3	3
METS	1	3.3	3.4
Ventilation			
f	12	27	33
$\dot{V}_E$ (BTPS)	8.020	21.220	22.630
$\dot{V}_A$ (BTPS)	4.17	11.671	12.447
V_T (BTPS)	0.668	0.768	0.686
V_D (BTPS)	0.321	0.350	0.309
V_D/V_T	0.48	0.45	0.45
Gas exchange			
$\dot{V}_{O_2}$	0.160	0.530	0.548
$\dot{V}_{CO_2}$	0.149	0.489	0.498
R	0.930	0.923	0.908
$\dot{V}_E/\dot{V}_{O_2}$	50.14	40.04	41.28
$\dot{V}_{O_2}$/HR	2.459	5.047	5.221
Blood gases			
pH	7.48	7.42	7.41
Pa_{CO_2}	34	39	37
Pa_{O_2}	74	60	63
Sa_{O_2}	94.9	89.9	91.0
$P(A\text{-}a)_{O_2}$	39	48	45
Hemodynamics			
HR	65	105	105
Systolic BP	160	212	250
Diastolic BP	80	100	102

Blood gas studies indicate a mild hypoxemia during exercise with an increased A-a gradient $(P(A-a)o_2)$. The Pa_{CO_2} rose slightly, and the pH changed accordingly, without evidence of anaerobic metabolism.

Her HR rose to 105/min, which is only 72% of the predicted maximum. The systolic BP rose dramatically from 160/80 to 250/102, at which point the test was terminated. There were no arrhythmias or S-T segment changes noted.

Impression. (1) Exercise limited by marked hypertension; (2) ventilatory reserve present despite moderately severe airway obstruction; (3) mild impairment of oxygenation during exercise, but not significantly limiting.

Discussion

J.Y. presents an example of an individual with well-documented airway obstruction in whom exercise limitation is caused primarily by an inappropriate cardiovascular response.

Comparison of her ventilation at the highest work load with her MVV (30.6 L/min) indicates the presence of a fair amount of ventilatory reserve. Her V_T, both at rest and during the mild exercise, remained relatively fixed near 700 ml. Since this volume was 50% to 60% of her VC, she increased her ventilation by increasing her rate (as might be expected). Her V_D/V_T ratio decreased only slightly, probably as a direct result of the fixed V_T. In instances in which both the V_T and V_D increase proportionately, the V_D/V_T ratio does not decrease. This pattern may be consistent with pulmonary vascular disorders but is probably not in evidence here, since neither the V_T nor the V_D increased significantly.

J.Y. has marked aerobic impairment as indicated by the low level of work tolerated $(\dot{V}o_2 = 0.548$ L/min) at 2 MPH and 0% grade on the treadmill. Her R appears to fall, perhaps because of the mild hyperventilation at the resting level. Her ventilation is inappropriately elevated for the work loads evaluated, as shown by the $\dot{V}E/\dot{V}o_2$. This is consistent with the increased V_D/V_T ratio (high ventilation required to maintain adequate $\dot{V}A$). The O_2 pulse $(\dot{V}O_2/HR)$ is slightly low at rest but increases normally during the mild exercise. The maximum O_2 pulse that might have been attained can be estimated by dividing her predicted $\dot{V}o_{2_{max}}$ by her predicted maximum HR ($\times$ 1000); in this case, $1.634/148$ ($\times$ 1000) = 11. J.Y. failed to increase her O_2 pulse because she was limited by other factors at an HR significantly lower than her predicted maximum. In this instance an inappropriate rise in systolic BP (to 250 mm Hg) led to termination of the test. Peripheral vasodilatation normally redirects the cardiac output to exercising muscles. The hypertensive response observed here indicates a failure of this mechanism. Both local lesions (as in claudication) and diffuse disease (as essential hypertension) can result in anaerobic metabolism at the muscle level with subsequent metabolic acidosis, stimulation of respiration, and dyspnea. J.Y. did not devolop a frank acidosis (pH of 7.41) or dyspnea during the test. Her presenting complaint of increasing shortness of breath may well have been related to both the hypertensive response and her pulmonary limitations.

Because of the results of the exercise evaluation and her slight hypertension at rest, the subject was referred for further evaluation of her hypertension.

CASE 9
History

C.J. is a 53-year-old office worker who was referred for evaluation of shortness of breath. She has a 44 pack/year history of smoking and continued to smoke up to the time of her test. She admits to a morning cough that produces thick white sputum, approximately

50 to 100 ml per day. Her chest x-ray film shows increased vascular markings and mild hyperinflation. She was taking no medications at the time of the test. No familial history of lung disease or cancer was found, and she has no unusual environmental exposure.

Pulmonary function tests

A. Personal data

Sex: Female
Age: 53 yr
Height: 65 in
Weight: 131 lb

B. Spirometry

	Before drug	Predicted	%	After drug	%
FVC	3.24	3.35	97	3.34	100
FEV_1 (L)	1.49	2.53	59	1.56	62
$Fev_{1\%}$ (%)	46	75	—	47	—
$FEF_{25\%-75\%}$ (L/sec)	0.79	2.86	27	1.19	42
$\dot{V}_{max\ 50}$ (L/sec)	1.99	4.24	47	2.25	53
$\dot{V}_{max\ 25}$ (L/sec)	0.68	1.86	37	0.99	53
MVV (L/min)	52	97.90	53	55	56
Raw (cm H_2O/L/sec)	2.22	0.6-2.4	—	2.10	—

C. Lung volumes (by plethysmograph)

	Before drug	Predicted	%
VC (L)	3.27	3.35	98
IC (L)	1.80	2.31	78
ERV (L)	0.99	1.04	95
FRC (L)	3.54	2.88	123
RV (L)	2.55	1.84	136
TLC (L)	5.82	5.20	112
RV/TLC (%)	44	35	—

D. Diffusing capacity

	Before drug	Predicted	%
$DL_{CO}SB$ (ml CO/min/mm Hg)	8.8	20.0	44

E. Blood gases (FI_{O_2} 0.21)

pH   7.38
$Paco_2$ 43
Pao_2 59
Sao_2 85.1%
COHb   5.7

Interpretation (pulmonary function study)

Spirometry shows a moderately severe obstructive process, predominantly in the small airways with a well-preserved FVC.

Lung volumes by plethysmography show a mildly increased FRC and moderately increased RV consistent with air trapping. The TLC is within normal limits, so that there is only mild hyperinflation.

The $DL_{CO}SB$ is severely reduced. Arterial blood gases with the subject breathing room air show moderate hypoxemia, which is complicated by an elevated COHb.

Impression. Moderately severe obstructive disease with air trapping and severely reduced DL_{CO}. Exercise evaluation for desaturation is recommended.

Interpretation (exercise evaluation)

Three days later a treadmill exercise test was performed with an arterial catheter in place; the test was repeated with oxygen supplementation. Gas with an $F_{I_{O_2}}$ of 0.28 was prepared in a meteorologic balloon for the portion of the exercise test on O_2 (see Table 12-3).

The exercise test was performed in two parts; the first part of the test was terminated because the subject's Pa_{O_2} fell to 46 mm Hg ($Sa_{O_2} = 77.3\%$). The second phase, with the subject breathing oxygen, was terminated because of shortness of breath on the part of the subject. The subject tolerated very low work loads even with supplementary oxygen.

Table 12-3. Exercise test—Case 9

	1	2	3	4	5
Exercise level	Air		Oxygen		
Work load					
MPH	0	1.5	0	1.5	2
% Grade	0	0	0	0	4
Duration	10	3	10	3	3
METS	1.48	4.00	1.34	3.11	4.73
Ventilation					
f	16	28	13	20	31
$\dot{V}_E$ (BTPS)	10.20	23.40	6.23	16.59	27.81
$\dot{V}_A$ (BTPS)	6.02	14.74	3.74	10.45	17.80
V_T (BTPS)	0.638	0.836	0.479	0.830	0.897
V_D (BTPS)	0.262	0.309	0.190	0.307	0.323
V_D/V_T	0.41	0.37	0.40	0.37	0.36
Gas exchange					
$\dot{V}_{O_2}$	0.310	0.835	0.279	0.649	0.986
$\dot{V}_{CO_2}$	0.303	0.743	0.251	0.617	0.976
R	0.98	0.89	0.90	0.95	0.99
$\dot{V}_E/\dot{V}_{O_2}$	32.90	28.00	22.33	25.50	28.20
V_{O_2}/HR	3.44	7.59	3.29	6.18	8.57
Blood gases					
pH	7.45	7.39	7.39	7.38	7.36
Pa_{CO_2}	34	39	44	45	46
Pa_{O_2}	61	47	84	71	66
Sa_{O_2}	87.4	77.3	91.4	88.9	87.0
COHb	5.1	4.7	4.8	4.7	4.6
$P(A\text{-}a)_{O_2}$	51	56	64	78	84
Hemodynamics					
HR •	90	110	92	105	115
Systolic BP	130	145	134	145	150
Diastolic BP	85	88	90	90	90

Ventilation was slightly elevated at rest but increased in a normal fashion. With the subject breathing oxygen, ventilation was slightly lower both at rest and at similar work loads. The VD/VT ratio was mildly elevated but decreased with exercise, with the subject breathing both air and oxygen. The subject's minute ventilation was lower than the observed MVV, indicating some ventilatory reserve.

The subject achieved a maximum $\dot{V}O_2$ or only 0.986 while breathing oxygen, which is 53% of her age-related predicted maximum (1.858), consistent with moderately severe exercise impairment. The ventilatory equivalent for O_2 is within normal limits, and the O_2 pulse increased normally, though not to maximal limits.

Blood gas analysis during exercise shows borderline hypoxemia at rest due to Pa_{O_2} of 61 mm Hg and an elevated COHb. The Pa_{O_2} fell markedly with only slight exertion to 47 mm Hg. With the subject breathing oxygen (FI_{O_2} = 0.28), the Pa_{O_2} improved to 84 mm Hg at rest but decreased with increasing work loads. The Pa_{CO_2} increased slightly during oxygen breathing, possibly as a result of respiratory depression. The COHb was elevated, probably because of the subject's continued smoking.

The HR and BP responses were appropriate for the work loads achieved with the subject breathing both air and oxygen. The low maximum HR suggests an exercise limitation other than cardiovascular pathology or deconditioning. The ECG was unremarkable.

Impression and recommendations. Moderately severe exercise impairment due primarily to desaturation during exercise. Some ventilatory limitation is probably present as well. The desaturation is aggravated by an elevated COHb. The subject should begin a formal effort to stop smoking and use oxygen at 1 to 2 L/min for exertion. A follow-up evaluation is recommended 1 to 3 months following smoking cessation.

Discussion

This subject typifies the subject with obstructive lung disease in whom derrangement of blood gases plays a larger role in exercise limitation than does impaired ventilation. C.J.'s ventilation and gas exchange are fairly normal at rest and at 1.5 MPH, 0% grade. The Po_2 is low, however, and falls precipitously with just a small increase in work load. In fact, the decrease is severe enough to warrant concern about the level of desaturation that might occur with simple daily activities or during sleep. The elevated carboxyhemoglobin further impairs O_2 delivery. Although an ear oximeter was used during the exercise test, it read spuriously high because of the elevated COHb. The pattern of desaturation follows what might be expected based on the poor diffusing capacity recorded on the pulmonary function studies.

To better elucidate the processes responsible for desaturation and to evaluate the efficacy of oxygen therapy, a controlled trial of walking while breathing supplementary O_2 was performed. The subject breathed from a balloon containing a gas analyzed to have an FI_{O_2} of 0.28. The most notable change was the increase in resting Pa_{O_2} from 61 to 84 mm Hg. The pattern of desaturation persisted, however, in that the O_2 tension fell dramatically, just as when the subject breathed room air. Because of the elevated baseline, the Pa_{O_2} remained above the level at which serious symptoms of hypoxemia might occur (approximately 55 mm Hg). Breathing supplementary oxygen may also be responsible for the decrease in total ventilation, at rest and during exercise, exhibited by the patient. The mild increase in Pa_{CO_2} might be further evidence of an increased sensitivity of the subject to hypoxemia, which becomes blunted when O_2 is breathed. Abnormal $\dot{V}/\dot{Q}$ is the most likely explanation of the pattern of desaturation observed in the subject, particularly in view of the bronchitic component of her obstructive disease.

The subject, while breathing oxygen, did not desaturate to the point where hypoxemia might be considered as a cause of the exercise limitation. Neither did she increase her ventilation to her maximum level. This might suggest that deconditioning was responsible for the low maximum work load achieved, but her heart rate and blood pressure did not rise to levels typically seen with significant deconditioning. Other possible causes for the low work load achieved while breathing oxygen might be inadequate subject effort, the development of bronchospasm, or greatly increased work of breathing.

The subject was referred for pulmonary rehabilitation, which included smoking cessation, bronchial hygiene, and exercise with supplementary oxygen.

SELECTED BIBLIOGRAPHY

Pulmonary function interpretation
Bates, D.V., Macklem, P.T., and Christie, R.V.: Respiratory function in disease, ed. 2, Philadelphia, 1971, W.B. Saunders Co.
Becklake, M.R., and Permutt, S.: Evaluation of tests of lung function for ''screening'' of early detection of chronic obstructive lung disease. In Macklem, P.T., and Permutt, S., editors: The lung in transition between health and disease, New York, 1979, Marcel Dekker, Inc.
Morris, A.H., et al.: Clinical pulmonary function testing, ed. 2, Salt Lake City, 1984, Intermountain Thoracic Society.
West, J.B.: Pulmonary pathophysiology—the essentials, ed. 2, Baltimore, 1983, Williams & Wilkins.

Exercise test interpretation
American College of Sports Medicine, Guidelines for graded exercise testing and exercise prescription, ed. 2, Philadelphia, 1980, Lea & Febiger.
Astrand, P.O., and Rodahl, K.: Textbook of work physiology, ed. 2, New York, 1977, McGraw-Hill Book Co.
Bell, C.W.: Pulmonary rehabilitation and exercise testing. In Wilson, P.K., Bell, C.W., and Norton, A.C., editors: Rehabilitation of the heart and lungs, Fullerton, Calif., 1980, Beckman Instruments.
Jones, N.L.: Exercise testing in pulmonary evaluation: rationale, methods, and the normal respiratory response to exercise, N. Engl. J. Med. 293:541, 1975.
Jones, N.L., et al.: Clinical exercise testing, ed. 2, Philadelphia, 1983, W.B. Saunders Co.
Kattus, A.A.: Exercise testing and training of apparently healthy individuals, New York, 1972, American Heart Association.
Spiro, S.G.: Exercise testing in clinical medicine, Br. J. Dis. Chest. 71:145, 1977.
Wasserman, K., and Whipp, B.J.: Exercise physiology in health and disease, Am. Rev. Respir. Dis. 112:219, 1975.

Appendix

SYMBOLS AND ABBREVIATIONS USED IN PULMONARY FUNCTION TESTING

General symbols

P	Pressure, blood or gas
V	Gas volume
$\dot{V}$	Gas-volume per unit time, or flow
F	Fractional concentration of gas
I	Inspired
E	Expired
A	Alveolar
T	Tidal
D	Dead space
Q	Blood volume
$\dot{Q}$	Blood flow
C	Content in blood
S	Saturation
a	Arterial
c	Capillary
v	Venous
$\bar{v}$	Mixed venous
BTPS	Body temperature, pressure, saturated with water vapor
ATPS	Ambient temperature, pressure, saturated with water vapor
STPD	Standard temperature, pressure, dry (0° C, 760 mm Hg, dry)

Lung volumes

VC	Vital capacity
IC	Inspiratory capacity
IRV	Inspiratory reserve volume
ERV	Expiratory reserve volume (FRC − RV)
FRC	Functional residual capacity (ERV + RV)
RV	Residual volume
TLC	Total lung capacity (VC + RV)
RV/TLC (%)	Residual volume/total lung capacity ratio expressed as a percentage
CV	Closing volume
CV/VC (%)	Closing volume/vital capacity ratio expressed as a percentage
CC	Closing capacity
CC/TLC (%)	Closing capacity/total lung capacity ratio expressed as a percentage
V_T	Tidal volume

SYMBOLS AND ABBREVIATIONS USED IN PULMONARY FUNCTION TESTING—cont'd

Lung volumes—cont'd

V_A	Alveolar volume
V_D	Dead space volume
V_L	Actual lung volume

Ventilation and gas exchange

$\dot{V}_E$	Expired volume per minute (BTPS)
$\dot{V}_A$	Alveolar ventilation per minute (BTPS)
$\dot{V}_D$	Dead space ventilation per minute (BTPS)
$\dot{V}_{O_2}$	Oxygen consumption per minute (STPD)
METS	Multiples of the resting oxygen uptake
$\dot{V}_{CO_2}$	Carbon dioxide production per minute (STPD)
f	Respiratory rate per minute
V_D/V_T	Ratio of dead space to tidal volume
MSVC	Maximum sustainable ventilatory capacity
P_{100}	Pressure in the first 100 msec of an occluded breath

Spirometry

FVC	Forced vital capacity with maximal expiratory effort
FIVC	Forced inspiratory vital capacity with maximal inspiratory effort
FEV_T	Forced expiratory volume for a specific interval T
FEV_T/FVC (%)	Forced expiratory volume/forced vital capacity ratio expressed as a percentage
FEF_x	Forced expiratory flow related to some specific portion of the FVC, denoted as x, referring to the amount of FVC already exhaled at the time of measurement
$FEF_{200-1200}$	Forced expiratory flow between 200 ml and 1200 ml of the FVC (formerly the MEFR)
$FEF_{25\%-75\%}$	Forced expiratory flow during the middle half of the FVC (formerly the MMF)
PEFR	Peak expiratory flow rate
MEFV	Maximum expiratory flow-volume curve
$\dot{V}_{max\ X}$	Forced expiratory flow related to the actual volume of the lungs denoted by x, which refers to the amount of lung volume remaining when measurement is made
$Viso\dot{V}$	Volume of isoflow
MVV_X	Maximum voluntary ventilation as the volume of air expired in a specified interval, denoted by x (formerly MBC)

Mechanics

C	Compliance, volume change per unit of pressure change
Cdyn	Dynamic compliance, measured during breathing
Cst	Static compliance, measured during periods of no airflow
C/V_L	Specific compliance
FDC	Frequency dependence of compliance (Cdyn/Cst $\times$ 100)
Raw	Airway resistance, pressure per unit of flow
Gaw	Airway conductance, flow per unit of pressure (1/Raw)

Mechanics—cont'd

Raw/V_L	Specific resistance
Gaw/V_L	Specific conductance
MEP	Maximum expiratory pressure
MIP	Maximum inspiratory pressure
KPM	Kilopond-meters, a unit of power output

Distribution

$N_{2750\text{-}1250}$ — Change in percent N_2 over the 750 to 1250 ml portion of the SBN_2 test

SBN_2 — Single-breath nitrogen elimination

Slope of Phase III — Slope of best-fit line through alveolar portion of the SBN_2 from 30% of VC to onset of Phase IV

IDI — Index of distribution of inspired gas (from 7-minute N_2 test)

Diffusion

$D_{L_{CO}}$	Diffusing capacity for carbon monoxide
1/Dm	Diffusion resistance of the alveolocapillary membrane
1/ΘVc	Diffusion resistance of the red cell and Hb reaction rate
D_L/V_A	Specific diffusion per unit of alveolar lung volume

Blood gases

$P_{A_{O_2}}$	Alveolar oxygen tension
Pa_{O_2}	Arterial oxygen tension
Sa_{O_2}	Arterial oxygen saturation
Ca_{O_2}	Arterial oxygen content
$P\bar{v}_{O_2}$	Mixed venous oxygen tension
$C\bar{v}_{O_2}$	Mixed venous oxygen content
$P_{A_{CO_2}}$	Alveolar carbon dioxide tension
Pa_{CO_2}	Arterial carbon dioxide tension
$C(a-\bar{v})o_2$	Arterial-venous O_2 content difference
$P(a-\bar{v})o_2$	Alveolar-arterial O_2 tension difference
pH	Negative logarithm of the H^+ concentration used as a positive number
HCO_3^-	Plasma bicarbonate concentration

TYPICAL VALUES FOR PULMONARY FUNCTION TESTS
(values are for a healthy young man, 1.7 m² body surface area)

Test	Value
Lung volumes (BTPS)	
IC	3600 ml
ERV	1200 ml
VC	4800 ml
RV	1200 ml
FRC	2400 ml
V_{TG}	2400 ml
TLC	6000 ml
(RV/TLC) × 100	20%

TYPICAL VALUES FOR PULMONARY FUNCTION TESTS—cont'd

Test	Value
Ventilation (BTPS)	
V_T	500 ml
f	12 breaths/min
$\dot{V}_E$	6 L/min
V_D	150 ml
$\dot{V}_A$	4200 ml/min
Pulmonary mechanics	
FVC	4800 ml
$FEV_{0.5\%}$	60%
$FEV_{1.0\%}$	83%
$FEV_{2.0\%}$	94%
$FEV_{3.0\%}$	97%
$FEF_{200-1200}$	6 L/sec
$FEF_{25\%-75\%}$	4.7 L/sec
MVV	170 L/min
C_L	0.2 L/cm H_2O
C_{LT}	0.1 L/cm H_2O
Airway resistance (Raw)	1.6 cm H_2O/L/sec
Distribution	
SBN_2	Less than 1.5% N_2
7-minute N_2	Less than 2.5% N_2
IDI (ideal lung = 1.0)	1.8
Diffusion	
DL_{CO}	25 ml CO/min/mm Hg
DL_{O_2}	31 ml O_2/min/mm Hg
Blood gases and related tests	
$\dot{V}_A/\dot{Q}_C$	0.8
$\dot{Q}s/\dot{Q}_T$	Less than 7%
V_D/V_T	0.3
Pa_{CO_2}	40 mm Hg
pH	7.40
Pa_{O_2}	95 mm Hg
Sa_{O_2}	97%
COHb	1.5%

USING PREDICTED VALUES

Predicted values for each of the many components of pulmonary function testing are derived from statistical analysis of a population of ''normal'' subjects. The subjects are usually classified as normal on the basis of the absence of history or symptoms of lung disease in themselves and their families. In addition, minimal exposure to risk factors (smoking, environmental pollution, etc.) is usually considered in selecting ''normals.'' In some older studies smokers were included as normals, and this most likely affected the resulting predicted values.

All pulmonary function parameters vary in the normal population, some much more than others. The arterial pH and Pa_{CO_2} have a very narrow range in normal subjects, unlike the $FEF_{25\%-75\%}$, which may vary by almost 2 L/sec. This variability must be taken into account in the interpretation of individual pulmonary function parameters, when a measured value is compared with a predicted normal. Most parameters "regress" (i.e., vary) in a predictable fashion in relation to one or more physical factors. The physical characteristics that most influence pulmonary function are:

Age
Sex
Height
Race or ethnic origin
Weight or body surface area

The altitude at which subjects reside also influences their lung function development. By analyzing each parameter in regard to the subject's physical characteristics, regression equations can be generated in order to predict the "normal" value. Most regression analyses presume that lung function changes are *linearly* related to the physical characteristics (age, height, etc.), but this may not always be the case, particularly in subjects at the extremes (very old or young, very tall or short).

Several methods of using predicted values are in common use:
1. Tables of normal values
2. Nomograms
3. Graphs
4. Regression equations

In instances where a calculator or computer is unavailable or not practical, tables, nomograms, or graphs may be used. However, the widespread use of calculators and computers allows the employment of even complex regression equations, as well as analysis of a measured value in relation to the predicted value in terms of variability.

Establishing a lower limit of normal is commonly done in one of several ways. Many clinicians use a fixed percent of the predicted value (measured/predicted × 100) to determine the degree of abnormality, usually with ± 20% as the limit of normal. Even if different "cut-off" percentages are used for each different parameter, this method has little statistical validity. A more precise approach is to define a lower limit based on the predicted value and the variability. Assuming that the lung function parameter varies in normal fashion, the mean ± 1.96 SD defines the 95% confidence limit. Statistically, 95% of the normal population falls within 1.96 SD of the mean; therefore if a subject's measured value is outside of the range (mean ± 1.96 SD), there is less than a 5% chance that the parameter is normal. Certain pulmonary function parameters require consideration of only the *lower* limit of normal (below the mean); in these cases 1.65 SD may be used to define the exact value below which there is less than a 5% chance of normality. Those parameters that can be abnormal by being either too high or too low (RV, TLC, Pa_{CO_2}, etc.) must use the 1.96 SD method. A more sophisticated means of representing the abnormality is to express the difference between the predicted value and the subject's measured value in terms of confidence intervals (CI). In this method the difference between predicted and measured is divided by the value representing the confidence interval (either 1.96 or 1.65 SD as noted above) and expressing the result as a ratio:

$$\frac{\text{Predicted} - \text{Measured}}{\text{CI}}$$

Using this scheme, a normal value is always less than or equal to 1.00, whereas abnormal values are greater. The degree of abnormality can also be quantified by relating the confidence interval to the degree of obstruction or restriction. For example, the $FEV_{1\%}$ may be evaluated in terms of confidence intervals:

Normal	1 CI
Mild obstruction	1-2 CI
Moderate obstruction	2-4 CI
Severe obstruction	4 CI

Degrees of abnormality are not always expressed in terms of whole units of confidence intervals. Parameters that display a wide variability ($FEF_{25\%-75\%}$, etc.) may have confidence intervals that in some instances are larger than the expected value, resulting in a lower limit of normal that is zero or even negative; though statistically valid, the use of the CI does not adequately describe the functional status in every situation.

In selecting predicted values, individual laboratories should attempt to choose studies that closely approximate the type of population that will be tested. The following factors may be considerations in selecting values to be used as normals:

1. What type of equipment was used for the population study? Does it comply with the American Thoracic Society recommendations (see Chapter 11)?
2. Were the methodologies used in the population study similar to those to be employed, particularly for lung volumes and DL_{CO}?
3. How large was the sample population? What age range was included? Did the study generate different regressions for different ethnic origins? Did the study include smokers as normals?
4. Is the standard deviation or standard error of estimate available, so that confidence intervals can be employed?
5. Was the study performed at a different altitude?
6. Do predicted values generated using the study's regressions differ markedly from other published reports?

Although there is no universally accepted set of predicted values, several excellent studies are available to provide a diverse combination of regressions so that many of the above considerations can be satisfied. The predicted values included here represent some of the more widely used regressions and compare favorably with other published studies. Other acceptable studies are included with the references.

PREDICTION REGRESSIONS FOR PULMONARY FUNCTION TESTS
(all values BTPS unless otherwise stated)*

Test	Formula	SD	Source
SVC (L)			
Males	$0.148H - 0.025A - 4.24$	0.58	1
Females	$0.115H - 0.024A - 2.85$	0.52	1
FRC (L)			
Males	$0.130H - 5.16$	—	2
Females	$0.119H - 4.85$	—	2
RV (L)			
Males	$0.069H + 0.017A - 3.45$	—	3
Females	$0.081H + 0.009A - 3.90$	—	3
Derived lung volumes			
	TLC (L) = SVC + RV		
	IC (L) = TLC − FRC		
	ERV (L) = VC − IC		
FVC (L)			
Males	(Same as SVC)		1
Females	(Same as SVC)		1
$FEV_{0.5}$ (L)			
Males	$0.24 + 0.02H - 0.024A$	0.51	4
FEV_1 (L)			
Males	$0.092H - 0.032A - 1.260$	0.55	1
Females	$0.089H - 0.024A - 1.93$	0.47	1
$FEF_{200-1200}$ (L/sec)			
Males	$0.109H - 0.047A + 2.010$	1.66	1
Females	$0.145H - 0.036A - 2.532$	1.19	1
$FEF_{25\%-75\%}$ (L/sec)			
Males	$0.047H - 0.045A + 2.513$	1.12	1
Females	$0.060H - 0.030A + 0.551$	0.80	1
PEFR (L/sec)			
Males	$0.144H - 0.024A + 0.225$	—	5
Females	$0.090H - 0.018A + 1.130$	—	5
$\dot{V}_{max\ 75}$ (L/sec)			
Males	$0.090H - 0.020A + 2.726$	—	5
Females	$0.069H - 0.019A + 2.147$	—	5
$\dot{V}_{max\ 50}$ (L/sec)			
Males	$0.065H - 0.030A + 2.403$	—	5
Females	$0.062H - 0.035A + 1.426$	—	5
$\dot{V}_{max\ 25}$ (L/sec)			
Males	$0.036H - 0.041A + 1.984$	—	5
Females	$0.023H - 0.035A + 2.216$	—	5

*H is height in inches; A is age in years; P_B is barometric pressure.

PREDICTION REGRESSIONS FOR PULMONARY FUNCTION TESTS—cont'd

Test	Formula	SD	Source
MVV (L/min)			
Males	$3.03H - 0.816A - 37.9$	—	5
Females	$2.14H - 0.685A - 4.87$	—	5
CV/VC (%)			
Males	$0.357A + 0.562$	4.15	6
Females	$0.293A + 2.812$	4.90	6
CC/TLC (%)			
Males	$0.496A + 14.878$	4.09	6
Females	$0.536A + 14.420$	4.43	6
Viso$\dot{V}$/FVC (%)			
All ages	$0.450A + 4.69$	5.27	7
<50 years	$0.303A + 13.43$	4.31	7
$DL_{CO}SB$ (ml CO/min/ mm Hg)			
Males	$0.250H - 0.177A + 19.93$	—	8
Females	$0.284H - 0.177A + 7.72$	—	8
Maximum expiratory pressure (cm H_2O)			
Males	$268 - 1.03A$	—	9
Females	$170 - 0.53A$	—	9
Maximum inspiratory pressure (cm H_2O)			
Males	$143 - 0.55A$	—	9
Females	$104 - 0.51A$	—	9
$\dot{V}O_{2\,max}$ (L/min)			
Males	$4.2 - 0.032A$	0.4	10
Females	$2.6 - 0.014A$	0.4	10
HR_{max}			
Males and females	$210 - 0.65A$	10-15	10
PA_{O_2}			
Males and females	$-0.279A + 0.113P_B + 14.632$	—	11

1. Morris, J.F., Koski, A., and Johnson, L.C.: Spirometric standards for healthy nonsmoking adults, Am. Rev. Respir. Dis. **103**:57, 1971.
2. Bates, D.V., Macklem, P.T., and Christie, R.V.: Respiratory function in disease, ed. 2, Philadelphia, 1971, W.B. Saunders Co.
3. Goldman, H.I., and Becklake, M.R.: Respiratory function tests: normal values at median altitudes and the prediction of normal results, Am. Rev. Tuberculosis **79**:457, 1959.
4. Kory, R.C., Callahan, R., and Syner, J.C.: The veterans administration—army cooperative study of pulmonary function. I. Clinical spirometry in normal men, Am. J. Med. **30**:243, 1961.
5. Cherniack, R.M., and Raber, M.D.: Normal standards for ventilatory function using an automated wedge spirometer, Am. Rev. Respir. Dis. **106**:38, 1972.
6. Buist, S.A., and Ross, B.B.: Predicted values for closing volumes using a modified single breath nitrogen test, Am. Rev. Respir. Dis. **111**:405, 1975.
7. Gelb, A.F., et al.: Sensitivity of volume of isoflow in the detection of mild airway obstruction, Am. Rev. Respir. Dis. **112**:401, 1975.
8. Gaensler, E.A., and Wright, G.W.: Evaluation of respiratory impairment, Arch, Environ. Health **12**:146, 1966.
9. Black, L.F., and Hyatt, R.E.: Maximal respiratory pressures: normal values and relationship to age and sex, Am. Rev. Respir. Dis. **99**:696, 1969.
10. Jones, N.L., et al.: Clinical exercise testing, ed. 2, Philadelphia, 1983, W.B. Saunders Co.
11. Morris, A.H., et al.: Clinical pulmonary function testing, ed. 2, Salt Lake City, 1984, Intermountain Thoracic Society.

ADDITIONAL RECOMMENDED SOURCES FOR PULMONARY FUNCTION PREDICTED VALUES

Spirometry

Crapo, R.O., Morris, A.H., and Gardner, R.M.: Reference spirometric values using techniques and equipment that meets ATS recommendations, Am. Rev. Respir. Dis. **123**:659, 1981.
Knudson, R.J., Slatin, R.C., and Lebowitz, M.D.: The maximal expiratory flow-volume curve: normal standards, variability, and effects of age, Am. Rev. Respir. Dis. **113**:587, 1976.

Lung volumes

Crapo, R.O., et al.: Lung volumes in healthy non-smoking adults, Bull. Eur. Physiopathol. Respir. **18**:419, 1982.
Grimby, G., and Soderholm, B.: Spirometric studies in normal subjects. III. Static lung volumes and maximum voluntary ventilation in adults with a note on physical fitness, Acta. Med. Scand. **173**:199, 1963.

Diffusing capacity

Bates, D.V., Macklem, P.T., and Christie, R.V.: Respiratory function in disease, Philadelphia, 1971, W.B. Saunders Co.
Crapo, R.O., and Morris, A.H.: Standardized single breath normal values for carbon monoxide diffusing capacity, Am. Rev. Respir. Dis. **123**:185, 1981.

Pediatric pulmonary function

Hsu, K.H.K., et al.: Ventilatory functions of normal children and young adults—Mexican-American, white, and black. I. Spirometry, J. Pediatr. **95**:14, 1979.
Polgar, G., and Promadhat, V.: Pulmonary function testing in children: techniques and standards, Philadelphia, 1971, W.B. Saunders Co.

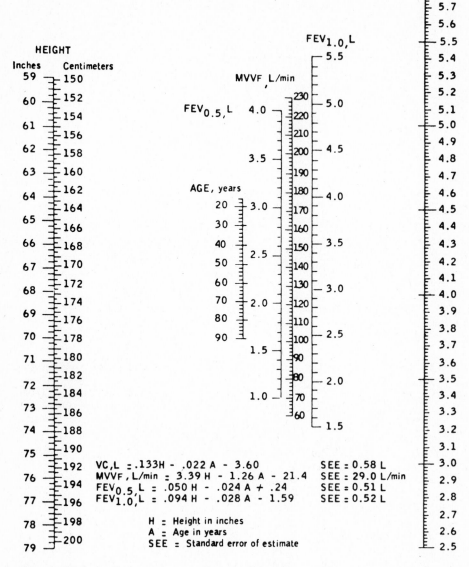

V.A. COOPERATIVE STUDY
Spirometry in normal males
Prediction nomograms

VC,L

HEIGHT

FEV₁.₀,L

MVVF, L/min

FEV₀.₅,L

AGE, years

VC,L = .133H - .022 A - 3.60   SEE = 0.58 L
MVVF, L/min = 3.39 H - 1.26 A - 21.4   SEE = 29.0 L/min
FEV₀.₅ L = .050 H - .024 A + .24   SEE = 0.51 L
FEV₁.₀,L = .094 H - .028 A - 1.59   SEE = 0.52 L

H = Height in inches
A = Age in years
SEE = Standard error of estimate

Fig. 1. Clinical spirometry in normal men, (From Kory, R.C., et al.: Am. J. Med. **30**:243, 1961.)

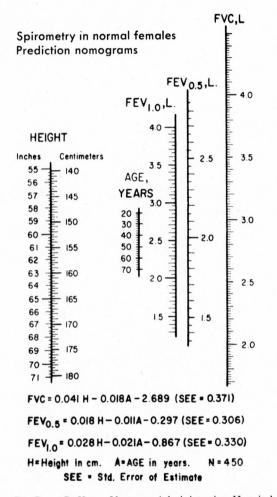

Spirometry in normal females
Prediction nomograms

FVC = 0.041 H − 0.018A − 2.689 (SEE = 0.371)

$FEV_{0.5}$ = 0.018 H − 0.011A − 0.297 (SEE = 0.306)

$FEV_{1.0}$ = 0.028 H − 0.021A − 0.867 (SEE = 0.330)

H = Height in cm.   A = AGE in years.   N = 450
SEE = Std. Error of Estimate

Fig. 2. (Courtesy Dr. Ross C. Kory, Veterans Administration Hospital, Tampa, Fla.)

Spirometric standards for normal males (BTPS)

Males

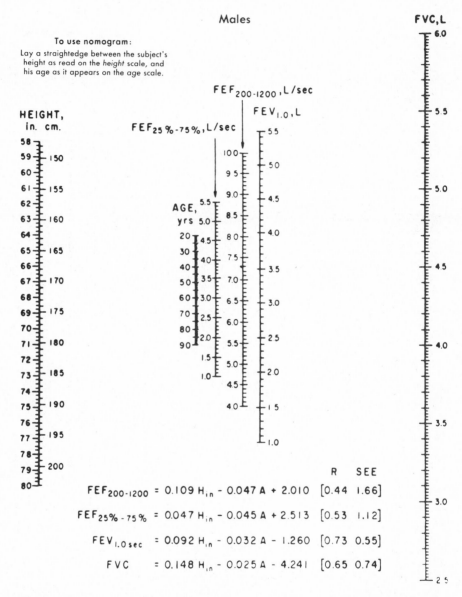

To use nomogram:
Lay a straightedge between the subject's
height as read on the *height* scale, and
his age as it appears on the *age* scale.

$$FEF_{200-1200} = 0.109\ H_{in} - 0.047\ A + 2.010\quad [0.44\ 1.66]$$

$$FEF_{25\%-75\%} = 0.047\ H_{in} - 0.045\ A + 2.513\quad [0.53\ 1.12]$$

$$FEV_{1.0sec} = 0.092\ H_{in} - 0.032\ A - 1.260\quad [0.73\ 0.55]$$

$$FVC = 0.148\ H_{in} - 0.025\ A - 4.241\quad [0.65\ 0.74]$$

Fig. 3. Prediction nomograms (BTPS), spirometric values in normal males. (From Morris, J.F., Koski, W.A., and Johnson, L.D.: Am. Rev. Respir. Dis. **103**(1):57, 1971.)

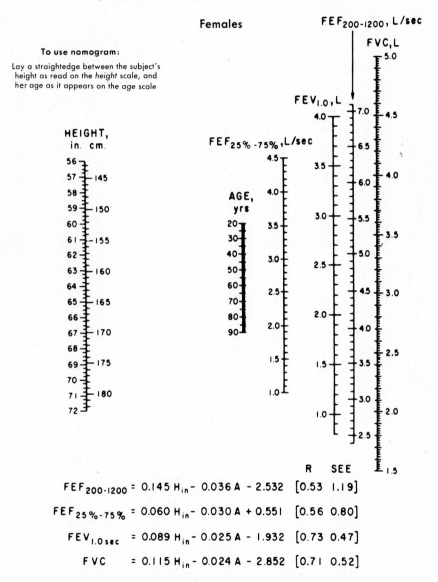

Spirometric standards for normal females (BTPS)

Females   FEF$_{200-1200}$, L/sec

FVC, L

To use nomogram:

Lay a straightedge between the subject's
height as read on the *height* scale, and
her age as it appears on the age scale

$$FEF_{200-1200} = 0.145\,H_{in} - 0.036\,A - 2.532 \quad [0.53 \quad 1.19]$$

$$FEF_{25\%-75\%} = 0.060\,H_{in} - 0.030\,A + 0.551 \quad [0.56 \quad 0.80]$$

$$FEV_{1.0\,sec} = 0.089\,H_{in} - 0.025\,A - 1.932 \quad [0.73 \quad 0.47]$$

$$FVC = 0.115\,H_{in} - 0.024\,A - 2.852 \quad [0.71 \quad 0.52]$$

Fig. 4. Prediction nomograms (BTPS), spirometric values in normal females. (From Morris, J.F., Koski, W.A., and Johnson, L.D.: Am. Rev. Respir. Dis. **103**(1):57, 1971.)

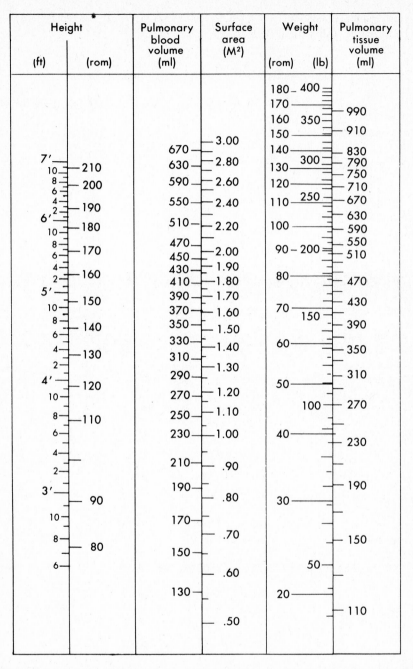

Fig. 5. Pulmonary tissue/blood volume nomogram (for use with the radiologic method of estimating TLC [see Chapter 1]). (From Ferris, B.G.: Am. Rev. Respir. Dis. **118**(suppl.):109, 1978.)

NORMAL VALUES FOR PULMONARY FUNCTION STUDIES IN CHILDREN   (all values BTPS)*

Test	Formula	SD	Source
(Children 42-59 inches, 5-17 years)			
FVC (L)			
Males	$0.094H - 3.04$	0.176	1
Females	$0.077H - 2.37$	0.171	1
FEV$_1$ (L)			
Males	$0.085H - 2.86$	0.159	1
Females	$0.074H - 2.48$	0.166	1
FEF$_{25\%\text{-}75\%}$ (L)			
Males	$0.094H - 2.61$	0.388	1
Females	$0.087H - 2.39$	0.347	1
PEFR (L/Sec)			
Males	$0.161H - 5.88$	0.451	1
Females	$0.130H - 4.51$	0.487	1
MVV (L/Min)			
Males and females	$3.81H - 134$	—	1
(Children 60-78 inches, 5-17 years)			
FVC (L)			
Males	$0.174A + 0.164H - 9.43$	0.354	1
Females	$0.102A + 0.117H - 5.87$	0.287	1
FEV$_1$ (L/Sec)			
Males	$0.126A + 0.143H - 7.86$	0.303	1
Females	$0.085A + 0.100H - 4.94$	0.290	1
FEV$_{25\%\text{-}75\%}$ (L/Sec)			
Males	$0.126A + 0.135H - 6.50$	0.612	1
Females	$0.083A + 0.093H - 3.50$	0.621	1
PEFR (L/Sec)			
Males	$0.205A + 0.181H - 9.54$	0.780	1
Females	$0.139A + 0.100H - 4.12$	0.798	1
MVV (L/Min)			
Males and females	$3.81H - 134$	—	1
SVC (L)			
Males	(Same as FVC)		1
Females	(Same as FVC)		1
FRC (L)			
Males and females	$0.067 \times e^{0.05334H}$	—	2

*H is height in inches; A is age in years.

NORMAL VALUES FOR PULMONARY FUNCTION STUDIES IN CHILDREN—cont'd

Test	Formula	SD	Source
RV (L)			
Males and females	$0.033 \times e^{0.05334H}$	—	2
Derived lung volumes (L)			
	TLC = VC + RV		
	IC = TLC − FRC		
	ERV = VC − IC		
$D_{L_{CO}}SB$ *(ml CO/min/mm Hg)*			
Males and females	$0.693H - 20.13$	—	3

1. Dickman, M.L., Schmidt, C.D., and Gardner, R.M.: Spirometric standards for normal children and adolescents (ages 5 years through 18 years), Am. Rev. Respir. Dis. **104:**680, 1971.
2. Weng, T.R., and Levison, H.: Standards of pulmonary function in children, Am. Rev. Respir. Dis. **99:**879, 1969.
3. Gaensler, E.A., and Wright, G.W.: Evaluation of respiratory impairment, Arch. Environ. Health **12:**146, 1966.

(See also Additional Recommended Sources for Pulmonary Function Predicted Values.)

SUMMARY CURVES FOR PREDICTING NORMAL VALUES IN CHILDREN

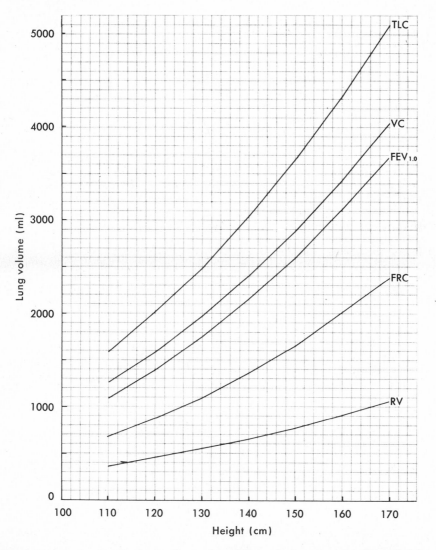

Fig. 6. Summary curves for lung volumes, in milliliters, for *boys,* as a function of height in centimeters. Summary curves are derived from regression equations from several different studies. (From Polgar, G., and Promadhat, V.: Pulmonary function testing in children, Philadelphia, 1971, W.B. Saunders Co.)

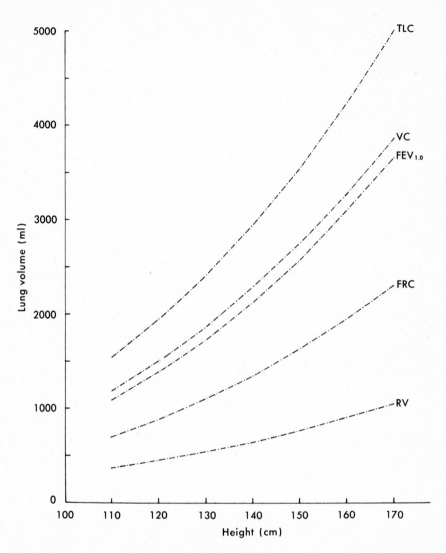

Fig. 7. Summary curves for lung volumes, in milliliters, for *girls,* as a function of height in centimeters. Summary curves are derived from regression equations from several different studies. (From Polgar, G., and Promadhat, V.: Pulmonary function testing in children, Philadelphia, 1971, W.B. Saunders Co.)

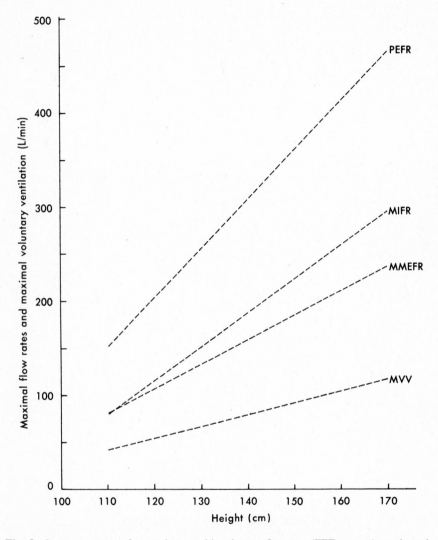

Fig. 8. Summary curves for maximum midexpiratory flow rate (FEF$_{25\%-75\%}$), peak expiratory flow rate (PEFR), maximum voluntary ventilation (MVV), and maximum inspiratory flow rate (MIFR) in liters per minute as a function of height for *boys and girls*. Summary curves are derived from regression equations from several different studies. (From Polgar, G., and Promadhat, V.: Pulmonary function testing in children, Philadelphia, 1971, W.B. Saunders Co.)

FACTORS FOR CONVERTING GAS VOLUMES FROM ATPS (ROOM TEMPERATURE) TO BTPS

$$\text{Volume (BTPS)} = \text{Volume (ATPS)} \times \frac{P_B - P_{H_2O}}{P_B - 47} \times \frac{310}{273 + T}$$

where

P_B = Barometric pressure, mm Hg
P_{H_2O} = Vapor pressure of water at spirometer temperature
T   = Temperature centigrade
47   = Vapor pressure of water at 37° C
310 = Absolute body temperature

Most of the factors of this equation can be combined to give an approximate value for a conversion factor; local P_B causes slight differences.

Conversion factor	Gas temperature (centigrade)
1.112	18
1.107	19
1.102	20
1.096	21
1.091	22
1.085	23
1.080	24
1.075	25
1.068	26
1.063	27
1.057	28
1.051	29
1.045	30
1.039	31
1.032	32
1.026	33
1.020	34
1.014	35
1.007	36
1.000	37

FACTORS FOR CONVERTING FROM ATPS (ROOM TEMPERATURE) TO STPD

$$\text{Volume (STPD)} = \text{Volume (ATPS)} \times \frac{P_B - P_{H_2O}}{760} \times \frac{273}{273 + T}$$

where

P_B = Barometric pressure
P_{H_2O} = Water vapor pressure at spirometer temperature
T   = Temperature of the spirometer
760 = Standard barometric pressure at sea level
273 = Absolute temperature equal to 0° C

USEFUL EQUATIONS
Alveolar air equation

It is often necessary to ascertain the composition of alveolar gas. Estimations of the partial pressure of CO_2, N_2, and H_2O can be done rather easily, but the P_{AO_2} is somewhat more difficult to obtain. The most practical application of the alveolar air equation is determination of P_{AO_2} as required for calculation of the percent of shunt. The formula for the alveolar equation is as follows:

$$P_{AO_2} = [F_{IO_2} \times (P_B - 47)] - Pa_{CO_2}(F_{IO_2} + \frac{1 - F_{IO_2}}{R})$$

where

F_{IO_2} = Fractional concentration of O_2 inspired
P_B = Barometric pressure
47   = Partial pressure of water vapor at $37°$ C
Pa_{CO_2} = Arterial CO_2 tension, presumed equal to alveolar CO_2 tension
R   = Respiratory exchange ratio ($\dot{V}_{CO_2}/\dot{V}_{O_2}$)

If the fraction of inspired O_2 is 1.0, the entire factor in parentheses becomes one and can be deleted. R usually varies between 0.70 and 1.00 and can usually be assumed to be about 0.80.

Poiseuille's law

Poiseuille's law describes the flow of gas through a tube. The law has many application in pulmonary physiology, notably insofar as it applies to gas flow through the conducting airways and as it is used in pneumotachography. The law is stated thus:

$$\Delta P = \frac{\dot{V}8\eta l}{\pi r^4}$$

where

ΔP = Change in pressure from one end of the tube to the other
$\dot{V}$ = Flow through the tube
η = Coefficient of viscosity of the gas
l   = Length of the tube
r   = Radius of the tube

The equation can be rearranged thus:

$$\frac{\Delta P}{\dot{V}} = \frac{8\eta l}{\pi r^4}$$

Here the relationship between the pressure difference at the ends of the tube and the flow through the tube, which defines *resistance,* is equated to the remaining variables, notably the length and radius of the tube. It should be noted that the resistance varies directly with the length of the conducting tube and inversely with the radius. A twofold increase in the length of the tube doubles the resistance, whereas a reduction of the radius by half increases the pressure differential

16 times. In the airways abnormal narrowing by mucous secretions or functional lesions can cause significant increases in airway resistance. Since Poiseuille's law holds true for any round tube in which laminar flow is possible, the principle of pneumotachography is based directly on this law. Because the length and radius of a pneumotachometer flow tube remain constant and the viscosity of respiratory gases varies only slightly, all the variables in Poiseuille's equation can be reduced to a constant except P and $\dot{V}$. By rearranging:

$$\dot{V} = \frac{\Delta P}{K_R}$$

where

K_R = Resistance constant

From this equation it is obvious that all that is necessary to measure the $\dot{V}$ is a means of determining the pressure differential; this is easily accomplished by means of pressure transducers.

Thoracic gas volume equation

Measurement of the V_{TG} with the body plethysmograph is based on Boyle's law:

$$P_1 V_1 = P_2 V_2$$

or

$$P_1 V_1 = (P_1 + \Delta P)(V_1 + \Delta V)$$

Simplifying

$$P_1 \Delta V + V_1 \Delta P + \Delta V \Delta P = 0$$

where

P_1 = Initial pressure change in the lungs (713 mm Hg or 970 cm H_2O)
V_1 = V_{TG} or thoracic gas volume
ΔV = Change in lung volume
ΔP = Change in lung pressure

Solving for V_1:

$$V_1 = -\frac{\Delta V}{\Delta P}(P_1 + \Delta P)$$

Since ΔP is small compared with P_1, $P_1 + \Delta P \approx P_1$, and therefore:

$$V_1 = -\frac{P_1(\Delta V)}{\Delta P}$$

In terms of the plethysmographic method (and disregarding the sign):

$$V_{TG} = 970 \frac{(\Delta V)}{(\Delta P)}$$

The slope recorded on the oscilloscope is the change in mouth pressure per unit change in box volume, $(\Delta P)/(\Delta V)$ or λ VTG, as the subject breathes against an occluded airway. The equation then becomes:

$$VTG = \frac{970}{\lambda VTG}$$

This is the working form of the equation after box pressure calibrations have been included. Simple measurements of the slope of the trace allows rapid calculation of VTG.

Fick's law of diffusion (modified)

In reference to gas exchange across a membrane, Fick's law states that:

$$\dot{V}_{gas} = \frac{A}{T} \times D \times (P_1 - P_2)$$

where

A	= Area of the membrane
T	= Thickness of the membrane
$P_1 - P_2$	= Pressure gradient across the membrane
D	= Diffusion constant

D is related to the molecular weight and solubility of the gas to which it refers by:

$$D \propto \frac{\text{Solubility}}{\sqrt{\text{Mol. wt.}}}$$

Since A and T remain constant in the lung system:

$$DL \propto \frac{\dot{V}_{gas}}{PA - PC}$$

where

DL = Diffusion constant for the lung
PA = Alveolar gas pressure
PC = Capillary gas pressure

When DL is measured with CO, the capillary Partial pressure is assumed to be zero; thus:

$$DL = \frac{\dot{V}CO}{PACO}$$

All of the CO methods of measuring DL use this basic equation. The single-breath and steady-state methods differ in that the former measures $\dot{V}CO$ during breath-holding, and the latter measures it during "normal" breathing. The steady-state methods vary by the way in which they measure PACO.

Fick principle (cardiac output determination)

The Fick principle relates $\dot{V}_{O_2}$ to arteriovenous O_2 content difference $(C[a-\bar{v}]_{O_2})$ to determine cardiac output $(\dot{Q})$:

$$\dot{Q}_T = \frac{\dot{V}_{O_2}}{Ca_{O_2} - C\bar{v}_{O_2}}$$

This equation forms the basis for determining various fractions of the cardiac output, namely, the shunt fraction $(\dot{Q}s)$ and the fraction participating in ideal gas exchange $(\dot{Q}c)$. The relationship between $\dot{Q}s$ and the total cardiac output $(\dot{Q}_T)$ can be expressed as a ratio using the concept of O_2 content differences:

$$\frac{\dot{Q}s}{\dot{Q}_T} = \frac{Cc_{O_2} - Ca_{O_2}}{Cc_{O_2} - C\bar{v}_{O_2}}$$

where

$Cc_{O_2} - Ca_{O_2}$ = Content differences between pulmonary end-capillary blood, Cc_{O_2}, and arterial blood, Ca_{O_2}, which increases when blood passes through the pulmonary system without coming into contact with alveolar gas (a shunt)

$Cc_{O_2} - C\bar{v}_{O_2}$ = Content difference between blood returning to the lungs by way of the pulmonary artery and the pulmonary end-capillary blood; the total change reflecting the arterialization of mixed venous blood

In a system in which all blood equilibrates with alveolar gas, Cc_{O_2} and Ca_{O_2} become identical, no matter what the value of the denominator, so that the ratio becomes zero and the shunt must be zero. As more blood fails to equilibrate, the numerator becomes larger in relation to the denominator and is reflected by an increased $\dot{Q}s/\dot{Q}_T$.

Since true pulmonary end-capillary O_2 content, Cc_{O_2}, is practically impossible to sample and represents a mathematical entity rather than an actual phenomenon, a modified form of the equation is used clinically (as described in Chapter 6):

$$\frac{\dot{Q}s}{\dot{Q}_T} = \frac{(P_{A_{O_2}} - Pa_{O_2})(0.0031)}{(C[a-\bar{v}]_{O_2}) + (P_{A_{O_2}} - Pa_{O_2})(0.0031)}$$

where

$P_{A_{O_2}} - Pa_{O_2}$ = *Tension* difference of O_2 between the alveoli and arterial blood

0.0031 = Solubility factor to convert O_2 tension to volume percent

The equation is implemented by having the subject breath 100% O_2 long enough to completely saturate the Hb (Pa_{O_2} greater than 150 mm Hg). Therefore the only difference between pulmonary end-capillary blood (assumed to be in equilibrium with the $P_{A_{O_2}}$) and arterial blood exists in the difference in O_2 content in the dissolved form. Again, this is related to the normal a-$\bar{v}$ content difference $(C[a-\bar{v}]_{O_2})$ plus the actual dissolved content difference, denoted by the same term in both numerator and denominator. A ratio is thus derived between the content difference of shunted blood and the total difference, in this case determined by using dissolved O_2 differences. $P_{A_{O_2}}$ is determined by the alveolar air equation outlined previously.

Calculated bicarbonate (HCO_3^-)

The bicarbonate concentration in plasma can be calculated from the Henderson-Hasselbalch equation if the pH and P_{CO_2} are known:

$$pH = pK + \log \frac{(HCO_3^-)}{(H_2CO_3)}$$

The working form of the equation becomes:

$$(HCO_3^-) = 0.0306 \times P_{CO_2} \times 10^{[(pH - 6.161)/0.9524]}$$

where

HCO_3^- = Bicarbonate concentration, mEq/L
0.0306 = Solubility coefficient for CO_2
6.161 = pK for carbonic acid
0.9524 = Empirically determined constant

The total CO_2 concentration can then be determined by summing the HCO_3^- and the dissolved CO_2:

$$\text{Total } CO_2 = 0.0306 \times P_{CO_2} + (HCO_3^-)$$

Calculated oxygen saturation

Although it is preferable to actually measure saturation (see Chapter 6), the saturation of Hb with O_2 can be calculated if the pH and P_{O_2} are known. Assuming that the Hb is normal (i.e., having a P_{50} of 26.6), the saturation may be calculated:

$$\text{Saturation} = \frac{Z^{2.60}}{(26.6)^{2.60} + Z^{2.60}} \times 100$$

where

$$Z = P_{O_2} \times 10^{[-0.48(7.40 - pH)]}$$

where

P_{O_2} = Partial pressure of O_2 in the sample
pH   = Hydrogen ion concentration ($-$ log) in the sample
-0.48 = Bohr factor (normal blood)

Because of the assumptions concerning normality of the hemoglobin as well as its P_{50}, calculated saturations may be in error if the true factors are unknown.

SAMPLE CALCULATIONS
Open-circuit FRC determination (N_2 washout) (see p. 4)

FRC:	Unknown
% $N_{2_{final}}$:	6% (0.06 as a fraction)
% $N_{2_{alveolar\ 1}}$:	76% (0.76 as a fraction)
% $N_{2_{alveolar\ 2}}$:	1% (0.01 as a fraction)
Vol. expired:	27.5 L
Test time (T):	7 min
Blood/tissue N_2 washout factor:	0.04 L/min (correction factor)
Spirometer temperature:	24° C

1. $FRC = \dfrac{[\% \ N_{2_{final}} \times (V_E + V_D)] - (T \times N_2 \ \text{correction})}{\% \ N_{2_{alveolar\ 1}} - \% \ N_{2_{alveolar\ 2}}}$

2. $= \dfrac{[0.06 \times (27.5 + 1.0 \ \text{L})] - (7.0 \ \text{min} \times 0.04 \ \text{L/min})}{0.76 - 0.01}$

3. $= \dfrac{(0.06 \times 28.5) - (0.28 \ \text{L})}{0.75}$

4. $= \dfrac{1.71 \ \text{L} - 0.28 \ \text{L}}{0.75}$

5. $= \dfrac{1.43}{0.75}$

6. FRC = 1.91 L (ATPS)

This value is ATPS and must be corrected to BTPS. The spirometer temperature was 24° C; thus using the appropriate correction factor from p. 272:

7. FRC (BTPS) = 1.91 × 1.08
8. FRC (BTPS) = 2.06

Closed-circuit FRC determination (helium dilution) (see p. 6)

FRC:	Unknown
He added:	0.5 L
% $He_{initial}$:	9.5% (0.095 as a fraction)
% He_{final}:	5.5% (0.055 as a fraction)
He absorption correction:	0.1 L
Spirometer temperature:	24° C

1. $FRC = \left[\dfrac{(\% \ He_{initial} - \% \ He_{final})}{\% \ He_{final}} \times \text{Initial volume} \right] - \text{He correction}$

2. Initial volume = $\dfrac{\text{He added}}{\% \ \text{He}_{\text{initial}}}$
   (spirometer +
   circuitry)

$$= \dfrac{0.5 \ \text{L}}{0.095}$$

$$= 5.26 \ \text{L}$$

3. FRC $= \left[\dfrac{(0.095 - 0.055)}{0.055} \times 5.26 \ \text{L} \right] - 0.1 \ \text{L}$

4. $= (0.73 \times 5.26 \ \text{L}) - 0.1 \ \text{L}$

5. $= 3.84 \ \text{L} - 0.1 \ \text{L}$

6. FRC $= 3.74 \ \text{L (ATPS)}$

Correcting to BTPS with appropriate correction factor from p. 272:

7. FRC (BTPS) $= 3.74 \times 1.08$
8. FRC (BTPS) $= 4.04 \ \text{L}$

Single-breath $D_{L_{CO}}$ (see Chapter 5)

Vol. inspired:	4.0 L
$F_{I_{CO}}$:	0.3% (0.003 as a fraction)
$F_{A_{CO_{t2}}}$:	0.125% (0.00125 as a fraction)
$F_{I_{He}}$:	10.0% (0.10 as a fraction)
$F_{E_{He}}$:	7.5% (0.075 as a fraction)
P_B:	760 mm Hg
Breath-hold time (t2 − t1):	10.0 sec
Spirometer temperature:	25° C

1. $D_{L_{CO}}SB = \dfrac{V_A \times 60}{(P_B - 47)(t2 - t1)} \times Ln \dfrac{(F_{A_{CO_{t1}}})}{(F_{A_{CO_{t2}}})}$

2. $V_A \quad = \dfrac{\text{Vol. inspired}}{F_{E_{He}}/F_{I_{He}}}$

   $= \dfrac{4.0 \ \text{L}}{0.075/0.10} = 5.33 \ \text{L (5333 ml)}$

3. $F_{A_{CO_{t1}}} = F_{I_{CO}} \times F_{E_{He}}/F_{I_{He}}$

   $= 0.003 \times 0.075/0.10 = 0.0025$

4. $D_{L_{CO}}SB = \dfrac{5333 \ \text{ml} \times 60}{(713) \times (10.0)} \times Ln \dfrac{(0.0025)}{(0.00125)}$

5. $= \dfrac{319.980}{7130} \times Ln \ (2.0)$

6. $= 44.9 \ \text{ml/min/mm Hg} \times (0.6931)$

7. $= 31.10 \ \text{ml CO/min/mm Hg (ATPS)}$

This value is ATPS and is normally converted to STPS (0° C, 760 mm Hg, dry).

8. $\dfrac{373}{273 + T° C} \times \dfrac{P_B - P_{H_2O} \ T° C}{760} = $ Correction factor

where

$\quad$ T° C $\qquad$ = Spirometer temperature

$\quad$ P_{H_2O} T° C = Partial pressure of water vapor at the spirometer temperature (in this case: 24 mm Hg at 25° C)

9. $\dfrac{273}{273 + 25} \times \dfrac{760 - 24}{760} = $ Correction factor

10. $0.916 \times 0.968 = 0.887$

11. $(31.10 \ \text{ml CO/min/mm Hg}) \times (0.887) = 27.6 \ \text{ml CO)/min/mm Hg (STPD)}$

Thoracic gas volume (V_{TG}) (see Chapter 1)

V_{TG}*:	Unknown
V_{TG} tangents:	0.71 (angle 35.4)
	0.73 (angle 36.1)
	0.73 (angle 36.1)
P_B:	755 mm Hg
Subject weight:	71 Kg
P_{mouth} calibration:	10 cm H_2O/cm
P_{box} calibration:	30 ml/cm
Dead space correction:	100 ml
Plethysmograph volume:	530 L

1. Average V_{TG} tangent

$\quad$ 0.71
$\quad$ 0.73
$\underline{+0.73}$
$\quad$ 2.17/3 = 0.72 (avg.)

2. Pressure correction

$\quad$ P_B corr = $(P_B - 47) \times 1.36$
$\qquad\qquad$ = (755 mm Hg − 47 mm Hg) × 1.36
$\qquad\qquad$ = 963 cm H_2O

3. Subject volume correction (K)

$$K = \frac{[\text{Pleth volume} - (\text{Subject weight}/1.07)]}{\text{Pleth volume}}$$

$$0.874 = \frac{[530 \ \text{L} - (71 \ \text{Kg}/1.07)]}{530 \ \text{L}}$$

---

*Data for V_{TG} and Raw (see calculation on p. 281) are from the same subject.

4. V_{TG} $= \left(\dfrac{\text{PB corr}}{\text{TAN}} \times \dfrac{\text{P}_{\text{box}} \text{ cal}}{\text{P}_{\text{mouth}} \text{ cal}} \times \text{K} \right) - \text{Dead space}$

$= \left(\dfrac{963}{0.72} \times \dfrac{30}{10} \times 0.874 \right) - 100$

$= (1338 \times 3 \times 0.874) - 100$

$= 3510 \text{ ml or } 3.51 \text{ L}$

Airway Resistance (RAW) (see Chapter 3)

Raw:	Unknown
$\text{P}_{\text{m}}/\text{P}_{\text{box}}$ TAN:	0.61 (angle = 31)
$\dot{\text{V}}/\text{P}_{\text{box}}$ TAN:	3.0 (angle = 72)
P_{mouth} calibration:	10 cm H_2O/cm
P_{box} calibration:	30 ml/cm
$\dot{\text{V}}$ calibration:	1.0 L/sec/cm
R_{sys}:	0.25 cm H_2O/L/sec

1. $\text{Raw} = \left(\dfrac{\text{P}_{\text{m}}/\text{P}_{\text{box}} \text{ TAN}}{\dot{\text{V}}/\text{P}_{\text{box}} \text{ TAN}} \times \dfrac{\text{P}_{\text{mouth}} \text{ cal}}{\dot{\text{V}} \text{ cal}} \right) - \text{R}_{\text{sys}}$

2. $= \left(\dfrac{0.61}{3.0} \times \dfrac{10}{1.0} \right) - 0.25$

3. $= (0.203 \times 10) - 0.25$

4. $= 1.78 \text{ cm } H_2O\text{/L/sec}$

Normally several repetitions of the maneuver are performed; unlike the V_{TG} however, the tangents are not averaged. Since the flow and volume tangents influence each other, the Raw is calculated and then averaged. To calculate the Gaw/V_{L} (specific airway conductance), the volume at which each Raw maneuver was performed is calculated as for the V_{TG}, using the $\text{P}_{\text{mouth}}/\text{P}_{\text{box}}$ tangent from the specific maneuver. For the above example:

1. $\text{Gaw}/\text{V}_{\text{L}} = (1/\text{Raw})/\text{V}_{\text{TG}}$

2. $\text{V}_{\text{TG}} = \left(\dfrac{963}{0.61} \times \dfrac{30}{10} \times 0.874 \right) - 100$

3. $= (1579 \times 3 \times 0.874) - 100$

4. $= 4039 \text{ ml or } 4.04 \text{ L}$

Calculating the Gaw/V_{L}:

5. $= (1/1.78)/4.04$

6. $= 0.14 \text{ cm } H_2O\text{/L/sec/L}$

The average of several maneuvers is normally reported, again after the SGaw for individual efforts has been calculated.

EXERCISE STUDY*

Volume exhaled (V):	20.0 L (ATPS)
Collection time (sec):	60 sec
Temperature (T):	24° C
FE_{O_2}:	17.0% (0.17 as a fraction)
FE_{CO_2}:	3.0% (0.03 as a fraction)
f:	25/min
HR:	100/min
Pa_{O_2}:	95 mm Hg
Pa_{CO_2}:	35 mm Hg
P_B:	750
Mechanical V_D:	18 ml (0.018 L)
Subject's weight:	55 Kg

The first step is to calculate conversion factors to correct ventilation and gas exchange measurements to BTPS and STPD (this STPD factor is for conversion from BTPS), respectively:

1. BTPS factor
$$= \frac{P_B - P_{H_2O}}{P_B - 47} \times \frac{273 + 37}{273 + T}$$
$$= \frac{721}{703} \times \frac{310}{297}$$
$$= 1.07$$

2. STPD factor
$$= \frac{P_B - 47}{760} \times \frac{273}{273 + 37}$$
$$= \frac{703}{760} \times 0.881$$
$$= 0.815$$

Next parameters of ventilation may be calculated:

3. $\dot{V}_E$ (BTPS)
$$= \frac{V \text{ exhaled} \times 60}{\text{Collection time (sec)}} \times \text{BTPS factor}$$
$$= \frac{20.0 \text{ L} \times 60}{60} \times 1.07$$
$$= 21.4 \text{ L (BTPS)}$$

4. V_T (BTPS)
$$= \frac{\dot{V}_E \text{ (BTPS)}}{f}$$
$$= \frac{21.4}{25}$$
$$= 0.856 \text{ L (BTPS)}$$

---

*Values as might be obtained at a submaximal level using either a treadmill or bicycle ergometer.

5. V_D (BTPS) $= V_T \text{ (BTPS)} \times \left[1 - \dfrac{F_{ECO_2} \times (P_B - 47)}{Pa_{CO_2}} \right] - V_{D_{mech}}$

$= 0.856 \times \left[\dfrac{1 - 0.03 \times 703}{35} \right] - 0.018$

$= .856 \times [1 - 0.603] - 0.018$

$= (0.856 \times 0.397) - 0.018$

$= 0.340 - 0.018$

$= 0.322 \text{ L (BTPS)}$

6. $\dot{V}_A$ (BTPS) $= \dot{V}_E \text{ (BTPS)} - [f \times V_D \text{ (BTPS)}]$

$= 21.4 - [25 \times 0.322]$

$= 21.4 - 8.05$

$= 13.4 \text{ L (BTPS)}$

7. V_D/V_T $= \dfrac{0.322}{0.856}$

$= 0.38 \text{ (or 38\%)}$

Next, gas exchange parameters are computed:

8. $\dot{V}_E$ (STPD) $= \dot{V}_E \text{ (BTPS)} \times \text{STPD factor}$

$= 21.4 \times 0.815$

$= 17.4 \text{ L (STPD)}$

9. $\dot{V}_{O_2}$ (STPD) $= \left[\left(\dfrac{1 - F_{EO_2} - F_{ECO_2}}{1 - F_{IO_2}} \times F_{IO_2} \right) - F_{EO_2} \right] \times \dot{V}_E \text{ (STPD)}$

$= \left[\left(\dfrac{1 - 0.17 - 0.03}{1 - 0.2093} \times 0.2093 \right) - 0.17 \right] \times 17.4$

$= \left[\left(\dfrac{0.80}{0.79} \times 0.2093 \right) - 0.17 \right] \times 17.4$

$= [(1.01 \times 0.2093) - 0.17] \times 17.4$

$= [0.212 - 0.17] \times 17.4$

$= 0.042 \times 17.4$

$= 0.731 \text{ L (STPD)}$

10. $\dot{V}_{CO_2}$ (STPD) $= (F_{ECO_2} - 0.0003) \times \dot{V}_E \text{ (STPD)}$

$= (0.03 - 0.0003) \times 17.4$

$= 0.297 \times 17.4$

$= 0.517 \text{ L (STPD)}$

11. R $= \dfrac{\dot{V}_{CO_2} \text{ (STPD)}}{\dot{V}_{O_2} \text{ (STPD)}}$

$= \dfrac{0.517}{0.731}$

$= 0.71$

12. $\dot{V}_E/\dot{V}_{O_2}$ $= \dfrac{\dot{V}_E \text{ (BTPS)}}{\dot{V}_{O_2} \text{ (STPD)}}$

$= \dfrac{21.4}{0.731}$

$= 29.3 \text{ L/L } \dot{V}_{O_2}$

13. $\dot{V}_{O_2}/\text{HR}$ $= \dfrac{\dot{V}_{O_2} \text{ (STPD)}}{\text{HR}} \times 1000$

$= \dfrac{0.731}{100} \times 1000$

$= 7.31 \text{ ml } O_2/\text{beat}$

The calculation of energy expenditure at any particular work load is described by the term *METS*, for multiples of the resting $\dot{V}_{O_2}$; the MET level for any work load can be calculated by one of two methods. In each method:

14. METS $= \dfrac{\dot{V}_{O_2} \text{ (STPD) exercise}}{\dot{V}_{O_2} \text{ (STPD) rest}}$

but the means of estimating $\dot{V}_{O_2}$ (STPD) at rest differs. $\dot{V}_{O_2}$ (STPD) at rest can be measured, or it may be estimated as 0.0035 L/min/kg (3.5 ml/kg). Using the second method in this example:

METS $= \dfrac{0.731}{0.035 \times 55}$

$= 3.80$

If the subject's measured $\dot{V}_{O_2}$ at rest had been 0.225 L/min (STPD) then:

METS $= \dfrac{0.731}{0.225}$

$= 3.25$

Index

287